Biologics in Orthopaedic Surgery

Biologics in Orthopaedic Surgery

AUGUSTUS D. MAZZOCCA, MS, MD
Department of Orthopaedic Surgery
University of Connecticut Health Center
Farmington, CT, United States

ADAM D. LINDSAY, MD
Orthopedic Surgery
Uconn Health
Farmington, CT, United States

ELSEVIER

ELSEVIER

3251 Riverport Lane
St. Louis, Missouri 63043

Biologics in Orthopaedic Surgery   ISBN: 978-0-323-66207-9

Copyright © 2019 Elsevier, Inc. All rights reserved.

Notices

Practitioners and researchers must always rely on their own experience and knowledge in evaluating and using any information, methods, compounds or experiments described herein. Because of rapid advances in the medical sciences, in particular, independent verification of diagnoses and drug dosages should be made. To the fullest extent of the law, no responsibility is assumed by Elsevier, authors, editors or contributors for any injury and/or damage to persons or property as a matter of products liability, negligence or otherwise, or from any use or operation of any methods, products, instructions, or ideas contained in the material herein.

Publisher: Mica Haley
Acquisition Editor: Kayla Wolfe
Editorial Project Manager: Jennifer Horigan
Production Project Manager: Kiruthika Govindaraju
Cover Designer: Will be updated

Typeset by TNQ Technologies

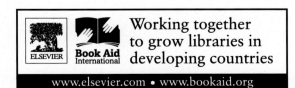

List of Contributors

Augustus D. Mazzocca, MS, MD
Department of Orthopaedic Surgery
University of Connecticut Health Center
Farmington, CT, United States

Xinning Li, MD
Orthopaedic Surgery
Boston University School of Medicine
Boston, MA, United States

Adam W. Anz, MD
Clinical Research
Andrews Institute
Andrews Research and Education Foundation
Gulf Breeze, FL, United States

Caleb O. Pinegar, DO, ATC
Orthopaedic Surgery
Andrews Research and Education Foundation
Gulf Breeze, FL, United States

Asheesh Bedi, MD
Harold W. and Helen L. Gehring Professor of
    Orthopaedic Surgery
Chief, Sports Medicine and Shoulder Surgery
Department of Orthopedic Surgery
University of Michigan
Ann Arbor, MI, United States

Anthony F. De Giacomo, MD
Orthopaedic Surgery
Sports Medicine
Kerlan Jobe Orthopaedic Clinic
Los Angeles, CA, United States

Mark A. Moore, PhD
Scientific Affairs
LifeNet Health
Virginia Beach, VA, United States

J.T. Tokish, MD
Tripler Army Medical Center
HI, United States

Adam Kwapisz, MD, PhD
Clinic of Orthopedics and Pediatric Orthopedics
Medical University of Lodz
Lodz, Poland

Sports Medicinem
PanAm Clinic
Winnipeg, MB, Canada

Jason P. Rogers, MD
Orthopedic Surgery
Steadman Hawkins Clinic of the Carolinas
Greenville, SC, United States

Matthew T. Provencher, MD, MC, USNR
Orthopaedic Clinic
Steadman Clinic
Vail, CO, United States

Anthony Sanchez, BS
Center for Outcomes-Based Orthopaedic Research
Steadman Philippon Research Institute
Vail, CO, United States

Bryan M. Saltzman, MD
Orthopedic Surgery
Rush University Medical Center
Chicago, IL, United States

David R. Christian, BS
Department of Orthopaedic Surgery
Rush University Medical Center
Chicago, IL, United States

Brian J. Cole, MD, MBA
Orthopedics
Rush University Medical Center
Chicago, IL, United States

Surgery
Rush Oak Park Hospital
Oak Park, IL, United States

Michael L. Redondo, MA, BS
Orthopaedic Surgery
Midwest Orthopaedics at Rush
Chicago, IL, United States

James P. Bradley, MD
Orthopaedic Surgery
University of Pittsburgh Medical Center
Pittsburgh, PA, United States

Katherine Coyner, MD
Orthopaedic Surgery
UConn Health
Farmington, CT, United States

Andreas H. Gomoll, MD
Orthopaedic Surgery
Harvard Medical School
Orthopaedic Surgery
Brigham and Women's Hospital
Boston, MA, United States

Joel Ferreira, MA, MD
Orthopaedic Surgery
UConn Health
Farmington, CT, United States

Ranjan Gupta, MD
Orthopaedic Surgery
UC Irvine
Orange, CA, United States

Isaac L. Moss, MD
Orthopeadic Surgery and Neurosurgery
UConn Health
Farmington, CT, United States

Adam D. Lindsay, MD
Orthopedic Surgery
Uconn Health
Farmington, CT, United States

Vinayak Sathe, MD, MS, FRCS
Orthopedic Surgery
University of Connecticut Health Center
Framington, CT, United States

John Playfair Ross, BS, MD
Orthopedic Surgery
UCONN
Farmington, CT, United States

Stephen L. Davis, MD
Orthopedic Surgery
Orthopedic Associates of Hartford
Hartford, CT, United States

Cato T. Laurencin, MD, PhD
Institute for Regenerative Engineering
The University of Connecticut
Farmington, CT, United States

Orthopaedic Surgery and Chemical, Materials and
    Biomolecular Engineering
The University of Connecticut
Farmington, CT, United States

Chief Executive Officer
Connecticut Institute for Clinical and Translational
    Science (CICATS)
The University of Connecticut
Farmington, CT, United States

Mary A Badon, MD, MBA
Connecticut Institute for Clinical and Translational
    Science
UConn Health
Farmington, CT, United States

Neil Bakshi, MD
Department of Orthopaedic Surgery
University of Michigan
Ann Arbor, MI, United States

Michael B. Banffy, MD
Kerlan Jobe Orthopaedic Clinic
Los Angeles, CA, United States

Samuel Baron, MD
Department of Orthopaedic Surgery
University of Connecticut
Farmington, CT, United States

Zachary Cavenaugh, MD
Orthopaedic Surgery Specialist
University of Connecticut Health Center John
    Dempsey Hospital
Farmington, CT, United States

Jorge Chahla, MD, PhD
Rush University Hospital
Chicago, IL, United States

Jeffrey Choi, BS
Boston University School of Medicine
Boston, MA, United States

Brian J. Cole, MD, MBA
Division of Sports Medicine
Department of Orthopedics
Rush University Medical Center
Midwest Orthopaedics, Chicago, IL, United States

Emily J. Curry, BA
Boston University School of Public Health
Boston, MA, United States

Neal S. Elattrache, MD
Kerlan Jobe Orthopaedic Clinic
Los Angeles, CA, United States

Jake A. Fox, BS
Steadman Philippon Research Institute
Vail, CO, United States

Jamie Friedman, MD
Orthopaedic Surgery
UConn Health
Farmington, CT, United States

Moin Khan, MD, MSc, FRCSC
Department of Orthopaedic Surgery
University of Michigan
Ann Arbor, MI, United States

Bert R. Mandelbaum, MD, DHL
Rush University Hospital
Chicago, IL, United States

Mary Beth R. McCarthy, BS
Research Associate and Translational Research
    Coordinator
Department of Orthopaedic Surgery
University of Connecticut
Farmington, CT, United States

Julie Mclean, PhD
Scientific Affairs
LifeNet Health
Virginia Beach, VA, United States

Colin P. Murphy, BA
Steadman Philippon Research Institute
Vail, CO, United States

Winnie A. Palispis, MD
Department of Orthopaedic Surgery
UCI
Peripheral Nerve Research Lab, Orange, CA, United
    States

Thierry Pauyo, MD, FRCSC
University of Pittsburgh Medical Center
Pittsburgh, PA, United States

Colin Pavano, BA
Orthopaedic Surgery
UConn Health
Farmington, CT, United States

Liam A. Peebles, BA
Steadman Philippon Research Institute
Vail, CO, United States

Craig M. Rodner, MD
Associate Professor of Orthopedic Surgery
UConn Health
UConn Musculoskeletal Institute
Farmington, CT, United States

Brian Samsell, BS
Scientific Affairs
LifeNet Health
Virginia Beach, VA, United States

Hardeep Singh, MD
UCONN Health
Department of Orthopaedic Surgery
Farmington, CT, United States

John M. Tokish, MD
Orthopedic Surgery Residency Program Director
Tripler Army Medical Center
Honolulu, HI, United States

Laura A. Vogel, MD
Orthopedic Surgery Sports Medicine Fellow
Department of Orthopaedic Surgery
University of Connecticut
Farmington, CT, United States

Ryu Yoshida, MD
Orthopaedic Surgeon
University of Connecticut Health Center
Farmington, CT, United States

Preface

Biologics in Orthopedic Surgery: Insights into the future of musculoskeletal medicine

The fields of orthopedic surgery and musculoskeletal medicine continue to evolve. Orthopedic surgeons are encountering new challenges and are presented with new solutions. Biologic interventions are showing potential in every subspecialty of orthopedic surgery. The goal of this text is three fold. The first is to review the basic science that supports the use of biologics in orthopedic surgery. The second is to demonstrate the successes and failures of biologic treatments in the different subspecialties of orthopedic medicine. The third, and likely the most important, is to expose the reader to work that we feel holds great potential for our patients in the future. Our hope is that this work will inspire readers to seek out new innovations and interventions that allow us to be better surgeons, providing better care for our patients.

ACKNOWLEDGEMENTS

We would like to thank all the authors who have contributed to the writing of this text. Their hard work, time, and ideas are greatly appreciated.

Dr Mazzocca

I would like to thank my wife Jennifer, Gus, Jillian, and Nicolo for all of their support. Without my family, this means nothing.

Dr Lindsay

First and foremost, I would like to thank my wife Britta for her patience and unwavering support. I am also very grateful to my mentors who have gained so much wisdom and let me borrow a little of it over the years.

Augustus D. Mazzocca MS, MD
Director of the UCONN Musculoskeletal Institute
Professor and Chairman, Department of
Orthopaedic Surgery
Director UCONN Orthopaedic Residency Program,
Gray-Gossling Endowed Chair of Orthopaedic Surgery
Orthopaedic Team Physician University
of Connecticut Athletics
Farmington CT 06030

Adam D. Lindsay, MD
Assistant Professor
Department of Orthopaedic Surgery
Division of Orthopaedic Oncology
UCONN Health Center
Farmington CT 06030

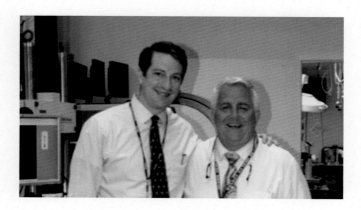

Contents

SECTION I
INTRODUCTION

1 **The Role of Orthobiologics in Orthopaedics,** *1*
Jeffrey Choi, BS, Emily J. Curry, BA, and Xinning Li, MD

2 **FDA Regulations and Their Impact,** *9*
Adam W. Anz, MD and Caleb O. Pinegar, DO, ATC

SECTION II
BASIC SCIENCE

3 **Growth Factors,** *19*
Neil Bakshi, MD, Moin Khan, MD, MSc, FRCSC, and Asheesh Bedi, MD

4 **Biologics in Orthopaedic Surgery,** *27*
Anthony F. De Giacomo, MD, Michael B. Banffy, MD, and Neal S. ElAttrache, MD

5 **Allograft Tissue Safety and Technology,** *49*
Mark A. Moore, PhD, Brian Samsell, BS, and Julie McLean, PhD

SECTION III
CLINICAL APPLICATIONS IN SPORTS MEDICINE

6 **Biologics in Sports Medicine—Introduction,** *63*
Laura A. Vogel, MD, Mary Beth R. McCarthy, BS, and Augustus D. Mazzocca, MS, MD

7 **Rotator Cuff Augmentation,** *69*
Jason P. Rogers, MD, Adam Kwapisz, MD, PhD, and John M. Tokish, MD

8 **Bone Loss in the Upper Extremity,** *75*
Matthew T. Provencher, MD, MC, USNR, Jake A. Fox, BS, Anthony Sanchez, BS, Colin P. Murphy, BA, and Liam A. Peebles, BA

9 **Preserving the Articulating Surface of the Knee,** *85*
Bryan M. Saltzman, MD, David R. Christian, BS, Michael L. Redondo, MA, BS, and Brian J. Cole, MD, MBA

10 **Orthobiologics in Osteoarthritis,** *101*
Thierry Pauyo, MD, FRCSC and James P. Bradley, MD

11 **Biologics in Orthopedic Surgery: Ligament Reconstruction in the Knee,** *105*
Katherine Coyner, MD, Jamie Friedman, MD, and Colin Pavano, BA

12 **Treating the Subchondral Environment and Avascular Necrosis,** *123*
Jorge Chahla, MD, PhD, Andreas H. Gomoll, MD, and Bert R. Mandelbaum, MD, DHL

SECTION IV
CLINICAL APPLICATIONS IN GENERAL ORTHOPAEDICS

13 **Biologics in Hand Surgery,** *135*
Ryu Yoshida, MD, Samuel Baron, BS, Craig Rodner, MD, and Joel Ferreira, MD

14 **Biologic Augmentation in Peripheral Nerve Repair,** *141*
Winnie A. Palispis, MD and Ranjan Gupta, MD

15 **Biologics in Spinal Fusion,** *165*
Hardeep Singh, MD and Isaac L. Moss, MD

16 Biologics in Foot and Ankle Surgery, *175*
Adam D. Lindsay, MD, Vinayak Sathe, MD, MS, FRCS, and John Playfair Ross, BS, MD

17 Biologics in Fracture Care, *185*
Stephen L. Davis, MD

18 Biologics in Musculoskeletal Oncology, *193*
Zachary Cavenaugh, MD and Adam D. Lindsay, MD

SECTION V
FUTURE DIRECTIONS

19 Regenerative Engineering in the Field of Orthopedic Surgery, *201*
Cato T. Laurencin, MD, PhD and Mary A. Badon, MD, MBA

INDEX, *215*

CHAPTER 1

The Role of Orthobiologics in Orthopaedics

JEFFREY CHOI, BS • EMILY J. CURRY, BA • XINNING LI, MD

The practice of medicine is ever-changing and with the exponential advancement of biotechnology, the field is developing and progressing faster than ever. We are continuously inundated by new medications, medical devices, and surgical equipment. The field of orthopaedic surgery is no exception, with constant improvements in arthroscopic techniques and implants for joint arthroplasty that provide more effective treatment options for patients. However, despite these advancements, daily challenges still exist in orthopaedics. For example, while total joint arthroplasty has been an extremely successful option for geriatric patients, owing to the limitations in long-term implant durability, it is a less desirable procedure for the younger and active patients. Instead, these patients will benefit from orthobiologic treatments that target cartilaginous healing or regeneration.

Due to an improved understanding of the role that particular cells and growth factors play in tissue healing and restoration, orthobiologics have emerged as a new class of substances that are intended to accelerate, improve, and augment biologic healing.[1] The use of orthobiologics is a novel way to treat many orthopaedic diseases. Orthobiologics function by harnessing or mimicking natural growth factors found within the body and redirecting their use to accelerate recovery and tissue healing.[1,2]

Over the past few decades, orthobiologics have evolved tremendously. The first generation of orthobiologics was composed of hyaluronic acid (HA) in the form of viscosupplementation.[3] It was then followed by platelet-rich plasma, the first autologous form of orthobiologics (Fig. 1.1).[3] More recently, cell therapies using stem cells have emerged as the third generation of orthobiologics.[3] However, the use of orthobiologics has outpaced its validation. In this chapter, we will explore the different roles of biologics in orthopaedics.

These topics will also be revisited in more detail in subsequent chapters.

Viscosupplementation was the first orthobiologic developed to treat joint arthritis. It was initially used in Europe and Asia and was approved by the U.S. Food and Drug Administration in 1997.[4] When conservative treatment modalities (such as a physical therapy, pain medications, and intraarticular steroids)[5] fail to manage symptoms of joint arthritis, viscosupplementation can be injected into the affected joint as another treatment option.[4] The HA found in these injections is derived from processed poultry combs and is intended to mimic hyaluronan, a gellike liquid found naturally in synovial fluid. HA works by lubricating the articular surfaces of a joint and absorbing shock to reduce joint loads.[6,7]

Intraarticular HA (IAHA) has been used for more than 20 years, especially for the management of knee osteoarthritis. HA injection has also been used off-label to treat shoulder and ankle arthritis. Nonetheless, the effectiveness of IAHA is still heavily debated.[8] While the Osteoarthritis Research Society International (OARSI) and the American College of Rheumatology (ACR) initially recommended IAHA to treat knee arthritis, they now only conditionally recommend it.[9-12] Furthermore, the American Academy of Orthopedic Surgeon Clinical Practice Guidelines do not recommend the use of HA for the symptomatic treatment of knee osteoarthritis.[13] Trigkilidas and Anand (2013) looked at 14 randomized controlled trials (RCTs), of which 12 studies compared HA with a placebo. Out of the 12 RCTs, five trials reported no statistically significant difference between the two groups.[14] The other seven studies suggested varying degrees of IAHA effect.[14] Consequently, there have been many systematic reviews and metaanalyses of the literature that have attempted to reach a definitive conclusion

Biologics in Orthopaedic Surgery. https://doi.org/10.1016/B978-0-323-55140-3.00001-1

about the efficacy of HA for knee arthritis. The conclusions from the reviews are controversial.[15] Of these, some reviews supported the use of viscosupplementation as opposed to placebo, acetaminophen, and

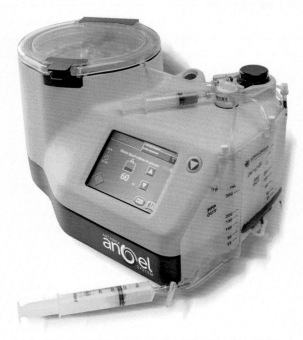

FIG. 1.1 Angel System by Arthrex (Naples, FL), which centrifuges whole blood from the patient to acquire platelet-rich plasma for the injections.

nonsteroidal antiinflammatory drugs (NSAIDs).[16–21] On the contrary, the other reviews state that viscosupplementation is not an effective therapy because of the marginal clinical benefit,[22,23] increased risk of adverse events,[24] and only recognizable short-term effects.[25]

PRP, also known as platelet-enriched plasma, platelet-rich concentrate, and autogenous platelet gel, is the plasma fraction of autologous blood that has a higher platelet concentration.[26] A platelet count of 4–5 times the baseline must be present to classify plasma as PRP,[1] and it is the first orthobiologic in the form of an autologous blood product. PRP was first used for open heart surgery by Ferrari et al. in 1987[27] and first applied in orthopaedic surgery for bone healing by Marx et al.[28] Since then, PRP has been used for numerous musculoskeletal conditions including decreasing symptoms in chronic conditions such as knee osteoarthritis and tendinopathies of the patellar tendon, elbow, and Achilles.[29] PRP has also been investigated for its use in accelerating fracture healing of nonunions and bone to tendon healing in anterior cruciate ligament (ACL) reconstruction and rotator cuff repair.[29]

PRP has its origins in autologous blood injections (ABI), which introduce the patient's own venous blood to the desired area (Fig. 1.2). However, the results of ABI had been inconsistent owing to the delivery of multiple blood components, such as red blood cells and white blood cells, which do not have healing properties.[1] However, the practice of using autologous blood to accelerate the healing process of damaged tissues continues to dramatically evolve as researchers

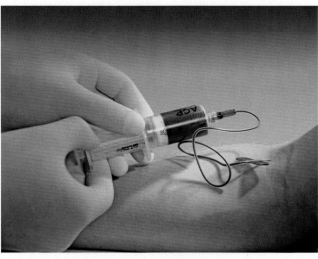

FIG. 1.2 First step in the autologous platelet-rich plasma preparation. Blood is taken from the patient before the centrifuge step.

gained a better understanding of the role of platelets not only in hemostasis but also in the regeneration of tissues.[30,31] The discovery of growth factors contained in the α-granules of platelets led to the use of concentrated platelets in the form of PRP.[1] There are approximately 50–80 α-granules and more than 30 different proteins in a mature platelet.[32] Some of the important proteins include platelet-derived growth factor (PDGF), transforming growth factor (TGF), epidermal growth factor (EGF), fibroblast growth factor (FGF), and vascular endothelial growth factor (VEGF).[26,33] The production and secretion of such growth factors directly influence the regenerative potential of PRP. Activated platelets quickly start releasing the proteins from α-granules within minutes and continue to generate and discharge these factors for the additional days of their life span.[26,34] There are many different preparations of PRP available including both leukocyte-rich and -poor concentrates that can be applied in two different ways: activated and nonactivated. However, there is no consensus on the standards of PRP preparation, which makes it difficult to compare available studies in the literature.[35–37] Two classification systems have been proposed based on different PRP preparations (Tables 1.1 and 1.2). Currently, PRP is being used in orthopaedic conditions that are commonly complicated by chronicity including osteoarthritis, lateral epicondylar tendinopathy, and patellar or Achilles tendinopathy.

PRP has become a new remedy for knee osteoarthritis due to the abundance of growth factors thought to reverse cartilage degeneration.[1] It is promising to know that most published randomized control trials have consistently demonstrated positive results with PRP injections for knee osteoarthritis compared with placebo and HA injections.[40,41] On the other hand, the results investigating the efficacy of PRP injections for chronic lateral epicondylar tendinopathy have been controversial, and further investigations should follow to find more evidence and reach a consensus.[42,43] Meanwhile, it might be worthwhile to try PRP injections in patients who have exhausted all other established conservative therapies before proceeding with surgery. Lastly, there is no current optimal nonsurgical management for patellar tendinopathy beyond eccentric exercise.[44–46] It led to trials that evaluated the use of PRP injections for chronic jumper's knee, which were supported by early promising results of PRP from in vitro models. Thus far, however, the experiments published have mostly been cohort or case series studies, and only one small RCT has been conducted.[47] With a good safety profile and optimistic clinical evidence, the use of PRP injections may play a major role in treating many orthopaedic conditions in the future.

TABLE 1.1
Sports Medicine Classification of Platelet-Rich Plasma

Type	Leukocyte	Activation of PRP	Platelet Concentration
1	Increased	No activation	A. = or > 5× B. < 5×
2	Increased	Activated	A. = or > 5× B. < 5×
3	Minimal/absent	No activation	A. = or > 5× B. < 5×
4	Minimal/absent	Activated	A. = or > 5× B. < 5×

Adapted from Mishra A, Harmon K, Woodall J, Vieira A. Sports medicine applications of platelet rich plasma. *Curr Pharm Biotechnol* 2012;13(7):1185–1195.

TABLE 1.2
Ehrenfest Platelet-Rich Plasma Classification[39]

Type	Leukocyte	Fibrin Network
Pure platelet-rich plasma (P-PRP)	Without	Low density
Leukocyte- and platelet-rich plasma (L-PRP)	With	Low density
Pure platelet-rich fibrin (P-PRF)	Without	High density
Leukocyte- and platelet-rich fibrin (L-PRF)	With	High density

Bone repair and fracture healing is another field that uses orthobiologics and is actively researched. There are four key elements that play a role in bone remodeling: osteogenic stem cells, osteoinductive growth factors, osteoconductive matrix, and vascular supply.[48] Growth factors, such as TGF, induce stem cells to differentiate into osteoblasts, which generate bone by using a scaffold made of matrix and blood supply.[49] A better understanding of these bone regeneration processes has allowed the emergence and use of other kinds of biologics, such as bone grafts, cellular-based therapies, and growth factors.[50]

Autologous bone grafting or "autograft" is used by transplanting osseous matter harvested from one location to another location of the same patient.[51] For example, the coracoid and iliac crest are two commonly harvested bone grafts for Latarjet anterior shoulder stabilization in shoulder surgery. Autologous bone grafting is considered the gold standard for healing nonunions and large bony defects owing to its complete histocompatibility, osteoinductive, osteoconductive, and osteogenic potentials.[52] The modern study of autologous bone grafting can be traced back to 1867 when Ollier demonstrated the osteogenic and osteoconductive properties of transplanted bone.[53] Since then, autologous bone grafts have been used in fracture nonunions of many different anatomic sites including the forearm, humerus, femur, and tibia; it has, however, produced mixed outcomes.[53] While recent studies have reported promising results, especially in femoral[54] and tibial[55] fracture nonunions, the harvesting process of bone has several limitations. Besides donor site pain (the most common complication), it can cause increased blood loss and operative time during the surgical procedure.[52] Most importantly, there is also a limited supply of graft for bridging large defects.[51]

Allografts are another type of graft that overcome some of the major limitations of autograft by harvesting osseous matter from human cadavers and prepared by ethanol, acids, and γ-irradiation to sterilize and eradicate viable cells (Fig. 1.3).[51] This resolves histoincompatibility, but at the same time, removes osteogenic potential.[56] Furthermore, the osteoinductive capacity of the allopathic bone graft is dependent on the preparation technique.[51] Demineralized bone matrix (DBM) is a highly processed allopathic bone graft derivative containing type-1 collagen, noncollagenous proteins, and osteoinductive growth factors.[51] DBM is highly osteoconductive due to its three-dimensional architecture to serve as a scaffold for bone regeneration.[57] Therefore, this material has become an attractive alternative treatment modality when autograft is not ideal, especially in the pediatric and osteoporotic population.[58] However, there have been insufficient human clinical data from case reports and uncontrolled retrospective reviews about the use of DBM, and most of the clinical trials involving DBM are those where it serves as an adjuvant to other therapies such as bone marrow aspirate or combination with autograft.[58,59] As such, DBM is now a popular adjunct for treating long bone fractures, nonunions, and spinal fusions.[51]

Synthetic bone grafts, such as calcium sulfate and calcium phosphate, were developed in the interest of creating an alternative osteoconductive porous material that can be implanted into bone. Even though synthetic bone grafts are strictly osteoconductive and therefore have a limited biological role in bone healing, they are widely available at relatively low cost and, most importantly, can be mixed with other adjuvants.[51,58] Calcium sulfate and calcium phosphate have been extensively used and evaluated for the management of distal radius and tibial plateau fractures, but beneficial evidence from clinical trials is limited.[60,61]

Synthetic bioactive growth factors have been used to treat bone injury based on their osteoinductive capacity. Bone morphogenetic proteins (BMPs), which belong to the TGF-β superfamily, are true osteoinducers, and are the most intensely researched osteogenic growth factors.[62] Among the many different types of BMP, which have shown significant osteogenic properties, BMP-2 and BMP-7 (osteogenic protein-1) are the most investigated.[50] Both BMP-2 and BMP-7 have demonstrated promising results in large randomized controlled studies, which have led to FDA approvals in certain clinical situations. Currently, BMP-2 is approved for use in acute, open tibial fractures as well as for insertion within a titanium tapered cage in anterior lumbar interbody fusion procedures.[58,63] BMP-7 is approved under the US FDA's Humanitarian Device Exemption for use as an alternative to autograft in long bone nonunions and revision posterior lumbar fusion procedures.[50] Other osteogenic growth factors, such as FGF and PDGF, have also been studied but have failed to show significant improvement in bone recovery.[64,65]

Stem cell–based therapy has quickly garnered great interest over the past decade in regenerative medicine owing to its unique ability to differentiate into various mature cell types. There are two types of stem cells:

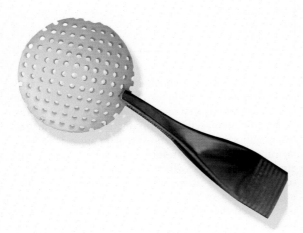

FIG. 1.3 Cartiform by Arthrex, which is an osteochondral allograft that is trimmable to match the defect size and contains chondrocytes, growth factors, and extracellular matrix proteins intended to promote healing.

embryonic stem cells (ESCs) and somatic/adult stem cells. ESCs have a potential to undergo infinite self-renewal and are truly pluripotent, with the ability to develop into any type of cell in the human body.[66,67] However, ESCs can only be collected from embryos because they are derived from the inner cell mass of blastocysts.[66,68] This has raised many ethical and legal concerns.[68] In addition, ESCs are forbidden for use in patients not only because of ethical and legal controversies but also due to their oncogenic potential of inducing teratomas.[66] Adult stem cells, on the other hand, are multipotent stem cells that can differentiate into cells of only one germ layer[69,70] and are isolated from postnatal animals, usually human beings.[71,72] Therefore, the application of adult stem cells has become a subject that has received great attention, as it is associated with less ethical concerns, a better safety profile, and nonimmunogenic property.[73] However, its applicability is limited by their multipotency. Among adult stem cells, mesenchymal stem cells (MSCs) harvested from adult mesenchymal tissues have held the most promise in orthobiologics.[66] In 1976, Friedenstein et al. first isolated MSCs from bone marrow, which is currently considered the gold standard.[74–76] For the last few years, there have been many attempts to isolate MSCs from other sources of the human body, including adipose tissue, peripheral blood, synovium, umbilical cord, and dental pulp.[74,76,77] These MSCs have an ability to differentiate into cartilage, bone, tendon, bone marrow stroma, and tendon,[78,79] which makes MSCs such an appealing candidate for use in the treatment of numerous orthopaedic diseases.

Bone marrow aspirate concentrate (BMAC), a type of autologous graft, was previously thought to contain a regenerative potential primarily owing to its high MSC concentration. However, it has been reported that only 0.001%–0.01% of mononuclear cells in bone marrow aspirates are MSCs.[71,80] It is still obscure as to where the beneficial effects originate from because BMAC also contains an abundance of growth factors and cytokines in addition to MSC. Nonetheless, osteogenic properties of BMAC have been demonstrated in the literature for treating many orthopaedic diseases, including osteoarthritis,[81] rotator cuff tears,[82] osteonecrosis,[83] and nonunions.[84]

Every year new types of biologics are developed, and their applications to treat different musculoskeletal disorders are expanding. For example, cell sheet technology has recently been introduced to augment tendon grafts. Tendon grafts wrapped with stem cell sheets have shown promising data especially for ACL reconstruction.[85] Gene therapy is another new technology that has been explored to overcome the inconvenience of growth factor treatment caused by repeated dosing owing to its short life span.[86] The insertion of genetic material into a target cell is expected to induce continuous production of growth factors or cytokines by the cell, and it has been intensely studied for rotator cuff repair.[87] There also have been many trials regarding synovial-derived stem cells for cartilage restoration because no clinical comparisons in the literature are available about the optimal source of MSC.[88] With greater chondrogenic potential than MSCs from other sources, the use of synovial-derived stem cells is gaining popularity as a treatment modality for cartilage defects.[88,89]

Besides musculoskeletal recovery, nerve regeneration has also benefited from the recent advancement of biologics. There has been an interest in using neurotrophic factors to speed peripheral nerve regeneration.[90] For instance, VEGF[91] and IGF[92,93] have demonstrated their potentials to improve Schwann cell formation and axonal outgrowth. Furthermore, cell-based therapies have been studied for augmenting peripheral nerve repair as MSCs have been shown to be able to differentiate into nonmesenchymal cells, such as Schwann cells, astrocytes, neurons, and oligodendrocytes. Furthermore, the application of MSCs has demonstrated increased myelin formation and nerve regeneration.[94,95] As recent studies have revealed that the central nerve system (CNS) is capable of a more robust healing than historically perceived,[96] CNS remodeling has also been approached with bioactive molecular, cell-based, and scaffold-based biologic modalities.[97]

Over the past decade, there has been growing attention and expanding attempts at using biologics for the treatment of various orthopaedic conditions. These treatments called orthobiologics have opened a new era of managing musculoskeletal injuries of intrinsically poor healing potential. In this book and the following chapters, we will provide an overview of the history, common uses, and potential future applications of many different kinds of orthobiologics in various topics of orthopaedics that will help address many different clinical scenarios. There is a paucity of clinical data available in terms of quality and quantity in human research studies supporting use of biologic materials in patients, demonstrating a great need to improve our understanding of the fundamental molecular and cellular mechanisms of musculoskeletal tissue regeneration to better tailor the use of biologic approaches. However, there is no doubt that biologics hold great promise and potential to reinforce healing of challenging orthopaedic tissue injuries. In the subsequent chapters, we will explore basic scientific backgrounds, the clinical applications in sports medicine, as well as other general orthopaedics, and future directions of orthobiologics.

REFERENCES

1. Dhillon MS, Behera P, Patel S, Shetty V. Orthobiologics and platelet rich plasma. *Indian J Orthop.* 2014;48(1):1–9.
2. *Helping Fractures Heal (Orthobiologics).* 2010. http://orthoinfo.aaos.org/topic.cfm?topic=A00525.
3. Sampson S, Gerhardt M, Mandelbaum B. Platelet rich plasma injection grafts for musculoskeletal injuries: a review. *Curr Rev Musculoskelet Med.* 2008;1(3–4):165–174.
4. Viscosupplementation Treatment for Knee Arthritis 2015. http://orthoinfo.aaos.org/topic.cfm?topic=a00217.
5. Adams ME. An analysis of clinical studies of the use of crosslinked hyaluronan, hylan, in the treatment of osteoarthritis. *J Rheumatol Suppl.* 1993;39:16–18.
6. Filardo G, Kon E, Di Martino A, et al. Platelet-rich plasma vs hyaluronic acid to treat knee degenerative pathology: study design and preliminary results of a randomized controlled trial. *BMC Musculoskelet Disord.* 2012;13:229.
7. Balazs EA, Denlinger JL. Viscosupplementation: a new concept in the treatment of osteoarthritis. *J Rheumatol Suppl.* 1993;39:3–9.
8. Richette P, Chevalier X, Ea HK, et al. Hyaluronan for knee osteoarthritis: an updated meta-analysis of trials with low risk of bias. *RMD Open.* 2015;1(1):e000071.
9. McAlindon TE, Bannuru RR, Sullivan MC, et al. OARSI guidelines for the non-surgical management of knee osteoarthritis. *Osteoarthr Cartil.* 2014;22(3):363–388.
10. Zhang W, Moskowitz RW, Nuki G, et al. OARSI recommendations for the management of hip and knee osteoarthritis, part II: OARSI evidence-based, expert consensus guidelines. *Osteoarthr Cartil.* 2008;16(2):137–162.
11. Recommendations for the medical management of osteoarthritis of the hip and knee: 2000 update. American College of Rheumatology Subcommittee on Osteoarthritis Guidelines. *Arthritis Rheum.* 2000;43(9):1905–1915.
12. Hochberg MC, Altman RD, April KT, et al. American College of Rheumatology 2012 recommendations for the use of nonpharmacologic and pharmacologic therapies in osteoarthritis of the hand, hip, and knee. *Arthritis Care Res Hob.* 2012;64(4):465–474.
13. Jevsevar DS, Brown GA, Jones DL, et al. The American Academy of Orthopaedic Surgeons evidence-based guideline on: treatment of osteoarthritis of the knee, 2nd edition. *J Bone Joint Surg Am.* 2013;95(20):1885–1886.
14. Trigkilidas D, Anand A. The effectiveness of hyaluronic acid intra-articular injections in managing osteoarthritic knee pain. *Ann R Coll Surg Engl.* 2013;95(8):545–551.
15. Campbell J, Bellamy N, Gee T. Differences between systematic reviews/meta-analyses of hyaluronic acid/hyaluronan/hylan in osteoarthritis of the knee. *Osteoarthr Cartil.* 2007;15(12):1424–1436.
16. Modawal A, Ferrer M, Choi HK, Castle JA. Hyaluronic acid injections relieve knee pain. *J Fam Pract.* 2005;54(9):758–767.
17. Wang CT, Lin J, Chang CJ, Lin YT, Hou SM. Therapeutic effects of hyaluronic acid on osteoarthritis of the knee. A meta-analysis of randomized controlled trials. *J Bone Joint Surg Am.* 2004;86-A(3):538–545.
18. Bellamy N, Campbell J, Robinson V, Gee T, Bourne R, Wells G. Viscosupplementation for the treatment of osteoarthritis of the knee. *Cochrane Database Syst Rev.* 2006;2:CD005321.
19. Bannuru RR, Natov NS, Dasi UR, Schmid CH, McAlindon TE. Therapeutic trajectory following intra-articular hyaluronic acid injection in knee osteoarthritis–meta-analysis. *Osteoarthr Cartil.* 2011;19(6):611–619.
20. Towheed TE, Maxwell L, Judd MG, Catton M, Hochberg MC, Wells G. Acetaminophen for osteoarthritis. *Cochrane Database Syst Rev.* 2006;1:CD004257.
21. Zhang W, Nuki G, Moskowitz RW, et al. OARSI recommendations for the management of hip and knee osteoarthritis: part III: changes in evidence following systematic cumulative update of research published through January 2009. *Osteoarthr Cartil.* 2010;18(4):476–499.
22. Arrich J, Piribauer F, Mad P, Schmid D, Klaushofer K, Mullner M. Intra-articular hyaluronic acid for the treatment of osteoarthritis of the knee: systematic review and meta-analysis. *CMAJ.* 2005;172(8):1039–1043.
23. Lo GH, LaValley M, McAlindon T, Felson DT. Intra-articular hyaluronic acid in treatment of knee osteoarthritis: a meta-analysis. *JAMA.* 2003;290(23):3115–3121.
24. Rutjes AW, Juni P, da Costa BR, Trelle S, Nuesch E, Reichenbach S. Viscosupplementation for osteoarthritis of the knee: a systematic review and meta-analysis. *Ann Intern Med.* 2012;157(3):180–191.
25. Medina JM, Thomas A, Denegar CR. Knee osteoarthritis: should your patient opt for hyaluronic acid injection? *J Fam Pract.* 2006;55(8):669–675.
26. Alsousou J, Thompson M, Hulley P, Noble A, Willett K. The biology of platelet-rich plasma and its application in trauma and orthopaedic surgery: a review of the literature. *J Bone Joint Surg Br.* 2009;91(8):987–996.
27. Ferrari M, Zia S, Valbonesi M, et al. A new technique for hemodilution, preparation of autologous platelet-rich plasma and intraoperative blood salvage in cardiac surgery. *Int J Artif Organs.* 1987;10(1):47–50.
28. Marx RE, Carlson ER, Eichstaedt RM, Schimmele SR, Strauss JE, Georgeff KR. Platelet-rich plasma: growth factor enhancement for bone grafts. *Oral Surg Oral Med Oral Pathol Oral Radiol Endod.* 1998;85(6):638–646.
29. Taylor DW, Petrera M, Hendry M, Theodoropoulos JS. A systematic review of the use of platelet-rich plasma in sports medicine as a new treatment for tendon and ligament injuries. *Clin J Sport Med.* 2011;21(4):344–352.
30. Anitua E, Sanchez M, Nurden AT, Nurden P, Orive G, Andia I. New insights into and novel applications for platelet-rich fibrin therapies. *Trends Biotechnol.* 2006;24(5):227–234.
31. Werner S, Grose R. Regulation of wound healing by growth factors and cytokines. *Physiol Rev.* 2003;83(3):835–870.
32. Harrison P, Cramer EM. Platelet alpha-granules. *Blood Rev.* 1993;7(1):52–62.
33. Sunitha Raja V, Munirathnam Naidu E. Platelet-rich fibrin: evolution of a second-generation platelet concentrate. *Indian J Dent Res.* 2008;19(1):42–46.

34. Kevy SV, Jacobson MS. Comparison of methods for point of care preparation of autologous platelet gel. *J Extra Corpor Technol.* 2004;36(1):28–35.

35. Dhurat R, Sukesh M. Principles and methods of preparation of platelet-rich plasma: a review and author's perspective. *J Cutan Aesthet Surg.* 2014;7(4):189–197.

36. Dragoo JL, Braun HJ, Durham JL, et al. Comparison of the acute inflammatory response of two commercial platelet-rich plasma systems in healthy rabbit tendons. *Am J Sports Med.* 2012;40(6):1274–1281.

37. McCarrel TM, Minas T, Fortier LA. Optimization of leukocyte concentration in platelet-rich plasma for the treatment of tendinopathy. *J Bone Joint Surg Am.* 2012;94(19): e143(141–148).

38. Mishra A, Harmon K, Woodall J, Vieira A. Sports medicine applications of platelet rich plasma. *Curr Pharm Biotechnol.* 2012;13(7):1185–1195.

39. Dohan Ehrenfest DM, Rasmusson L, Albrektsson T. Classification of platelet concentrates: from pure platelet-rich plasma (P-PRP) to leucocyte- and platelet-rich fibrin (L-PRF). *Trends Biotechnol.* 2009;27(3):158–167.

40. Cerza F, Carni S, Carcangiu A, et al. Comparison between hyaluronic acid and platelet-rich plasma, intra-articular infiltration in the treatment of gonarthrosis. *Am J Sports Med.* 2012;40(12):2822–2827.

41. Patel S, Dhillon MS, Aggarwal S, Marwaha N, Jain A. Treatment with platelet-rich plasma is more effective than placebo for knee osteoarthritis: a prospective, double-blind, randomized trial. *Am J Sports Med.* 2013;41(2):356–364.

42. Mishra AK, Skrepnik NV, Edwards SG, et al. Efficacy of platelet-rich plasma for chronic tennis elbow: a double-blind, prospective, multicenter, randomized controlled trial of 230 patients. *Am J Sports Med.* 2014;42(2): 463–471.

43. Krogh TP, Fredberg U, Stengaard-Pedersen K, Christensen R, Jensen P, Ellingsen T. Treatment of lateral epicondylitis with platelet-rich plasma, glucocorticoid, or saline: a randomized, double-blind, placebo-controlled trial. *Am J Sports Med.* 2013;41(3):625–635.

44. Jonsson P, Alfredson H. Superior results with eccentric compared to concentric quadriceps training in patients with jumper's knee: a prospective randomised study. *Br J Sports Med.* 2005;39(11):847–850.

45. Andres BM, Murrell GA. Treatment of tendinopathy: what works, what does not, and what is on the horizon. *Clin Orthop Relat Res.* 2008;466(7):1539–1554.

46. Peers KH, Lysens RJ. Patellar tendinopathy in athletes: current diagnostic and therapeutic recommendations. *Sports Med.* 2005;35(1):71–87.

47. Dragoo JL, Wasterlain AS, Braun HJ, Nead KT. Platelet-rich plasma as a treatment for patellar tendinopathy: a double-blind, randomized controlled trial. *Am J Sports Med.* 2014;42(3):610–618.

48. Lieberman JR. Orthopaedic gene therapy. Fracture healing and other nongenetic problems of bone. *Clin Orthop Relat Res.* 2000;(suppl 379):S156–S158.

49. Hannallah D, Peterson B, Lieberman JR, Fu FH, Huard J. Gene therapy in orthopaedic surgery. *Instr Course Lect.* 2003;52:753–768.

50. Virk MS, Lieberman JR. Biologic adjuvants for fracture healing. *Arthritis Res Ther.* 2012;14(6):225.

51. Roberts TT, Rosenbaum AJ. Bone grafts, bone substitutes and orthobiologics: the bridge between basic science and clinical advancements in fracture healing. *Organogenesis.* 2012;8(4):114–124.

52. Khan SN, Cammisa Jr FP, Sandhu HS, Diwan AD, Girardi FP, Lane JM. The biology of bone grafting. *J Am Acad Orthop Surg.* 2005;13(1):77–86.

53. Marino JT, Ziran BH. Use of solid and cancellous autologous bone graft for fractures and nonunions. *Orthop Clin North Am.* 2010;41(1):15–26.

54. Chapman MW, Finkemeier CG. Treatment of supracondylar nonunions of the femur with plate fixation and bone graft. *J Bone Joint Surg Am.* 1999;81(9): 1217–1228.

55. Wiss DA, Stetson WB. Tibial nonunion: treatment alternatives. *J Am Acad Orthop Surg.* 1996;4(5):249–257.

56. Bae DS, Waters PM, Gebhardt MC. Results of free vascularized fibula grafting for allograft nonunion after limb salvage surgery for malignant bone tumors. *J Pediatr Orthop.* 2006;26(6):809–814.

57. Kirk JF, Ritter G, Waters C, Narisawa S, Millan JL, Talton JD. Osteoconductivity and osteoinductivity of NanoFUSE((R)) DBM. *Cell Tissue Bank.* 2013;14(1):33–44.

58. Watson JT, Nicolaou DA. Orthobiologics in the augmentation of osteoporotic fractures. *Curr Osteoporos Rep.* 2015;13(1):22–29.

59. Hierholzer C, Sama D, Toro JB, Peterson M, Helfet DL. Plate fixation of ununited humeral shaft fractures: effect of type of bone graft on healing. *J Bone Joint Surg Am.* 2006;88(7):1442–1447.

60. Goff T, Kanakaris NK, Giannoudis PV. Use of bone graft substitutes in the management of tibial plateau fractures. *Injury.* 2013;44(suppl 1):S86–S94.

61. Kim JK, Koh YD, Kook SH. Effect of calcium phosphate bone cement augmentation on volar plate fixation of unstable distal radial fractures in the elderly. *J Bone Joint Surg Am.* 2011;93(7):609–614.

62. Chen D, Zhao M, Mundy GR. Bone morphogenetic proteins. *Growth Factors.* 2004;22(4):233–241.

63. Rihn JA, Gates C, Glassman SD, Phillips FM, Schwender JD, Albert TJ. The use of bone morphogenetic protein in lumbar spine surgery. *J Bone Joint Surg Am.* 2008;90(9):2014–2025.

64. Kawaguchi H, Oka H, Jingushi S, et al. A local application of recombinant human fibroblast growth factor 2 for tibial shaft fractures: a randomized, placebo-controlled trial. *J Bone Miner Res.* 2010;25(12): 2735–2743.

65. Digiovanni CW, Baumhauer J, Lin SS, et al. Prospective, randomized, multi-center feasibility trial of rhPDGF-BB versus autologous bone graft in a foot and ankle fusion model. *Foot Ankle Int.* 2011;32(4):344–354.

66. Schmitt A, van Griensven M, Imhoff AB, Buchmann S. Application of stem cells in orthopedics. *Stem Cells Int.* 2012;2012:394962.

67. Kotobuki N, Hirose M, Takakura Y, Ohgushi H. Cultured autologous human cells for hard tissue regeneration: preparation and characterization of mesenchymal stem cells from bone marrow. *Artif Organs.* 2004;28(1):33–39.

68. Thomson JA, Itskovitz-Eldor J, Shapiro SS, et al. Embryonic stem cell lines derived from human blastocysts. *Science.* 1998;282(5391):1145–1147.

69. Ehnert S, Glanemann M, Schmitt A, et al. The possible use of stem cells in regenerative medicine: dream or reality? *Langenbecks Arch Surg.* 2009;394(6):985–997.

70. Ahmad Z, Wardale J, Brooks R, Henson F, Noorani A, Rushton N. Exploring the application of stem cells in tendon repair and regeneration. *Arthroscopy.* 2012;28(7):1018–1029.

71. Pittenger MF, Mackay AM, Beck SC, et al. Multilineage potential of adult human mesenchymal stem cells. *Science.* 1999;284(5411):143–147.

72. Jiang Y, Jahagirdar BN, Reinhardt RL, et al. Pluripotency of mesenchymal stem cells derived from adult marrow. *Nature.* 2002;418(6893):41–49.

73. Javazon EH, Beggs KJ, Flake AW. Mesenchymal stem cells: paradoxes of passaging. *Exp Hematol.* 2004;32(5):414–425.

74. Hass R, Kasper C, Bohm S, Jacobs R. Different populations and sources of human mesenchymal stem cells (MSC): a comparison of adult and neonatal tissue-derived MSC. *Cell Commun Signal.* 2011;9:12.

75. Friedenstein AJ, Gorskaja JF, Kulagina NN. Fibroblast precursors in normal and irradiated mouse hematopoietic organs. *Exp Hematol.* 1976;4(5):267–274.

76. Nancarrow-Lei R, Mafi P, Mafi R, Khan W. A systemic review of the sources of adult mesenchymal stem cells and their suitability in musculoskeletal applications. *Curr Stem Cell Res Ther.* 2017;12(8):601–610.

77. Mafi R, Hindocha S, Mafi P, Griffin M, Khan WS. Sources of adult mesenchymal stem cells applicable for musculoskeletal applications - a systematic review of the literature. *Open Orthop J.* 2011;5(suppl 2):242–248.

78. Ohgushi H, Caplan AI. Stem cell technology and bioceramics: from cell to gene engineering. *J Biomed Mater Res.* 1999;48(6):913–927.

79. Zaidi N, Nixon AJ. Stem cell therapy in bone repair and regeneration. *Ann N Y Acad Sci.* 2007;1117:62–72.

80. Martin DR, Cox NR, Hathcock TL, Niemeyer GP, Baker HJ. Isolation and characterization of multipotential mesenchymal stem cells from feline bone marrow. *Exp Hematol.* 2002;30(8):879–886.

81. Yubo M, Yanyan L, Li L, Tao S, Bo L, Lin C. Clinical efficacy and safety of mesenchymal stem cell transplantation for osteoarthritis treatment: a meta-analysis. *PLoS One.* 2017;12(4):e0175449.

82. Ellera Gomes JL, da Silva RC, Silla LM, Abreu MR, Pellanda R. Conventional rotator cuff repair complemented by the aid of mononuclear autologous stem cells. *Knee Surg Sports Traumatol Arthrosc.* 2012;20(2):373–377.

83. Hernigou P, Poignard A, Zilber S, Rouard H. Cell therapy of hip osteonecrosis with autologous bone marrow grafting. *Indian J Orthop.* 2009;43(1):40–45.

84. Connolly JF, Guse R, Tiedeman J, Dehne R. Autologous marrow injection as a substitute for operative grafting of tibial nonunions. *Clin Orthop Relat Res.* 1991;266:259–270.

85. Mifune Y, Matsumoto T, Takayama K, et al. Tendon graft revitalization using adult anterior cruciate ligament (ACL)-derived CD34+ cell sheets for ACL reconstruction. *Biomaterials.* 2013;34(22):5476–5487.

86. Lu YF, Chan KM, Li G, Zhang JF. Tenogenic differentiation of mesenchymal stem cells and noncoding RNA: from bench to bedside. *Exp Cell Res.* 2016;341(2):237–242.

87. Murray IR, LaPrade RF, Musahl V, et al. Biologic treatments for sports injuries II think tank-current concepts, future research, and barriers to advancement, part 2: rotator cuff. *Orthop J Sports Med.* 2016;4(3):2325967116636586.

88. Zlotnicki JP, Geeslin AG, Murray IR, et al. Biologic treatments for sports injuries II think tank-current concepts, future research, and barriers to advancement, part 3: articular cartilage. *Orthop J Sports Med.* 2016;4(4):2325967116642433.

89. Nakamura T, Sekiya I, Muneta T, et al. Arthroscopic, histological and MRI analyses of cartilage repair after a minimally invasive method of transplantation of allogeneic synovial mesenchymal stromal cells into cartilage defects in pigs. *Cytotherapy.* 2012;14(3):327–338.

90. Fowler JR, Lavasani M, Huard J, Goitz RJ. Biologic strategies to improve nerve regeneration after peripheral nerve repair. *J Reconstr Microsurg.* 2015;31(4):243–248.

91. Mohammadi R, Ahsan S, Masoumi M, Amini K. Vascular endothelial growth factor promotes peripheral nerve regeneration after sciatic nerve transection in rat. *Chin J Traumatol.* 2013;16(6):323–329.

92. Mohammadi R, Esmaeil-Sani Z, Amini K. Effect of local administration of insulin-like growth factor I combined with inside-out artery graft on peripheral nerve regeneration. *Injury.* 2013;44(10):1295–1301.

93. Emel E, Ergun SS, Kotan D, et al. Effects of insulin-like growth factor-I and platelet-rich plasma on sciatic nerve crush injury in a rat model. *J Neurosurg.* 2011;114(2):522–528.

94. Ladak A, Olson J, Tredget EE, Gordon T. Differentiation of mesenchymal stem cells to support peripheral nerve regeneration in a rat model. *Exp Neurol.* 2011;228(2):242–252.

95. Keilhoff G, Goihl A, Langnase K, Fansa H, Wolf G. Transdifferentiation of mesenchymal stem cells into Schwann cell-like myelinating cells. *Eur J Cell Biol.* 2006;85(1):11–24.

96. David S, Aguayo AJ. Axonal elongation into peripheral nervous system "bridges" after central nervous system injury in adult rats. *Science.* 1981;214(4523):931–933.

97. Meng F, Modo M, Badylak SF. Biologic scaffold for CNS repair. *Regen Med.* 2014;9(3):367–383.

CHAPTER 2

FDA Regulations and Their Impact

ADAM W. ANZ, MD • CALEB O. PINEGAR, DO, ATC

INTRODUCTION

Progress of biologics in orthopaedic surgery, or ortho-biologics, currently faces a delicate balance involving providers sprinting to apply clinically and profit on unproven technologies and the marathon of technology development through translational medicine. Weighing the balance is the orthopedic community and government regulatory bodies, while aspiring to move the front lines of patient care forward in a safe and ethical manner. While early promising development of orthobiologics was in the hands of basic scientists, the next steps of translation require patient care and have stumbled upon regulatory hurdles and early clinical shortcomings, i.e., technologies not performing as well in clinical trials as they performed in laboratory and animal studies. These hurdles and shortcomings are part of the developmental process and should not be cause for concern. To overcome the hurdles, clinicians and scientists must develop a deeper understanding not only of cellular/molecular mechanisms but also of the entire development process, which requires regulation. One can consider the study and understanding of FDA regulation a lot like understanding the rules of a sport. Rules have been made, precedent has been set, and we as clinicians should understand how to use the rules to not only judge emerging technologies but also sort out how to use them in our clinical practice and clinical trials. As clinicians, we should consider ourselves the referees in this game, at times getting yelled at by industry on one sideline and our patients on the other. The more we know, the better we will perform at translational medicine and the more we can stay out of trouble from regulatory bodies and/or malpractice risk when treating our patients.

Orthobiologics to an orthopedic clinician represent any naturally derived product, which can be used to improve the biology of healing in an orthopaedic intervention, including procedures in clinic such as joint injections and surgical procedures in the operating room. To the Federal Food and Drug Association (FDA), biological products are a subset of drugs and "biological" refers to those medical products that are derived from living material, as opposed to chemically synthesized.[1] The FDA does not consider everything that clinicians consider orthobiologics as biological products. However, the FDA applies the *Federal Food, Drug and Cosmetic Act (FDC Act)* for the monitoring and regulation of many orthobiologics especially those involving cells.

Monitoring and regulation of orthobiologics is a double edge sword, important for patient safety and proof of worth on one side but stifling to progress at times on the other. Loose regulation encourages clinical experimentation, but raises concerns for patient safety, and does not force products to prove their value before clinicians set prices, market, and use them for patient treatments. Although rigid regulation stifles progress, it ensures patient safety and forces technologies to prove themselves through a developmental process. The latter requires a significant investment of time and money but produces clear indications and evidence for care. Although there is not currently an answer (or agreement) to how much freedom or regulation should be established in the development of biologics, the following will be a discussion regarding where we are today, how we got here, and where are we headed.

HISTORY OF THE FEDERAL FOOD AND DRUG ASSOCIATION

The Federal Food and Drug Association (FDA) is an entity that was created by the US government in order to protect the citizens of the United States from abuses in the consumer product marketplace.[2] Prior to 1930, it was known as the Department of Agriculture, but it is origin and history begins almost 100 years earlier.

In 1848, the United States Patent Office appointed Lewis Caleb Beck to analyze agricultural products by means of chemical testing. This marked the beginning of product monitoring and consumer protection in the United States. By 1862, demand had grown such that an entire department was created, the Department of Agriculture.[3] Near the turn of the 20th century, a chemist, Harvey Washington Wiley, worked within

Biologics in Orthopaedic Surgery. https://doi.org/10.1016/B978-0-323-55140-3.00002-3.

the department to prohibit the interstate trade of poor quality and misbranded foods and drugs. In 1906, 25 years of Wiley's work led to the passage of the "Pure Food and Drugs Act." The passage of this act set into motion the modern regulatory functions of the FDA, and it's stated mission today continues to be to protect and promote public health.

It was nearly 30 years after the passage of the Pure Food and Drugs Act that the next bill regarding product safety was passed. This occurred after multiple products came onto the market that resulted in serious reactions and even death to consumers. The worst involved a sulfa drug targeted to pediatric patients, which contained a harmful substance similar to a component of antifreeze. Over 100 people died as a result of exposure to the harmful drug, including children. On June 25th, 1938, Franklin D. Roosevelt approved the "Food, Drug, and Cosmetic Act," a law requiring product labels to include directions for safe use and premarket approval before a drug could be marketed and sold. This approval required that manufacturing companies provide evidence of a drug's safety before marketing and sales could be initiated.

As this new law was enforced and direct-to-consumer marketing emerged, it became evident that not all products could be safely marketed to and used by the public. It was decided that certain products would require a prescription from a physician for individual consumer use. Over ensuing years further legislation was required and evolved as the regulations demanded change to accommodate the growing marketplace of new products and developing technology. For example, as the available supply of nutritional supplements and medications flooded the consumer markets, the control of these products was challenged at the judicial level. Some manufacturers challenged the need for government regulation of their products, and in 1976, the FDA was prohibited from controlling the potency of dietary supplements after being challenged within the court system.

In that same year (1976), medical devices began to receive added attention under the jurisdiction of the FDA after an intrauterine device injured thousands of women. The "1976 Medical Device Amendments" demanded that new devices be placed into three classes, each of which required a different degree of control to ensure both safety and efficacy. The most regulated, Class III, are devices that support or sustain human life, associated with high risks of use. Class II are devices with moderate risk to humans. Class I are considered low-risk items and are not used in supporting or sustaining human life.

Over the last 20 years, many advancements in the regulation and duties of the FDA have been made,

and today the FDA is an agency within the US Department of Health and Human Services. Currently this department consists of the Office of the Commissioner and four directorates that specifically monitor the four core functions of the agency[4]: Medical Products and Tobacco, Food and Veterinary Medicine, Global Regulatory Operations and Policy, and Operations (see Fig. 2.1). While monitoring these core functions the FDA also has specific responsibilities. These responsibilities have been described in five basic categories: protecting the public health by assuring that foods are safe and properly labeled (a shared duty with the US Department of Agriculture) and ensuring that drugs, vaccines, and other biological products and medical devices intended for human use are safe and effective; protecting the public from electronic product radiation; assuring cosmetics and dietary supplements are safe and properly labeled; regulating tobacco products; advancing the public health by helping to speed product innovations (see Fig. 2.2).[5]

SAFETY AND EFFICACY

One of the FDA's most important roles (yet sometimes questioned in the realm of orthobiologics) is to ensure product safety and efficacy prior to marketing. "Safety" involves ensuring that in the course of administering a product in appropriate fashion the product does not cause harm, injury, or loss by the recipient in a direct or indirect manner. For safety, the FDA most concerns itself with the possible introduction, spread, and/or transmission of infectious disease as well as ensuring that treatments do not cause undue adverse events. Adverse events for which the FDA has raised concerns include the possibilities of immune reactions to biologic treatments, infections, the potential for neoplasms, and/or increasing the likelihood of a venous thromboembolic event. "Efficacy" generally involves the power of a treatment to produce a claimed effect. As new biologic treatments are emerging, the due diligence of safety and efficacy should preceed marketing and/or making claims regarding biologic treatments. If the medical community is not willing to police itself regarding safety and efficacy prior to making claims and marketing unproven treatments, the FDA was founded upon a responsibility to protect the public and likely sees this as their charge.[6] Since 2008, the reach of the FDA has extended into both industry and the practice of medicine regarding stem cells and orthobiologics. For this reason, it is important to understand the approval process and demands requested of these therapies.

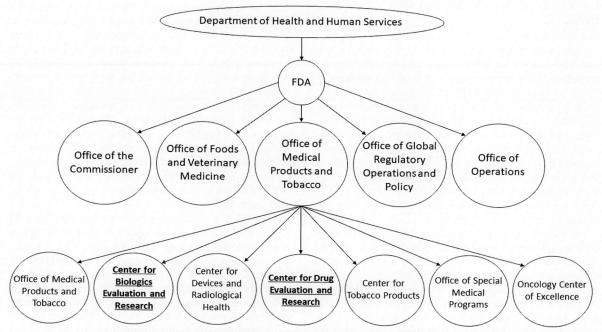

FIG. 2.1 Organization of the FDA. The CDER and CBER (bolded and underlined) have regulatory responsibility for therapeutic biological products, including premarket review and oversight. (Reprinted/adapted by permission from RightsLink Permissions Springer Customer Service Centre GmbH: Springer. Cartilage Restoration by Jack Farr, Andreas H. Gomoll. 2018.)

Responsibilities of the FDA

1. Protect public health by assuring the safety and efficacy of foods*, drugs, medical devices, and biologics.
2. Protect the public from electronic product radiation.
3. Assure proper labeling and safety of cosmetics and dietary supplements.
4. Regulate tobacco products.
5. Advance public health by helping speed product innovations.

FIG. 2.2 *Meat from livestock, poultry, and some egg products are regulated by the US Department of Agriculture and not the FDA.

LAYERED REGULATION: 351 VERSUS 361 PRODUCTS

The FDA derives its authority to regulate biologic products from the Public Health Service Act (PHSA), a federal law enacted in 1944, which outlines the federal government's duties to protect the health of the public. Section 351 of the PHSA (PHSA 351) addresses biological products defined as "virus, therapeutic serum, toxin, antitoxin, vaccine, blood, blood component or derivative, allergenic product, or analogous product,…applicable to the prevention, treatment, or cure of a disease or condition of human beings."[7] PHSA 351 established the authority for the FDA's oversight in the development of these products. Section 361 of the PHSA (PHSA 361) granted the FDA the authority to prevent the spread of communicable diseases.

As biologics have emerged in medicine, the FDA developed layered regulations, based upon perceived risk to the US public, which set the mechanisms of control and oversight established in PHSA 351 and PHSA 361. These regulations are set forth in the Code of Federal Regulations. The Code of Federal Regulations is a document produced yearly that depicts the rules published in the Federal Register. These rules are established by the executive departments and other agencies within the federal government. This document depicts the policies of the FDA and contains specific instructions to manufacturers, healthcare providers, and sponsors in the development/manufacture of products. Title 21 specifically focuses on the rules of the Food and Drug Administration. Part 1271 of Title 21 (21CFR1271) is titled: Human Cells, Tissues, and Cellular and Tissue-based Products, or HCT/Ps for short, and addresses "articles containing or consisting of human cells or tissues that are intended for implantation transplantation, infusion, or transfer into a human recipient."

21 CFR 1271 states that an HCT/P is regulated solely under 361 of the PHSA and must be manufactured to meet the requirements of 21 CFR 1271 alone if it meets four criteria: (1) the HCT/P is minimally manipulated; (2) the HCT/P is intended for homologous use only; (3) the manufacture of the HCT/P does not involve the combination of the cells or tissues with another article, except for water, crystalloids, or a sterilizing, preserving, or storage agent, provided that the addition of water, crystalloids, or the sterilizing, preserving, or storage agent does not raise new clinical safety concerns with respect to the HCT/P; and (4) either the HCT/P does not have a systemic effect and is not dependent upon the metabolic activity of living cells for its primary function or if the HCT/P does have a systemic

effect or is dependent upon the metabolic activity of living cells for its primary function, it is autologous or allogenic in a first-degree or second-degree blood relative (see Fig. 2.3). HCT/Ps that meet these four criteria are often termed "361 products." Although these HCT/P's are not subject to premarket FDA review requirements, 1271 does set forth clear requirements within six domains: (1) registration and listing with the FDA, (2) donor screening and testing, (3) current good tissue practices, (4) labeling, (5) adverse-event reporting, and (6) inspection and enforcement. HCT/Ps that are harvested, processed, and reinjected in the same surgical procedure are exempt from the requirements of CFR 1271; however, they are not exempt from overall regulation under PHSA 361 and/or 351.

HCT/Ps that do not meet criteria described in CFR 1271 are regulated as a drug under section 201(g) of the Federal Food, Drug, and Cosmetic Act, a device, and/or a biological product as outlined in PHSA 351 of the PHS Act. These products, often termed "351 products" are subject to premarket and postmarket development requirements and FDA approval before they can be marketed. In addition, their manufacture must comply with both current good tissue practices and current good manufacturing practices. Development requirements involve a series of steps, which is often called the "351 pathway," and start with preclinical laboratory and animal testing to show that investigational use would be safe in humans. Prior to initiating clinical studies in humans, an investigational New Drug Application (IND) must be in place as described in 21 CFR 312. Subsequent clinical trials prove safety and efficacy in a phased fashion, most often involving first small pilot human study (phase I), small single-site randomized controlled trial (phase II), and large multicenter randomized controlled trial (phase III). Results demonstrating safety and efficacy for an indication are submitted to the FDA as part of a biologics license application (BLA). Approval of a BLA is required prior to marketing or administration of the product in clinical practice. A number of milestones are recognized through the process, and the sponsor communicates with the FDA at multiple time points to guide the process (Fig. 2.4).

While orthopaedists may consider it a surgical procedure, the FDA considers the process of taking tissue from an individual, processing the tissue, and replacing the tissue as the manufacture of a product. It is important to highlight that[8] although PHSA 351 specifically states that blood or blood components are biologic products, the FDA has expressly stated that whole blood, blood components, and minimally

4 Criteria for HCT/P Regulation
Under PHSA 361 and 21 CFR 1271 Alone

1 **Minimal Manipulation:**
      The HCT/P is minimally manipulated

2 **Homologous Use:**
      The HCT/P is intended for homologous use only, as reflected by the labeling, advertising, or other indications of the manufacturer's objective intent;

3 **None Combination Product:**
      The manufacture of the HCT/P does not involve the combination of the cells or tissues with another article, except for water, crystalloids, or a sterilizing, preserving, or storage agent, provided that the addition of water, crystalloids, or the sterilizing, preserving, or storage agent does not raise new clinical safety concerns with respect to the HCT/P; and

4 **None Systemic Effect or Autologous:**
      Either:
        i   The HCT/P does not have a systemic effect and is not dependent upon the metabolic activity of living cells for its primary function; or
        ii   The HCT/P has a systemic effect or is dependent upon the metabolic activity of living cells for its primary function, and:
                a   Is for autologous use;
                b   Is for allogeneic use in a first-degree or second-degree blood relative; or
                c   Is for reproductive use.

FIG. 2.3 Regulation of human cells, tissues, and cellular and tissue-based products (HCT/Ps). (Reprinted/adapted by permission from RightsLink Permissions Springer Customer Service Centre GmbH: Springer: Cartilage Restoration by Jack Farr, Andreas H. Gomoll. 2018.)

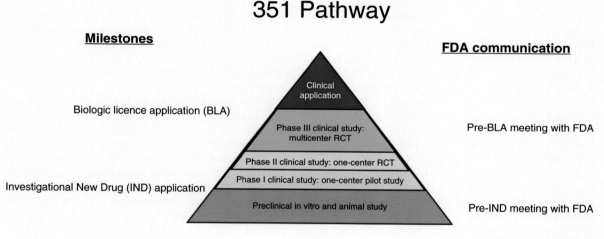

FIG. 2.4 351 product development pathway. *RCT*, randomized controlled trial. (Modified with permission from Am J Orthop. 2016;45(5):274-278, 318. Copyright Frontline Medical Communications Inc. 2016. All rights reserved.)

manipulated bone marrow for homologous use are not considered HCT/Ps in draft guidance documents and has no precedent of regulating the application of these products by clinicians. However, through Untitled Letters, Warning Letters, statements of the Tissue Reference Group (TRG), and draft guidance documents, the FDA has set precedent for adipose tissue, products derived from human placenta, allograft cell products, cultured cell products, and hematopoietic stem cells, suggesting that they regard these as 351 products.

PRECEDENT

Precedent is helpful when studying and applying both laws and regulation, as it provides real-world examples. FDA precedent is published on its website and includes the following: Untitled/Warning letters from the FDA to Industry/Clinicians, determinations of the TRG, and guidance documents from the FDA to Industry/Clinicians. Precedent is key to understanding risk and how the FDA has applied and acted upon the regulation they have created. For example, the criteria of minimal manipulation and homologous use have garnered controversial attention, as individual parties have different views and motivations when applying these principles. The perceived ability of an HCT/P to meet requirements may be dependent upon the perspective/bias of the individual making the determination. An industry representative may have one perspective of homologous use while a clinician, patient, patient's future lawyer, a jury, or FDA representative may have another. Precedent aids the clinician when ambiguity exists.

Untitled Letters and Warning Letters are legal documents from the FDA to a manufacturer, researcher, clinician, or development company depicting deviations or violations of rules. They are typically written in a pattern where they first identify when and how the violation was found, identify the product which is of concern, explain why and how the product is deviating from regulation, and contain options for corrective action. Letters often end with the phrase: "You should take prompt action to correct these deviations. Failure to promptly correct these deviations may result in regulatory action without further notice. Such actions include seizure and/or injunction." Once a Warning Letter has been issued, the FDA will follow up to ensure that the corrections are adequate.[9] As examples, letters have been delivered to two clinicians offering adipose-derived products, a clinician offering cultured bone marrow–derived cells, a company distributing allograft cells, and multiple companies manufacturing placenta-derived products. In each of these letters, the FDA states that these products are to be regulated not only by CFR 1271 but also as a drug under section 201(g) of the Federal Food, Drug, and Cosmetic Act and as biologic products under PHSA 351. For the cases involving adipose products, in 2012 and 2015 the FDA cited that the product did not meet the criteria of minimal manipulation or homologous use.[10,11] For an allograft stem cell product, in 2011 the FDA cited that the product did not meet the criteria because it was dependent upon metabolic activity and was not autologous or intended for a first- or second-degree relative. For amnionic/chorionic products, they cite that the products do not meet the criteria because processing is considered more than minimal manipulation and the products do not meet the homologous use criterion.[12,13] For cultured cells, the FDA cited more than minimal manipulation and nonhomologous use.[14] Other than minimally manipulated bone marrow aspirate, which is considered a primitive cell therapy, the FDA has set precedent of treating stem cell products as drugs.

Guidance documents from the FDA are meant to aid industry and clinicians by outlining the regulation, offering specific definitions, and describing the current interpretation of their policy by offering real-world examples. Released to clarify ambiguity, examples include documents on the controversial subjects of homologous use, minimal manipulation, and adipose products.[8,15,16] The FDA will often release these documents in draft form for comment by the public, i.e., industry and clinicians, before finalizing them on the website. While not binding as law, these clarify the current perspective of the FDA. As an example, the current draft guidance document for adipose was published in December of 2014. In the draft form, the document states: "Processing to isolate non-adipocyte or non-structural components from adipose tissue is generally consider more than minimal manipulation" and "Because adipose tissue does not perform this function in the donor, using HCT/P's from adipose tissue to treat bone and joint disease is generally considered a nonhomologous use." A complete review of the document leads one to believe that in their current thinking, the FDA considers mechanical processing of adipose tissue more than minimal manipulation and injection for orthopedic indications nonhomologous use.[15] This document was followed by an open forum of physicians and industry hosted by the FDA in the fall of 2016. To date a final document has not been released by the FDA.

It is important to consider that the FDA's guidance documents, as specifically stated by the FDA, do not establish legally enforceable responsibilities. Instead, these documents describe the Agency's current thinking on a topic and should be viewed only as recommendations, except when specific regulatory requirements are cited. In many instances the FDA uses the word "should" in guidance documents, and they state that this means that something is "suggested or recommended," but not required.

Recommendations of the TRG are also a source of precedent. The TRG was created in 1997 to provide a single reference point for product-specific questions regarding HCT/Ps. It is a working group within the FDA that provides review and recommendations upon inquiries from industry and clinicians. Annual reports of recommendations are updated on the FDA's website.[17] Industry and clinicians can petition the TRG in writing with an inquiry as well as review the annual reports in order to understand the application of 1271 and 351. Previous recommendations in 2015 specifically addressed a dehydrated chorioamniotic membrane product and an adipose tissue–derived product described as cells from subcutaneous fluid. The report stated that the dehydrated chorioamniotic membrane is regulated solely under section 361 and 1271 when used as a wound covering. The report also states that the adipose tissue–derived product was not regulated solely under section 361.[17]

FUTURE OF REGULATION

Historically, the FDA has been the global leader of regulation. Industrialized nations including but not limited to the European Union, Canada, and Australia have followed the lead by creating modern regulatory mechanisms. While a few clinicians have taken advantage of underdeveloped countries to offer products not available in the United States including cultured cells and cells from placenta tissue, this is not the norm outside of the United States in developed countries or in the global stem cell community. The developed world sees the need for regulation in this space to protect vulnerable patients from unproven technologies, and regulatory evolution is the key to translating these technologies to patient care. In 2014, Japan differentiated stem cell therapy from other pharmaceuticals by referring to these cell treatments as "regenerative medicine products." A new approval system was created and allowed early observed commercialization with reimbursement following a much less demanding safety and efficacy review. With this less demanding system, developing therapies can financially support some of the final most expensive clinical trials through early observed commercialization. With this change in regulation, Japan has positioned themselves to be leaders in this expanding field of research and development.

In March of 2016, an attempt to evolve the US approval system was made. The "Reliable and Effective Growth for Regenerative Health Options that Improve Wellness" (REGROW) Act was proposed both to the United States Senate and House of Representatives and proposed a change in regulation, which mirrored Japan's regulatory change. The REGROW Act proposed an addition to the Public Health Service Act, section 351B, to specifically address emerging technologies. Section 351B would have allowed for a conditional approval after certain developmental milestones. Specifically, following appropriate animal studies, completion of phase I testing, and early results of phase II testing, a conditional approval would have been granted to allow the sponsor of the therapy to treat patients and market the therapy during a 5-year trial period. At the end of the 5-year trial, the sponsor would apply for approval of the product as a biologic product. The goal of the addition would be to lower the initial financial hurdle of premarket development steps while still requiring the technologies to prove safety and efficacy.[18]

In late 2016, the discussion and direction of the REGROW Act became enveloped in the 21st Century Cures Act. The 21st Century Cures Act is a bill that was first introduced into the US House of Representatives in January of 2015, passed by the House in January 2016, passed by the Senate in October of 2016, and signed by President Barack Obama in December of 2016. This Act was supported and influenced by large pharmaceutical organizations and opposed by consumer organizations. Through the process, there was discussion about the creation of 351B; however, this was opposed by biopharmaceutical representatives. Instead of creating the 351B pathway, the 21st Century Cures Act created the Regenerative Medicine Advanced Therapy (RMAT) Designation. RMAT designation can be requested by technology sponsors concurrent with an IND application or as an amendment to an IND application. RMAT eligibility is based upon three conditions: (1) the product is a regenerative medicine therapy, which is defined as a cell therapy, therapeutic tissue engineering product, human cell and tissue product, or any combination product using such therapies or products, except for 316 products; (2) the product is intended to treat, modify, reverse, or cure a serious or life-threatening disease or condition; and (3) preliminary clinical evidence indicates that the drug has the potential to address unmet medical needs for such disease or condition. The FDA upon determination that the technology meets the requirements allows for the treatment to enter one of the FDA's four Expedited Programs for Serious Conditions.[19] Additionally, under certain circumstances, the act allows for companies to use observational studies, insurance claim data, patient input data, and level V evidence as opposed to traditional drug trial design.[20]

While the proposed intention of the 21st Century Cures Act was to advance the research and development of new therapies and diagnostics, the immediate results of the Act included a donation of $6.3 B in funding (mostly for research funding directed to the National Institutes of Health (NIH) on brain and cancer research), a grant to states for the fight on the growing opioid epidemic, the RMAT approval process, creation of waiver of research informed consent in certain research scenarios, regulation to bolster mental health parity, and a division addressing tax laws related to health plans for small employers. To provide the funding streams, the act orchestrated the sale of 15 million barrels of crude oil from the Strategic Petroleum Reserve. Time will determine whether the RMAT designation will improve the translation potential for orthobiologics; however, it is likely that the 21st Century Cures Act has missed the mark to effect productive change in the biologic regulation pathway, and future legislation or executive direction will be necessary.

During this time of regulatory confusion, the International Society for Stem Cell Research (ISSCR) has emerged as a global leader. In 2008, the ISSCR released guidelines for the clinical translation of stem cells, founded on principles of scientific, clinical, and ethical conduct for researchers, clinician–scientists, and regulators in the international community. The ISSCR described "an urgent need" regarding the marketing of unproven stem cell treatments directly to patients, citing clinics around the world exploiting patients' hopes and charging large sums of money. The principles of scientific rationale, transparency, oversight, and patient protection were touted. The guidelines provide recommendations to researchers and clinicians involving cell processing and manufacture, preclinical studies, and clinical research and were most recently updated in May of 2016.[21] The latest version involved a multidisciplinary group of 25 stem cell researchers, clinicians, ethicists, and regulatory officials from nine countries.

CONCLUSION

While the past is marked by murky regulation, the future of biologics within orthopedics is brighter and clearer with reformed regulation on the horizon. As the world collaborates on biologics, clear and practical regulation will emerge. Clinical practice should not outpace evidence regarding safety and efficacy. It is important to remember that the influencing forces in this space include hope, hype, logistics, and truth. The orthopedic community must remain grounded in evidence and truth, instead of seeking to profit on the vulnerability of patients by marketing unproven treatments. There is a thick gray area when applying biologics. To navigate, providers should review FDA guidance documents (even in draft form), Warning Letters, and TRG recommendations to understand the FDA's current perspective and actions, evaluate the evidence behind the application of these technologies, and lastly consider the physical risk to the patient and the judicial/regulator risk to the provider versus benefit of offering these technologies. As always, the endless pursuit of well-designed clinical trials and animal studies remain the future for our understanding. We should remain hungry, persistent, and resolute in the quest.

DISCLOSURE STATEMENT

Anz: Consultant for Arthrex; Pinegar: no disclosures.

REFERENCES

1. Frequently asked questions about therapeutic biological products. In: *Therapeutic Biologic Applications (BLA)*. 2017. Available from: https://www.fda.gov/drugs/developmentapprovalprocess/howdrugsaredevelopedandapproved/approvalapplications/therapeuticbiologicapplications/ucm113522.htm.
2. When and why was FDA formed?. In: *FDA Basics*. 2017. Available from: https://www.fda.gov/AboutFDA/Transparency/Basics/ucm214403.htm.
3. History. In: *What We Do*. 2015. Available from: https://www.fda.gov/AboutFDA/WhatWeDo/History/default.htm.
4. Basics. In: *Transparency*. 2016. Available from: www.fda.gov/AboutFDA/Transparency/Basics.ucm192695.htm.
5. What does FDA do?. In: *FDA Basics*. 2017. Available from: https://www.fda.gov/AboutFDA/Transparency/Basics/ucm194877.htm.
6. Inspections, compliance, enforcement, and criminal investigations. In: *Warning Letters*. 2012. Available from: https://www.fda.gov/ICECI/EnforcementActions/WarningLetters/ucm297245.htm.
7. Frequently asked questions about therapeutic biological products. In: *Therapeutic Biologic Applications (BLA)*. 2015. Available from: https://www.fda.gov/drugs/developmentapprovalprocess/howdrugsaredevelopedandapproved/approvalapplications/therapeuticbiologicapplications/ucm113522.htm.
8. Minimal manipulation of human cells, tissues, and cellular and tissue-based products: draft guidance. In: *Cellular & Gene Therapy Guidances*. 2015. Available from: https://www.fda.gov/biologicsbloodvaccines/guidancecomplianceregulatoryinformation/guidances/cellularandgenetherapy/ucm427692.htm.
9. Inspections, compliance, enforcement, and criminal investigations. In: *Warning Letters*. 2011. Available from: https://www.fda.gov/ICECI/EnforcementActions/WarningLetters/ucm278624.htm.
10. Inspections, Compliance, Enforcement, and Criminal Investigations. In: *2012*. 2012. Available from: https://www.fda.gov/ICECI/EnforcementActions/WarningLetters/2012/ucm297245.htm.
11. Irvine Stem Cell Treatment Center 12/30/15. In *2015*. 2016. Available from: https://www.fda.gov/ICECI/EnforcementActions/WarningLetters/2015/ucm479837.htm.
12. Amniotic Therapies LLC. 8/17/16. In: *2016*. 2016. Available from: https://www.fda.gov/ICECI/EnforcementActions/WarningLetters/2016/ucm517448.htm.
13. Surgical Biologics – Untitled Letter. *In: Untitled Letters (Biologics)*. 2013. Available from: https://www.fda.gov/biologicsbloodvaccines/guidancecomplianceregulatoryinformation/complianceactivities/enforcement/untitledletters/ucm367184.htm.
14. Regenexx. In: *2008*. 2012. Available from: http://www.casewatch.org/fdawarning/prod/2008/regenexx.shtml.
15. Human cells, tissues, and cellular and tissue-based products (HCT/Ps) from adipose tissue: regulatory considerations; draft guidance. In: *Tissue Guidance*. 2015. Available from: https://www.fda.gov/biologicsbloodvaccines/guidancecomplianceregulatoryinformation/guidances/tissue/ucm427795.htm.

16. Homologous use of human cells, tissues, and cellular and tissue-based products. In: *Tissues*. 2015. Available from: https://www.fda.gov/downloads/BiologicsBloodVaccines/ GuidanceComplianceRegulatoryInformation/Guidances/ Tissue/UCM469751.pdf.

17. Tissue Reference Group. In: *Regulation of Tissues*. 2017. Available from: https://www.fda.gov/biologicsbloodvacci nes/tissuetissueproducts/regulationoftissues/ucm152857 .htm.

18. S.2689 – REGROW Act. In: *114th Congress (2015-2016)*. 2016. Available from: https://www.congress.gov/bill/114th-congress/senate-bill/2689.

19. Guidance for industry expedited programs for serious conditions – drugs and biologics. In: *Guidances*. 2014. Available from: https://www.fda.gov/downloads/Drugs/ GuidanceComplianceRegulatoryInformation/Guidances/ UCM358301.pdf.

20. Inside the 21st Century Cures Act. In: *Spring 2017*. 2017. Available from: http://www.cancertodaymag.org/Spring 2017/Pages/Inside-the-21st-Century-Cures-Act.aspx.

21. Guidelines for Stem Cell Research and Clinical Translation. In: *ISSCR Guidelines*. Available from: http://www.isscr.org/ docs/default-source/guidelines/isscr-guidelines-for-stem-cell-research-and-clinical-translation.pdf?sfvrsn=2.

CHAPTER 3

Growth Factors

NEIL BAKSHI, MD • MOIN KHAN, MD, MSC, FRCSC • ASHEESH BEDI, MD

INTRODUCTION

There have been significant advancements over the last several decades in the field of orthopedic surgery with regard to our understanding of biomechanics, tissue healing, and the pathogenesis of musculoskeletal diseases. Biologics and regenerative medicine have received significant attention over the last decade with an aim to accelerate the healing process and potentially reverse degenerative processes. As research continues into current technologies such as bone marrow aspirate, platelet-rich plasma, and adult stem cells, newer biologic treatment options are on the horizon. This chapter will review the biological basis for healing as well as current biological treatment options and indications for orthopedic injuries.

THE HEALING CASCADE

Acute orthopedic injuries result from a single, traumatic event such as a fracture, muscle contusion, or ligament sprain/tear. Chronic bony and soft tissue injuries often result from repetitive mechanical stress, followed by a prolonged inflammatory state such as in the case of stress fractures or tendinopathies (e.g., rotator cuff tendinopathy and Achilles tendinopathy). Regardless of the type of injury, the general wound-healing process is shared, with differences in timing, duration of phases, and interactions between key mediators.[1,2]

The general healing cascade involves four overlapping phases: (1) hemostasis; (2) inflammation; (3) cellular and matrix proliferation, which begins within days of an injury and comprises the most important phase of healing; and (4) wound remodeling, the longest phase, which may involve scar tissue formation. Immediately after injury, capillary leak allows for the recruitment of hemostatic factors and inflammatory mediators. The coagulation cascade is activated leading to platelet aggregation, clot formation, and development of a provisional extracellular matrix construct. Platelets adhere to exposed collagen and circulating extracellular matrix proteins, which triggers the release of bioactive factors from platelet alpha granules. These bioactive actors include growth factors, chemokines, and cytokines, in addition to proinflammatory mediators. The inflammatory phase follows in a highly orchestrated fashion. Chemoattractant agents begin to recruit neutrophils to the injured site within 1–2 hours in the early inflammatory phase. Later, macrophages appear in the wound and play the leading role in wound debridement and regulation of inflammation. They are also involved in recruiting fibroblasts and endothelial cells. The cellular and matrix proliferation phase is arguably the most important phase of wound healing because the cells involved serve as a metabolic engine driving tissue repair. After 2–3 days of wound healing, macrophages and chemotactic, mitogenic, and angiogenic growth factors recruit fibroblasts and epithelial cells to infiltrate the site of injury. Once in the wound, fibroblasts synthesize collagen and facilitate wound contraction. Angiogenesis and the formation of granulation tissue are also important aspects during the proliferative phase of healing. The final phase of the healing process involves wound maturation and remodeling. During this phase, growth factors such as platelet-derived growth factors (PDGFs) and transforming growth factor-beta (TGF-β), and fibronectin stimulate fibroblasts proliferation, migration, and synthesis of the components of extracellular matrix. The remodeling phase is tightly regulated to maintain the balance between degradation and synthesis. Type I collagen replaces type III collagen, proteoglycan, and fibronectin to form a more robust matrix with increased tensile strength. The maturation phase varies in duration depending on the extent of the wound pathology, individual characteristics, as well as specific tissue-healing capabilities of the tissue involved. In addition, pathophysiological and metabolic factors can affect wound healing. They include local causes such as ischemia, tissue hypoxia, infection, and growth factor imbalance, as well as systemic causes such as metabolic disease and

Biologics in Orthopaedic Surgery. https://doi.org/10.1016/B978-0-323-55140-3.00003-5

nutritional status. In such unfavorable environments, PRP and other mediums rich in growth factors have been shown to be a viable therapeutic adjunct for acute and chronic orthopedic injuries.[1,2]

TYPES OF GROWTH FACTORS

PRP and other autologous blood products primarily function through the release of growth factors, such as PDGFs, epidermal growth factors, TGF-β1, vascular endothelial growth factor (VEGF), basic fibroblast growth factor, hepatocyte growth factor, and insulin-like growth factor 1 (IGF-1). These growth factors are released from the alpha granules of activated platelets and are involved in important cellular processes including mitogenesis, chemotaxis, differentiation, and metabolism.[3–7]

VEGF has received significant attention given its critical role in the formation and maturation of new blood vessels at the site of injury during the healing process. For this, VEGF acts by binding to its receptors VEGFR-1, VEGFR-2, and VEGFR-3, activating signaling cascades that promote the migration, proliferation, and survival of endothelial cells.[8]

PDGF has also been extensively studied due to the role it plays in regulating osteoblast replication and bone collagen degradation, controlling the proliferation of repair cells, and inducing cartilage and bone formation.[9] As a multiple mitogen, PDGF is released by platelets and facilitates blood clotting via the adhesion between platelets and blood vessels. Previous studies demonstrated that PDGF was a stimulator for bone fracture healing and was responsible for bone metabolism processes, including cell proliferation, migration, and apoptosis.[10,11] Nash et al.[12] reported in a rabbit model that bone marrow cavity volume and bone mineral density were markedly increased after injecting an isoform of recombinant human PDGF into rabbits with tibial fractures, indicating that PDGF participates in the stimulation of fracture healing. In addition, human cartilage cells cultured with PDGF and TGF-β1 exhibited a significantly higher proliferation rate in an in vitro study by Brandl et al.,[11] suggesting that PDGF participates in the proliferation of chondrocytes and plays a role in the repair of cartilage tissue.

TGF-β1 has been found to play a significant role in the osseous and soft tissue–healing processes but may have detrimental effects on tissue healing and regeneration. TGF is a superfamily of proteins that primarily functions to enhance the proliferative activity of fibroblasts, stimulates biosynthesis of type 1 collagen and fibronectin, induces deposition of bone matrix, and inhibits osteoclast function/bone resorption. This family of growth factors also includes bone morphogenetic proteins, which function to maintain tissue homeostasis, stimulate bone and cartilage formation, and promote vascular remodeling. Although these attributes of TGF-β growth factors can enhance tissue repair, they can also lead to extensive tissue fibrosis.[13] TGF-β has been implicated in the development of fibrosis in skeletal muscle, as well as other tissues, and may contribute to the association between PRP and muscle fibrosis through collagen deposition and conversion of skin fibroblasts to myofibroblast-like cells.[13,14] Furthermore, TGF-β has been found to inhibit myogenic differentiation, myoblast fusion, and expression of various muscle-specific proteins.[14] Owing to these characteristics of TGF-β, some have advocated the concomitant use of antifibrotic agents such as losartan or TGF-β neutralization antibodies with PRP injection (Table 3.1).[15]

PLATELET RICH PLASMA

Research into PRP has increased exponentially over the past decade with over 80 randomized controlled trials (RCTs) performed. This exponential increase in research coincides with a global market for PRP projected to exceed $451 million in the next decade.[16]

PRP is classically described as a volume of plasma that has a platelet count more than that of whole blood. In clinical use, platelet concentration is increased 4- to 10-fold the baseline levels. Platelets are irregularly shaped, non-nucleated cytoplasmic bodies derived from fragmentation of megakaryocyte precursors. As discussed previously, platelets serve as a natural reservoir of growth factors and are released from the alpha granules of activated platelets. Therefore the rationale for creating and using PRP is to increase platelet concentration in injured tissue, resulting in the exponential release of multiple bioactive factors, and to subsequently enhance/stimulate the natural healing process.[1,17]

To create PRP, autologous whole blood is collected in the presence of an anticoagulant that binds calcium and prevents the initiation of the clotting cascade by inhibiting the conversion of prothrombin to thrombin. PRP can be produced in the absence of an anticoagulant as well; however, the time required between blood draw and PRP injection must be significantly shortened. Although several anticoagulants are available, acid citrate dextrose-A, citrate phosphate dextrose, and sodium citrate are commonly used because of their ability to maintain the structural and functional integrity of platelets. Once the anticoagulated whole blood is collected, it is separated into its individual components using plasmapheresis, a 1- to 2-phase centrifugation process that separates blood

TABLE 3.1
Growth Factors and Their Cellular Effects[1]

Growth Factor	Cellular Effects
PDGF (platelet-derived growth factor)	• Macrophage activation and angiogenesis • Fibroblast chemotaxis and proliferative activity • Enhances collagen synthesis • Enhances bone cell proliferation
IGF-I (insulin-like growth factor I)	• Chemotactic for myoblast and fibroblasts and stimulates protein synthesis • Mediator in growth and repair of skeletal muscle • Enhances bone formation by proliferation and differentiation of osteoblasts
TGF-β (transforming growth factor-beta)	• Enhances the proliferative activity of fibroblasts • Stimulates biosynthesis of type I collagen and fibronectin • Induces deposition of bone matrix • Inhibits osteoclast formation and bone resorption • Regulation in balance between fibrosis and myocyte regeneration.
PDEGF (platelet-derived endothelial growth factor)	• Promotes wound healing by stimulating the proliferation of keratinocytes and dermal fibroblasts
PDAF (platelet-derived angiogenic factor)	• Induces vascularization by stimulating vascular endothelial cells
EGF (endothelial growth factor)	• Cellular proliferation • Differentiation of epithelial cells
VEGF (vascular endothelial growth factor)	• Angiogenesis • Migration and mitosis of endothelial cells • Creation of blood vessel lumen • Creation of fenestrations • Chemotactic for macrophages and granulocytes • Vasodilation (indirectly by release of nitrous oxide)
HGF (hepatocyte growth factor)	• Stimulates hepatocyte proliferation and liver tissue regeneration • Angiogenesis • Mitogen for endothelial cells • Antifibrotic

components based on their size and density. Owing to their inherent morphologic differences, centrifugation separates the whole blood into a clear plasma layer on top, a buffy coat layer consisting of the white blood cells (WBCs) and platelets in middle, and red blood cells (RBCs) at the bottom. If a two-phase centrifugation process is used, the second phase is performed to separate the platelet-poor plasma from the platelet-rich fraction (Table 3.2).[1,17,18]

Although the term PRP suggests a mixture of only platelets and plasma, it encompasses a broader group of products that may also include RBC and/or WBCs. In addition, there can be significant variations in PRP preparations with regard to the volume of whole blood, concentration of platelets in plasma, amount of growth factors, volume of PRP, the presence and/or concentration of RBCs and/or WBCs, the presence of platelet activators, and pH of the solution. More than 40

commercial PRP systems are available, and each product may contain differing concentrations of platelets, leukocytes, and growth factors.[19] Owing to this variation, the success of specific PRP products cannot be generalized to all preparations, limiting the ability to evaluate the clinical efficacy of PRP for various indications.[1,17]

PRP can be activated via platelet activators such as thrombin or calcium chloride which results in a rapid release of the growth factors. Ninety percent of the growth factors contained within the platelets will be released within the first 10 minutes after activation. Many growth factors have very short half-lives, suggesting platelet activation should be performed at the time of injection or just before injection to be most efficacious. Owing to this, most commercial PRP kits for use in soft tissue do not activate PRP. Using unactivated PRP results in a more physiologic activation by the tissue into which it is injected or applied.[20]

TABLE 3.2
Platelet-Rich Plasma Two-phase Preparation Steps[17]
Platelet-Rich Plasma Two-Phase Preparation
1. Obtain whole by venipuncture in acid citrate dextrose (ACD) tubes
2. Do not cool the blood at any time before or during platelet separation
3. Centrifuge the blood using a "soft" spin (spin phase 1)
4. Transfer the supernatant plasma containing platelets into another sterile tube (without anticoagulant)
5. Centrifuge tube at a higher speed (a hard spin) to obtain a platelet concentrate (spin phase 2)
6. The lower one-third is PRP and upper two-third is platelet-poor plasma (PPP). At the bottom of the tube, platelet pellets are formed.
7. Remove PPP and suspend the platelet pellets in a minimum quantity of plasma (2–4 mL) by gently shaking the tube.

CLASSIFICATION OF PLATELET-RICH PLASMA (PRP)

PRP is categorized into four general groups: (1) pure platelet-rich plasma (P-PRP), (2) leukocyte- and platelet-rich plasma (L-PRP), (3) pure platelet-rich fibrin (P-PRF), and (4) leukocyte- and platelet-rich fibrin (L-PRF).[21] Further research is required to ascertain if certain formulations have improved therapeutic effects over others.

1. P-PRP products are preparations without leukocytes and with a low-density fibrin network. All the products of this family can be used as liquid solutions or in an activated gel form through the use of thrombin or calcium chloride. P-PRP can be injected for use in muscle/tendon injuries or placed during gelling on a skin wound or suture.[21]

2. L-PRP products are preparations with a high concentration of leukocytes and with a low-density fibrin network after activation. As with P-PRP, it can be used in liquid solution or activated gel form and can be injected at the site of injury or placed during gelling on a skin wound or suture. Controversy exists over the presence of leukocytes (neutrophils, monocytes, macrophages, and lymphocytes) having potentially beneficial or detrimental effects on the injured tissue. Leukocytes stimulate an immune response against infections and promote chemotaxis, proliferation, and differentiation of cells. However, leukocytes also release inflammatory cytokines such as interleukin-1 beta and tumor necrosis factor-alpha, as well as reactive oxygen species, which are suggested to potentially result in detrimental effects on the treated tissues.[21] The literature does not conclusively support the use of one formulation over another.

3. P-PRFs are preparations without leukocytes and with a high-density fibrin network. Owing to its inherent characteristics, P-PRF products only exist in a strongly activated gel form and cannot be injected as a result. However, because of their strong fibrin matrix, these products can be handled as solid materials for other applications in orthopedic surgery.[21] They have been used for hemostasis and have been shown to improve healing of articular cartilage defects at the femoral condyles, as demonstrated by Kazemi et al.[22] Others have attempted to use P-PRF mixed with autologous bone marrow cells during posterior spinal fusions.[23] He et al. demonstrated with rat models that P-PRF released autologous growth factors gradually and expressed stronger and more durable effect on proliferation and differentiation of rat osteoblasts than PRP in vitro.[24] The main inconvenience of this technique, however, remains its cost and relative complexity in preparation.[21]

4. L-PRF products are preparations with leukocytes and with a high-density fibrin network. Similar to the P-PRF, these products only exist in a strongly activated gel form and cannot be injected or used like traditional fibrin glues. However, because of a strong fibrin matrix, they can be handled as solid material for other applications. It has most commonly been used in dentistry and periodontics to stimulate wound healing and bone regeneration.

Mishra et al. introduced a sports medicine classification system for platelet-rich plasma, which involves four types of formulations.[20] Type 1 PRP contains an increased concentration of platelets and white blood cells over baseline and is not activated by an exogenous activator such as thrombin or calcium. Type 2 is activated with thrombin and or calcium and contains both increased platelets and white blood cells. This type of PRP is also known as platelet-leukocyte gel. Type 3 PRP contains only an increased concentration of platelets without any white blood cells, and it is not activated before application. This type is sometimes known as platelet concentrate. Type 4 is activated with thrombin and or calcium and contains only an increased platelet concentration. This type of PRP may also be called platelet gel in the literature. Subtype A contains an increased platelet concentration at or above five times the baseline concentration. Subtype B contains an increased platelet concentration less than five times the baseline concentration. If no concentration is reported, no subtype is noted.[20]

PRP APPLICATION IN ORTHOPEDIC SURGERY/SPORTS MEDICINE

The application of PRP preparations in orthopedic and sports medicine has only been formally investigated in recent years. The use of PRP has been evaluated for the treatment of a variety of pathologies in orthopedics, most notably tendinopathies, rotator cuff tears, muscle injuries, ligament tears/reconstruction, and osteoarthritis.

Tendinopathy

As the pathogenesis of tendinopathy is primarily degenerative, treatment modalities that attempt to initiate the body's own regenerative mechanisms would seem to be beneficial. Tendon healing is characterized by an initial inflammatory response associated with the influx of growth factors such as PDGF and TGF-β within 2 days, resulting in subsequent angiogenesis and collagen synthesis. Because PRP contains these critical growth factors, administering PRP in the setting of acute or chronic tendinopathy may promote body's healing and regenerative capacity.

In particular, the use of PRP for elbow tendinopathy has been well studied and appears to be very promising compared with other anatomic areas. Mishra and Pavelko first published regarding the use of PRP for chronic severe elbow tendinosis in a prospective, controlled pilot study.[25] They reported significant improvement in pain and elbow scores after PRP injection compared with a control group treated with bupivacaine/epinephrine injection. They found a 60% improvement in pain scores for PRP-treated patients versus a 16% improvement in control patients 8 weeks after treatment ($P = .001$). At the final follow-up (mean, 25.6 months; range, 12–38 months), the PRP patients reported 93% reduction in pain. Peerbooms et al. confirmed these beneficial effects by comparing the use of PRP with corticosteroid injection in the treatment of lateral epicondylitis in 100 patients.[26] They reported significantly improved outcomes in the PRP group with regard to pain and function. They also reported that the benefits of the corticosteroid were transient, whereas PRP patients progressively improved.

Rotator Cuff

The use of PRP has also been studied with regard to rotator cuff pathology. It has been examined as an adjunct to arthroscopic rotator cuff repair with conflicting results. Randelli et al. performed a prospective randomized trial of 53 patients who underwent arthroscopic rotator cuff repair and reported on the clinical efficacy of PRP in this population.[27] They demonstrated significantly improved pain up to 1 month postoperatively and significantly improved physical examination and outcome scores at 3 months postoperatively. Others, however, have demonstrated less promising results. Weber et al. performed a prospective randomized trial of 60 patients who underwent arthroscopic rotator cuff repair to evaluate the benefits of adjunctive PRF use. They reported no differences in outcomes at 3 months in terms of residual defects or perioperative morbidity.[28] Saltzman et al. performed a systematic review in 2016 of meta-analyses and determined administering PRP at the time of rotator cuff repair did not result in significantly lower retear rates or improved clinical outcome scores.[29]

Muscle Injuries

PRP has also been used for the treatment of muscle injuries in an attempt to accelerate the recovery period. Limited and conflicting evidence has been reported regarding its clinical efficacy. Bubnov et al. performed a randomized comparative trial in 30 male professional athletes with acute muscle injuries and demonstrated faster pain relief, muscle function, and return to sport (22 vs. 10 days) in the PRP group.[30] However, they reported no differences between the PRP and control groups at 28 days. Wetzel et al. reported on a case series of 15 patients with proximal hamstring injuries and found no benefit to PRP compared with the control treatment in terms of pain scores and return to sport.[31] Finally, Reurink et al. performed a randomized, double-blind, controlled trial of 80 athletes with acute hamstring muscle injuries and demonstrated no difference in time to return to sport with PRP injection compared with placebo.[32]

Osteoarthritis

PRP has also shown some promising results in the treatment of osteoarthritis. PRP contains factors that are critical for joint repair, including TGF-β1, thrombospondin-1, and IGF-1.[16] A study of 78 patients with bilateral knee osteoarthritis who were randomized to receive a single WBC-filtered PRP injection, 2 PRP injections at 3-week intervals, or a single saline injection shows that outcomes of the PRP groups are significantly better than those of the control groups 6 months after treatment.[33] An RCT of 120 patients found that outcomes were significantly better 24 weeks after a local injection of PRP than those after an injection of hyaluronic acid.[34] Another recent study compared PRP injections with hyaluronic acid injections for the treatment of knee osteoarthritis.[35] In this study, Montanez-Heredia et al. demonstrated that while short-term pain-relieving effects were comparative between the 2 treatments, a greater number of participants in the PRP group had more significant improvements in functionality and maintained these improvements in greater numbers at 3-month postinjection follow-up compared with the hyaluronic acid group.[35] Meheux et al.[36] performed a systematic review and reported intraarticular PRP results in significant clinical improvements up to 12 months after injection. PRP resulted in improved clinical outcomes as assessed by WOMAC scores in comparison to hyaluronic acid injections at 3–12 months of follow-up.

Conclusion

The use of growth factors and PRP in orthopedic surgery is a rapidly expanding area of research with a wide array of possible clinical applications. PRP and other autologous blood products primarily function through the release of growth factors from the alpha granules of activated platelets. These growth factors are important for cellular processes such as mitogenesis, chemotaxis, differentiation, and metabolism, all of which are important to healing and regeneration after musculoskeletal injury. Further high-quality evidence is required for PRP and biologics to identify areas of efficacy, specific indications, and formulations for which a treatment effect exists in orthopedic surgery.

REFERENCES

1. Middleton KK, Barro V, Muller B, Terada S, Fu FH. Evaluation of the effects of platelet-rich plasma (PRP) therapy involved in the healing of sports-related soft tissue injuries. *Iowa Orthop J.* 2012;32:150–163.
2. Glat PM, Gibbons LM. Wound healing. In: Aston SJ, Beasley RW, Thorne CH, eds. *Grabb and Smith's Plastic Surgery.* 5th ed. Philadelphia: Lippincott-Raven; 1997:3–12.
3. Zhang J, Wang JH. Platelet-rich plasma releasate promotes differentiation of tendon stem cells into active tenocytes. *Am J Sports Med.* 2010;38:2477–2486.
4. Fu SC, Rolf C, Cheuk YC, Lui PP, Chan KM. Deciphering the pathogenesis of tendinopathy: a three-stages process. *Sports Med Arthrosc Rehabil Ther Technol.* 2010;2:30.
5. Bielecki TM, Gazdzik TS, Arendt J, Szczepanski T, Krol W, Wielkoszynski T. Antibacterial effect of autologous platelet gel enriched with growth factors and other active substances: an in vitro study. *J Bone Joint Surg Br.* 2007;89:417–420.
6. Connell DA, Ali KE, Ahmad M, Lambert S, Corbett S, Curtis M. Ultrasoundguided autologous blood injection for tennis elbow. *Skeletal Radiol.* 2006;35:371–377.
7. Mishra A, Harmon K, Woodall J, Vieira A. Sports medicine applications of platelet rich plasma. *Curr Pharm Biotechnol.* 2012;13(7):1185–95.
8. Ferrara N, Gerber HP, LeCouter J. The biology of VEGF and its receptors. *Nat Med.* 2003;9(6):669–676.
9. Yang D, Chen J, Jing Z, Jin D. Platelet-derived growth factor (PDGF)-AA: a self-imposed cytokine in the proliferation of human fetal osteoblasts. *Cytokine.* 2000;12:1271–1274.
10. Filardo G, Kon E, Di Martino A, Iacono F, Marcacci M. Arthroscopic second-generation autologous chondrocyte implantation: a prospective 7-year follow-up study. *Am J Sports Med.* 2011;39:2153–2160.
11. Brandl A, Angele P, Roll C, Prantl L, Kujat R, Kinner B. Influence of the growth factors PDGF-Bb, TGF-beta1 and bFGF on the replicative aging of human articular chondrocytes during in vitro expansion. *J Orthop Res.* 2010;28:354–360.
12. Nash TJ, Howlett CR, Martin C, Steele J, Johnson KA, Hicklin DJ. Effect of platelet-derived growth factor on tibial orteotomies in rabbits. *Bone.* 1994;15:203–208.
13. Border WA, Noble NA. Transforming growth factor beta in tissue fibrosis. *N Engl J Med.* 1994;331:1286–1292.
14. Li H, Hicks JJ, Wang L, et al. Customized platelet-rich plasma with transforming growth factor β1 neutralization antibody to reduce fibrosis in skeletal muscle. *Biomaterials.* May 2016;87:147–156.
15. Terada S, Ota S, Kobayashi M, et al. Use of an antifibrotic agent improves the effect of platelet-rich plasma on muscle healing after injury. *J Bone Joint Surg Am.* 2013;95:980–988.
16. GlobalData. *Platelet Rich Plasma (PRP) Market - Global Industry Analysis, Size, Share, Growth, Trends and Forecast 2016-2024*; 2016:1–5.
17. Navani A, Li G, Chrystal J. Platelet rich plasma in musculoskeletal pathology: a necessary rescue or a lost cause? *Pain Physician.* 2017;20(3):E345–E356.
18. Sweeny J, Grossman BJ. Blood collection, storage and component preparation methods. In: Brecher M, ed. *Technical Manual.* 14th ed. Bethesda, MD: American Association of Blood Banks (AABB); 2002:955–958.
19. Khan M, Bedi A. Cochrane in CORR®: platelet-rich therapies for musculoskeletal soft tissue injuries (review). *Clin Orthop Relat Rese.* 2015;473(7):2207–2213.
20. Mishra A, Harmon K, Woodall J, Vieira A. Sports medicine applications of platelet rich plasma. *Curr Pharm Biotechnol.* 2012;13(7):1185–1195.

21. Ehrenfest DD, Andia I, Zumstein MA, Zhang CQ, Pinto NR, Bielecki T. Classification of platelet concentrates (Platelet-Rich Plasma-PRP, Platelet-Rich Fibrin-PRF) for topical and infiltrative use in orthopedic and sports medicine: current consensus, clinical implications and perspectives. *Muscles Ligaments Tendons J*. 2014;4(1):3–9.

22. Kazemi D, Fakhrjou A, Dizaji VM, Alishahi MK. Effect of autologous platelet rich fibrin on the healing of experimental articular cartilage defects of the knee in an animal model. *Biomed Res Int*. 2014:1–10.

23. Vadalà G, Di Martino A, Tirindelli MC, Denaro L, Denaro V. Use of autologous bone marrow cells concentrate enriched with platelet-rich fibrin on corticocancellous bone allograft for posterolateral multilevel cervical fusion. *J Tissue Eng Regen Med*. 2008;2(8):515–520.

24. He L, Lin Y, Hu X, Zhang Y, Wu H. A comparative study of platelet-rich fibrin (PRF) and platelet-rich plasma (PRP) on the effect of proliferation and differentiation of rat osteoblasts in vitro. *Oral Surg Oral Med Oral Pathol Oral Radiol Endod*. 2009;108(5):707–713.

25. Mishra A, Pavelko T. Treatment of chronic elbow tendonosis with buffered platelet-rich plasma. *Am J Sports Med*. 2006;34(11):1774–1778.

26. Peerbooms JC, Sluimer J, Bruijn DJ, et al. Platelet-rich plasma versus corticosteroid injection with a 1-year follow-up. *Am J Sports Med*. 2010;38:255–262.

27. Randelli P, Arrigoni P, Cabitza P. Autologous platelet rich plasma for arthroscopic rotator cuff repair. A pilot study. *Disabil Rehabil*. 2008;00:1–6.

28. Weber SC, Kauffman JI, Parise C, Weber SJ, Katz SD. Platelet-rich fibrin matrix in the management of arthroscopic repair of the rotator cuff: a prospective, randomized, double-blinded study. *Am J Sports Med*. 2013;41(2):263–270.

29. Saltzman BM, Jain A, Campbell KA, et al. Does the use of platelet-rich plasma at the time of surgery improve clinical outcomes in arthroscopic rotator cuff repair when compared with control cohorts? A systematic review of meta-analyses. *Arthroscopy*. 2016;32(5):906–918.

30. Bubnov R, Yevseenko V, Semeniv I. Ultrasound guided injections of platelets rich in plasma for muscle injury in professional athletes: comparative study. *Med Ultrasound*. 2013;15(2):101–105.

31. Wetzel RJ, Patel RM, Terry MA. Platelet-rich plasma as an effective treatment for proximal hamstring injuries. *Orthopedics*. 2013;36(1):e64–e70. https://doi.org/10.3928/01477447-20121217-20.

32. Reurink G, Goudswaard GJ, Moen MH, et al. Platelet rich plasma injections in muscle injury. *N Engl J Med*. 2014;370(26):2546–2547.

33. Patel S, Dhillon MS, Aggarwal S, Marwaha N, Jain A. Treatment with platelet-rich plasma is more effective than placebo for knee osteoarthritis: a prospective, double-blind, randomized trial. *Am J Sports Med*. 2013;41:356–364.

34. Cerza F, Carnì S, Carcangiu A, et al. Comparison between hyaluronic acid and platelet-rich plasma, intra-articular infiltration in the treatment of gonarthrosis. *Am J Sports Med*. 2012;40:2822–2827.

35. Montañez-Heredia E, Irízar S, Huertas PJ, et al. Intra-articular injections of platelet-rich plasma versus hyaluronic acid in the treatment of osteoarthritic knee pain: a randomized clinical trial in the context of the Spanish National Health Care System. *Int J Mol Sci*. 2016;17:1064.

36. Meheux CJ, McCulloch PC, Lintner DM, Varner KE, Harris JD. Efficacy of intra-articular platelet-rich plasma injections in knee osteoarthritis: a systematic review. *Arthroscopy*. 2016;32(3):495–505.

FURTHER READING

1. Aspenberg P, Virchenko O. Platelet concentrate injection improves Achilles tendon repair in rats. *Acta Orthop Scand*. 2004;75:93–99.

CHAPTER 4

Biologics in Orthopaedic Surgery

ANTHONY F. DE GIACOMO, MD • MICHAEL B. BANFFY, MD • NEAL S. ELATTRACHE, MD

BONE MARROW ASPIRATE CONCENTRATE

Bone marrow aspirate concentrate (BMAC) is derived from fluid obtained from bone marrow.[1,2] Given the source of origin, BMAC contains a composition of cells—mesenchymal stem cells (MSCs), hematopoietic stem cells, endothelial progenitor cells, white blood cells, and red blood cells. Equally important, BMAC, along with a strong source of cells, also contains platelets, cytokines, and growth factors such as bone morphogenic proteins (BMPs), platelet-derived growth factor (PDGF), transforming growth factor-B, vascular endothelial growth factor (VEGF), interleukin-B, and interleukin-1 receptor antagonist (Fig. 4.1).[3] This combination of cells and growth factors from BMAC allows a single source to support cell growth and recovery following injury to musculoskeletal tissue.[4]

The Importance of Concentrating Bone Marrow Aspirate

Without concentration techniques, bone marrow aspirate alone has a low percentage of MSCs of only 0.001%–0.01% of nucleated cells.[5] For this reason, centrifugation is used to concentrate bone marrow aspirate in order to increase the percentage of MSCs.[6] In bone marrow aspirate, the predominant cell type is neutrophils and erythrocytes. With this in mind, there have been gender differences noted in the predominant cell type among bone marrow aspirate with male aspirate containing more erythroblasts and female aspirate containing more neutrophils.[7] In general, the cellular composition of BMAC is 28.1% erythroblasts, 32.7% neutrophils, 13% lymphocytes, 2.2% eosinophils, 1.3% monocytes, and 0.1% basophils.[7] In comparison to platelet-rich plasma (PRP), the cellular composition of BMAC has 11.8 times the amount of white blood cells, 19.4 times the amount of neutrophils, and 2.5 times the amount of platelets.[8] Similar to PRP, BMAC contains a comparable concentration of monocytes, lymphocytes, eosinophils, and basophils.[8]

The importance of concentrating bone marrow aspirate into BMAC has been highlighted by several studies supporting a direct correlation of the number of cells with healing potential and optimal outcomes. [4,9-11] With this in mind, the minimum number needed, to induce biologic healing, is 1000 progenitors/cm^3 of BMAC.[9] In like manner, a study on bone healing of nonunions showed a statistically significant lower rate of union in patients who received a BMAC with less than 1000 progenitors/cm^3 and less than 30,000 progenitor cells in total.[12] At the same time, this study found a positive correlation between the number and concentration of osteoprogenitor cells delivered in the bone marrow aspirate with the volume of mineralized callus present at the sites of bone healing. All things considered, Hernigou et al. concluded that 1 mL of bone marrow aspirate contained a competent concentration of cells to form 1 cm of bone in areas of nonunion.[9] Further emphasis has been placed on the critical concentration of certain cellular elements, such as MSCs, rather than the total cell count of the entire composition of cells contained within BMAC.[13] As can be seen, the concentration of bone marrow aspirate is imperative to obtain the optimal volume of the essential cellular elements, i.e., MSCs, recommended to expedite the biologic healing response; yet, BMAC also provides a source of growth factor therapy to enhance treatment.

Growth Factors and Cytokines Contained in Bone Marrow Aspirate Concentrate

Growth factors are biologically active polypeptides that can be applied to stimulate cell growth and enhance both chondrogenesis and osteogenesis.[8,14] Commonly encountered growth factors, pertinent to healing of musculoskeletal tissue, are transforming growth factor-β2 (TGF-β2), PDGF, fibroblast growth factors (FGFs), VEGF, interleukins (ILs), Insulin-like growth factor-1 (IGF-1), and BMPs (Table 4.1). BMAC, not to mention, has an increased concentration of growth

Biologics in Orthopaedic Surgery. https://doi.org/10.1016/B978-0-323-55140-3.00004-7

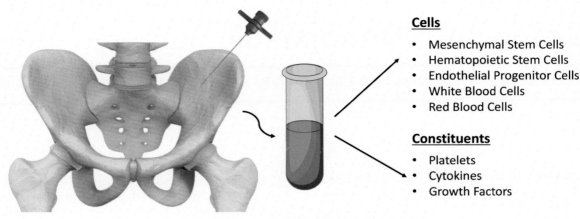

Cells

- Mesenchymal Stem Cells
- Hematopoietic Stem Cells
- Endothelial Progenitor Cells
- White Blood Cells
- Red Blood Cells

Constituents

- Platelets
- Cytokines
- Growth Factors

FIG. 4.1 Contents of Bone Marrow Aspirate.

TABLE 4.1
Growth Factors and Cytokines in Bone Marrow Aspirate Concentrate

Growth Factor/ Cytokine	Function
TGF-β1, TGF-β2, TFG-β3	Chondrogenesis via SMAD
PDGF	Wound healing, collagen synthesis, enhanced BMP signaling, promotes cartilage formation
FGF-2, FGF-18	Chondrogenic differentiation, MSC chemotaxis
VEGF	Angiogenesis, supports bone/cartilage growth
IL-1, IL-8	Inflammatory response, MSC chemotaxis to injury site
IGF-1	↑ metabolism, ↑ proteoglycan synthesis, ↑ collagen synthesis
BMP-2	Osteogenesis/chondrogenesis, matrix synthesis
BMP-7	Cartilage matrix synthesis, ↑ extracellular matrix

BMP, bone morphogenic protein; *FGF*, fibroblast growth factor; *IGF*, insulin growth factor; *IL*, interleukin; *PDGF*, platelet-derived growth factor; *SMAD*, suppressor of mother against decapentaplegic; *TGF-β*, transforming growth factor-β; *VEGF*, vascular endothelial growth factor.

factors due to the substantial number of platelets with α-granules. Specifically, the α-granules of platelets contain TGF-β2, PDGF, VEGF, FGF, BMP, and IGF. In comparison to PRP, BMAC has a significantly increased

supply of growth factors with 172.5 times more VEGF, 78 times more IL-8, 4.6 times more IL-1B, 3.4 times more TGF-β2, and 1.3 times more PDGF.[8] Each of these aforementioned growth factors has specific functions to stimulate healing in select tissues important in orthopaedics. As an illustration, the most common growth factor used to stimulate chondrogenesis is TGF-β2, which stimulates extracellular matrix synthesis and chondrogenesis in the synovial lining all while decreasing the catabolic activity of IL-1.[8] Explicitly, the proliferation and differentiation of chondrocytes by TGF-β2 is via phosphorylation of SMAD (Suppressor of Mothers Against Decapentaplegic) proteins that transduce extracellular signals to the nucleus to active downstream gene transcription for chondrogenesis.[8,14] In the same fashion, BMPs have been shown to stimulate, through autocrine signaling, both osteogenesis and chondrogenesis. In particular, BMP-2 has been used to stimulate bone growth in the setting of fracture healing, while BMP-7 has been used to stimulate cartilage matrix synthesis by inhibiting catabolic factors of matrix metalloproteinases.[14,15] ILs, involved in the initial inflammatory response to injury, aid in cell migration to the site of injury while increasing production of other favorable factors, such as VEGF. In the same fashion, VEGF promotes angiogenesis to provide transport of necessary products for healing and growth of mesenchymal tissue. Further healing is augmented with PDGF as a chemotactic factor for mesenchymal cells and suppressor of IL-1β, which induces cartilage degradation by downregulation of nuclear factor-κβ.[5] PDGF, at the same time, stimulates wound healing and collagen synthesis and promotes formation of cartilage.[14] Another growth factor, commonly contained in BMAC, is IGF-1 that increases collagen and proteoglycan synthesis, increases metabolic activity, and helps maintain the integrity of articular cartilage.[5] A large family of growth factors is FGFs with special emphasis for FGF-2 and FGF-18, both of which are involved in chemotaxis of MSCs and chondrogenic differentiation. Taken together, the growth factors and stem cells contained in BMAC are individually important in augmenting the biologic healing of musculoskeletal tissue.

Sources of Bone Marrow Aspirate

The aspiration of bone marrow can be performed at various locations throughout the human body. Despite the different anatomic locations available for bone marrow aspiration, all sites of aspiration do not provide the same proportion of BMAC. In fact, the quantity of progenitor cells, from bone marrow aspirate, decreases from axial to appendicular skeleton as well as from proximal to distal in the appendicular skeleton.[3] The highest quantity of progenitor cells in bone marrow aspirate has been found in the vertebral bodies.[16] Although this may be true, aspiration of bone marrow from the vertebral body is not as practical as other available anatomic sites for aspiration. More reasonable locations for aspiration have been obtained from bone near the site of surgery or the iliac crest, which is based on both accessibility and percentage yield of progenitor cells. In like manner, a study comparing sites to harvest BMAC from the iliac crest, tibia, and calcaneus found that the highest concentration of progenitor cells resided in the iliac crest.[17] Equally important, this study demonstrated that all anatomic sites of harvest, even the proximal tibia and calcaneus, are both safe and amenable to achieve adequate amounts of progenitor cells.[17] By the same token, no difference in cell yield was noted with demographics of age or sex or with comorbidities of smoking and diabetes.[17] Given the accessibility of the iliac crest, this anatomic site is one of the most commonly used locations for obtaining bone marrow aspirate. For this reason, Pierini and colleagues further evaluated the yield of progenitor cells from either the anterior or posterior iliac crest.[18] In comparison to both sites of the iliac crest, the highest yield of colony-founding connective tissue progenitor cells was aspirated from the posterior iliac crest. However, no difference in the biologic potential in terms of viability or differentiation of MSCs was noted between the anterior or posterior iliac crest.[18] In spite of this study, another study by Marx and colleagues found no significant difference in the yield of either stromal stem cells or hematopoietic stem cells between the anterior

or posterior iliac crest.[19] Rather, both the anterior and posterior iliac crest harvest provided twice the amount of stromal and hematopoietic stem cells than harvest from the tibial plateau.[19] As can be seen, the iliac crest is the preferred anatomic location for aspiration of bone marrow, yet other anatomic sites, near the area of surgery, may be able to provide the principal BMAC preparation required for healing.

The Bone Marrow Aspirate Concentrate Technique

The technique of harvesting BMAC can be applied to most anatomic locations. For simplicity, the technique will be further described in reference to the iliac crest, which is the most commonly used site for aspiration of bone marrow. The technique begins with a percutaneous stab incision placed over the iliac crest. Without delay, a Jamshidi needle is directed parallel to the iliac wing between the inner and outer tables of the crest. With use of the Jamshidi needle two starting holes are made, with one hole used to collect the first 30 mL of aspirate and the second hole used to collect the second 30 mL of aspirate. To begin with, 5 mL of marrow is aspirated, and then the Jamshidi needle is rotated 45 degrees to begin the next aspiration. After the next 5 mL of bone marrow is aspirated, the Jamshidi needle is advanced 1–2 cm, and then the process is repeated with another 5 mL aspiration followed by a 45-degree rotation of the needle. With each advancement and reposition of the needle, the obturator is reinserted into the needle in order to clear the bore of the needle from debris. Importantly, the vacuum aspiration of bone marrow occurs in conjunction with anticoagulation via heparin/ACD-A solution (8 mL of anticoagulant per 60 mL of bone marrow aspirate). In due time, with aspiration of the desired volume of bone marrow, the fluid is concentrated with use of a centrifuge system. Straightaway processing and concentration of bone marrow aspirate takes place with density gradient centrifugation using an automatic microprocessor-controlled centrifuge system. Following about 15 minutes of centrifugation, the erythrocytes, nucleated cells, and plasma are separated into a second chamber. Completion of the centrifugation process yields approximately 7–10 mL of BMAC available for injection into the designated area to augment biologic healing.

Several studies have investigated multiple methods to optimize the technique of harvesting bone marrow aspirate. These studies have evaluated the needle advancement, the syringe size, the aspirate volume, and the different commercial systems available for

TABLE 4.2
Techniques to Increase Yield With BMAC

Technique Optimization	Comment
LOCATION	
1. Vertebral body 2. Illiac crest 3. Site near surgery	1. Highest quantity of osteogenic progenitor cells 2. Posterior illiac crest > anterior illiac crest 3. Lower yield than illiac crest but may be sufficient for treatment site
VOLUME	
1. Syringe size 2. Aspirate amount	1. 10mL > 50mL syringe, higher cell yield with small syringe 2. Small volume > large volume, higher cell yield in first 1mL aspirate than with first 5mL, multiple small volume aspirates ↑ yeild
NEEDLE PLACEMENT	
1. Advancement 2. Rotation	1. Needle advancement by 5mm increments with aspiration ↑ MSCs 2. 45° rotation of Jamshidi needle with obturator reinsertion clears channel for MSC collection
CENTRIFUGATION SYSTEM	
1. System selection	1. Not all centrifuge systems are the same, some studies support certain systems for higher % yield of MSCs

BMAC, bone marrow aspirate concentrate; *MSC*, mesenchymal stem cell.

BMAC harvest (Table 4.2). With attention to needle placement, movement of the needle throughout the aspiration process provides a higher yield than a stationary needle. Peters and colleagues demonstrated that multiple needle advancements resulted in a higher concentration of MSCs.[20] In particular, needle advancement of 5 mm up to 3 times throughout the procedure increases the proportion of MSCs.[20] Not to mention, the size of the syringe used for vacuum aspiration of the bone marrow matters in regard to cell yield. In a study by Hernigou et al.,[21] a 10 and 50 mL syringe were compared during bilateral aspiration of bone marrow from the iliac crest. In comparison, there was a 300% higher cell yield with a 10 ml syringe, and equally important, there were significantly more cells in the first 1 mL aspirate of the 10 mL syringe as opposed to the first 5 mL of the 50 mL

syringe.[21] As a result, the more efficient technique to optimize aspiration of bone marrow is by aspirating smaller volumes in small syringes. By the same token, larger volumes of aspirate appear to dilute the concentration of bone marrow. As small a difference as 2 mL of bone marrow aspirate can produce a drastic difference in the amount of MSCs.[22] Indeed, Muschler and colleagues demonstrated a difference between 2 and 4 mL of bone marrow aspirate from the anterior iliac crest of patients with the number of MSCs decreasing by 50% from the higher volume of aspirate.[23] In like manner, a study by Bacigalup et al.[24] determined that harvest of bone marrow using multiple small volume aspirations decreased the dilution with peripheral blood, thus resulting in a higher yield of MSCs. Multiple commercial companies provide systems for harvesting of bone marrow aspirate. A study comparing different systems to harvest BMAC included the following systems: Harvest SmartPRep2, Biomet BioCUE, and Arteriocyte Magellan.[25] In comparison of these systems, the Harvest system showed significantly greater concentration of connective tissue progenitors both before and after centrifugation in comparison to the Biomet BioCUE system. In a similar fashion, the Harvest system showed significantly higher percent yield of connective tissue progenitor cells after centrifugation in comparison to the Arteriocyte Magellan system. Under these circumstances, the difference between systems, in harvest of bone marrow aspirate, is believed to be due to differences in the centrifugation device that leads to a variation in yield of concentrated progenitor cells.[25]

The Application of Bone Marrow Aspirate Concentrate

The utility of BMAC has been applied to address numerous pathologies of the musculoskeletal system. As an illustration, BMAC has been used to induce and increase bone formation.[12,26,27] In an analysis of basic science evidence for long bone healing, Gianakos et al., summarized that several studies support BMAC significantly increasing the amount of bone formation.[27] To demonstrate this finding, imaging showed significant increases in bone formation by an increase in bone volume, callus formation, and union of healing bone. At the same time, on microcomputed tomography of animal subjects receiving BMAC, there was an 81% reported significant increase in the bone area of these study subjects. Under closer observation, histologic and histomorphometric assessment of BMAC subjects showed a 90% significant improvement in earlier bone healing. The increased bone formation, in bone defects treated with BMAC, translated into a higher torsional stiffness of 78%.[27] In like manner, BMAC, in addition to adding bone, has also exhibited the ability to add cartilage and augment cartilage healing.[28–30] Must be remembered, BMAC contains MSCs that have been validated to increase aggrecan content and tissue firmness that together compliment the cartilage repair. In a goat model by Saw and colleagues, surgically created cartilage defects when treated with BMAC, along with hyaluronic acid (HA), promoted the healing of cartilage with more glycosaminoglycan and a higher content and a better organization of hyaline cartilage.[30] In an equine model by Fortier and colleagues, cartilage defects were treated with either microfracture alone or microfracture along with BMAC.[31] In comparison of both groups, the addition of BMAC resulted in increased glycosaminoglycan, increased type II collagen, improved collagen orientation, and improved filling of cartilage defects.[31] Important to realize, the remarkable results in animal models has translated into optimized outcomes in human patients. In a study by Gobbi et al., BMAC was compared with matrix-induced autologous chondrocyte implantation (MACI) for treatment of patellofemoral chondral lesions. Although both groups of patients reported significant improvements, patients treated with BMAC showed significantly greater improvements in functional outcome scores.[32] Summation of clinical studies of BMAC, through a systematic review by Chahla et al., has synthesized good to excellent overall outcomes with treatment of BMAC for both knee osteoarthritis and knee chondral defects.[28] Another key point, from this systematic review, was that BMAC has better outcomes for treatment of cartilage lesions in patients younger than 45 years, with smaller size of chondral lesions, and with a fewer number of lesions.[33] Even though there is a broad range of clinical applications for BMAC from healing of fractures to treatment of osteoarthritis or cartilage defects, future studies are warranted to further elucidate the exact mechanisms and particular patients that would most benefit from augmentation of biologic healing with BMAC.

Safety of Bone Marrow Aspirate Concentrate

As with all treatment inventions, the safety and risk of potential complications must be weighed against the benefits of the BMAC procedure. The use of BMAC requires harvesting the bone marrow from a donor site of the patient; this entails an additional area of interruption and potential increased morbidity from the surgical technique. For fear of morbidity, the safety of autologous BMAC was evaluated by Hendrich et al., in the initial experiences in 101 patients.[34] After an average of 14 months, upon reexamination of all the patients, no major morbidity or mortality was directly due to the BMAC treatment. In particular, there were no noted infections, no induction of tumor formation, and no noted complications at the harvest site of the iliac crest.[34] Given the contents of BMAC containing stem cells, there is concern of cancerous formation from these pluripotent cells. With this in mind, the risk of cancer was explored by Hernigou et al., in patients treated for orthopaedic diseases with autologous bone marrow cell concentrate.[35] At a mean of 12.5 years of follow-up, there was 1873 patients treated with BMAC, and after reviews of more than 7300 magnetic resonance images (MRIs) and 52,000 radiographs, there were only 53 cancers diagnosed and not one of these cancers occurred in areas of the body that received an injection of BMAC.[35] On a less severe scale of complications, one of the most common adverse events reported, after BMAC treatment, were swelling and pain at either the harvest site or the site of injection. As an illustration, these common complications of swelling and pain were noted in the majority of the 75 degenerative knees that received BMAC for osteoarthritis.[36] On the contrary, in another study by Centeno and colleagues, after 840 BMAC procedures for knee osteoarthritis, no severe adverse events post procedure were due directly from the BMAC technique.[37] In detail, symptoms after BMAC treatment were 6% for those patients who only received BMAC and 8.9% for those patients who received BMAC with adipose graft with the majority of these symptoms being mostly self-limited pain and swelling.[37] As a result, the consensus of these studies conclude that BMAC treatment has no significant increase risk of cancer, limited harvest site morbidity, and the most common complications being self-limited symptoms without severe consequence.

CHONDROCYTE IMPLANTATION

Articular cartilage, one of the five forms of cartilage, functions to decrease friction and distribute loads across a joint. The composition of cartilage is cells, primarily chondrocytes, and extracellular matrix, with the majority of the matrix consisting of water and type II collagen. Of course, this composition of articular cartilage is arranged into three zones and a tidemark, which are established by the shape of the chondrocytes

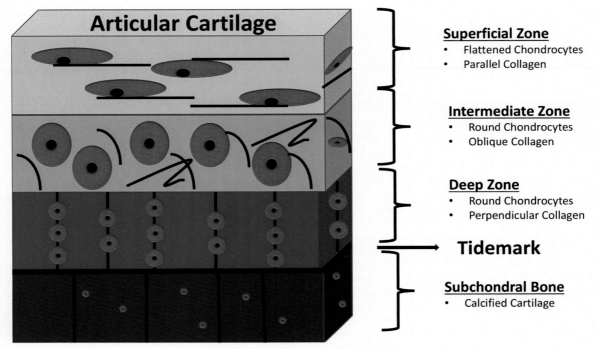

FIG. 4.2 Zones of Articular Cartilage.

and the orientation of the type II collagen (Fig. 4.2). In correspondence, the three zones are the superficial tangential zone, the intermediate zone, and the deep basal zone (Fig. 4.2). In the first place, the superficial tangential zone contains flattened chondrocytes with the type II collagen orientation parallel to the joint to resist shear forces. The next zone, intermediate zone, is the thickest layer with round chondrocytes and type II collagen oriented oblique to the joint. The last zone, deep basal zone, contains round chondrocytes with type II collagen orientation perpendicular to the joint to resist compressive forces. Below the deep basal zone is the tidemark that divides the superficial uncalcified cartilage from the deeper calcified cartilage. Perforation of the tidemark, such as with an awl in microfracture, allows marrow elements to extricate and eventually end up filling the cartilage defects as fibrocartilage.

Injury to Articular Cartilage
Articular cartilage is an avascular structure that receives nourishment at the surface from synovial fluid. Given the avascular nature of articular cartilage, there is limited ability for healing of defects created in the surface. Furthermore, the number of chondrocytes in the articular cartilage is limited, and these chondrocytes have

limited migratory ability that together further limit the healing potential of cartilage.[38] Often, injury to the articular cartilage occurs from acute high-impact loading to a joint or from repetitive shear and torsional loads to the superficial zone of the articular cartilage. When this injury penetrates past the tidemark into the underlying subchondral bone, MSCs, through a bleeding response, fill the injured area of articular cartilage with fibrocartilage.[38] However, fibrocartilage possesses different properties than articular cartilage with a higher coefficient of friction.[39] To help understand the severity of injury to the articular cartilage and to help guide treatment for defects to this surface, classification systems, with the most commonly referenced being the Outerbridge grading system and the International Cartilage Repair Society (ICRS) grading system, have been established (Table 4.3).[40,41] In accordance, the Outerbridge arthroscopic grading system consists of the following grades: grade 0—normal cartilage; grade I—softening and swelling; grade II—superficial fissures; grade III—deep fissures without exposed bone; grade IV—exposed subchondral bone. In a similar fashion, the ICRS grading system follows the following format: grade 0—normal cartilage; grade 1—superficial lesions; grade 2—lesions <50% of cartilage depth;

TABLE 4.3
Classifications Systems for Articular Cartilage Injury

	Outerbridge Grading System	International Cartilage Repair Society (ICRS) Grading System
Grade 0	Normal cartilage	Normal cartilage
Grade 1	Softening/swelling	Superficial lesions
Grade 2	Superficial fissures	Lesions <50% cartilage depth
Grade 3	Deep fissures without exposed bone	Lesions >50% cartilage depth
Grade 4	Exposed subchondral bone	Through subchondral bone

grade 3—lesions >50% of cartilage depth; grade 4—lesions extending into subchondral bone. With these classifications systems in mind, the proper indications for patient treatment selection and the prevalence of cartilage injuries can be communicated.

Injury to the articular cartilage, especially in the knee, is common. In a retrospective review of 31,516 knee arthroscopies, the prevalence of chondral lesions was 63%.[42] In particular, grade III lesions of articular cartilage were most common on the patella and grade IV lesions were most common on the medial femoral condyle with an average of 2.7 lesions per knee.[42] In another study of 1000 consecutive knee arthroscopies, the prevalence of chondral or osteochondral lesions were found in 61% of patients.[43] By location, the main injury to the articular cartilage was found on the medial femoral condyle in 58%, patella in 11%, lateral tibia in 11%, lateral femoral condyle in 9%, trochlea in 6%, and medial tibia in 5% with an overall average area of injury to the surface of 2.1 cm².[43] The size of the chondral defect helps guide treatment approaches to address the articular cartilage. For contained cartilage lesions less than 2 cm², an acceptable initial procedure is microfracture, such as that described by Steadman, where an awl is used to penetrate pass the tidemark into subchondral bone in order to release MSCs that eventually form fibrocartilage.[44] For contained cartilage lesions greater than 2 cm², but less than 12 cm², an acceptable procedure to perform is autologous chondrocyte implantation (ACI). Indeed, ACI is ideal for treatment of ICRS grade 3 or grade 4 lesions, especially

along the regions of the femoral condyle or the femoral trochlea. ACI is a staged procedure where the initial procedure involves a biopsy of articular cartilage that is followed by expansion of cultured chondrocytes that are then reimplanted in a second procedure to fill the defect in the surface of the cartilage. The technique of ACI was explored early in a rabbit model by Grande and colleagues, where autologous chondrocytes grown in vitro were labeled prior to grafting with a nuclear tracer then replanted into defects in the articular cartilage.[45] From this implantation, 82% of the articular cartilage was found to be reconstituted and the nuclear labeled chondrocytes were found to be incorporated into the repaired matrix of cartilage.[45] By all means, the evidence from the animal models led to translation of ACI used in humans. The initial experience of ACI in humans was reported by Brittberg et al., in 1994, where 23 patients with full-thickness cartilage defects had healthy chondrocytes from an uninjured area of the knee harvested, cultured, and then transplanted via injection into the injured area of cartilage.[46] After transplantation, patients reevaluated with arthroscopy were found to have transplants with the same macroscopic appearance, as the surrounding healthy cartilage and biopsy of the transplanted area, under microscopic examination, showed hyaline cartilage.[46]

The Autologous Chondrocyte Implantation Technique

The initial stage of the ACI technique requires obtaining a biopsy specimen from an uninvolved healthy area of articular cartilage. At the initial stage of the procedure, the defect in cartilage is closely evaluated for not only size of involvement but also for signs of any significant bone loss. If no subchondral bone is present in the area of the articular cartilage defect, then bone grafting may be required during this foremost part of the procedure. Also, sizing up the lesion allows the ordering of cells, prior to implantation, to be determined. Most commonly, the biopsy specimens are obtained from either the superomedial or superolateral edge of the femoral trochlea or from the lateral aspect of the intercondylar notch (Fig. 4.3). In total, biopsy specimens should contain both the entire surface of articular cartilage as well as a small portion of the underlying subchondral bone. Total weight of the biopsy specimen should be 200–300 mg. Within this weight range, the biopsy specimen should contain between 200,000 and 300,000 cells.[38] After obtaining the biopsy specimen, the harvested cells are maintained at 4°C until processing. Typically, one vial of cells is sufficient to supply distinct defects up to 6 cm², assuming that each vial contains approximately

Superolateral Trochlear Ridge   **Superomedial Trochlear Ridge**

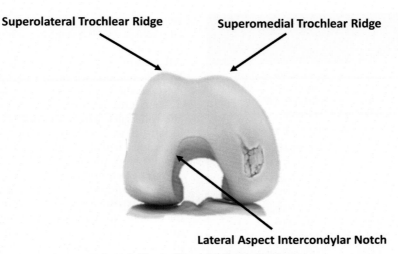

Lateral Aspect Intercondylar Notch

FIG. 4.3 Biopsy Sites of Articular Cartilage.

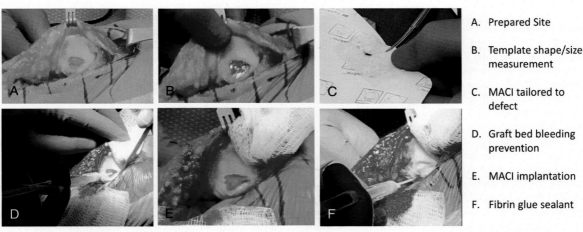

A. Prepared Site

B. Template shape/size measurement

C. MACI tailored to defect

D. Graft bed bleeding prevention

E. MACI implantation

F. Fibrin glue sealant

FIG. 4.4 Stages of Autologous Chondrocyte Implantation (ACI) Technique with Matrix-Induced ACI (MACI).

12 million cells along with 0.3–0.4 mL of Ham F-12 medium with serum supplementation.[38] Therefore, larger defects (>6 cm^2) or multiple defects may require additional vials; for this reason, determining the size of the cartilage lesion and presence of multiple defects in the cartilage should be closely observed and measured at the time of biopsy. During processing, the biopsy of cartilage is digested with enzymes with intention to release chondrocytes from the collagen matrix. For approximately 30 days, the chondrocytes are expanded in a suspension culture to obtain approximately 15–20 million cells.

In due time, the second stage of the ACI technique is performed to implant the cultured chondrocytes into the desired defect (Fig. 4.4). Inaugural techniques of ACI were performed with a medially or laterally based mini arthrotomy. Subsequent and more recent generations of ACI techniques are performed, without arthrotomy, using only arthroscopic techniques. In certain instances, a one-stage application of minced articular cartilage may even be a potential procedure to perform. Regardless of the technical approach being performed, the defect in the articular cartilage has to be prepared prior to receipt of the cultivated chondrocytes. Preparation of the defect begins with debridement, back until normal vertical margins of articular cartilage are achieved. Any cartilage that is not normal, with delamination or defibrillation, is removed. During preparation of the graft bed, any bone deficiency greater than 6 mm requires grafting until an even and established graft bed is recreated. Care is taken during graft bed preparation to prevent penetration into the underlying subchondral bone in order to prevent hemorrhage throughout the implantation technique. If bleeding is encountered, potential options include using thrombin spray or 1:1000 epinephrine–normal saline solution mixture in cotton pledges to obtain hemostasis. To begin with, the first generation of ACI techniques used a periosteal graft to create a seal over the prepared defect, prior to injection of the chondrocytes. Normally, the periosteum consists of an outer fibrogenic layer and an inner cambium layer with the principal harvest site for the periosteal graft being the proximal–medial aspect of the tibia just distal to the pes anserinus or semitendinosus tendon insertion. Importantly, to preserve cells in the cambium layer of the periosteum, no electrocautery is used during the patch harvest. After obtaining the periosteum, the graft is secured in place, over the recipient bed, with 6-0 vicryl suture approximately 2 mm from the surface and extending peripherally approximately 4 mm from the defect edge. Once, each corner of the periosteal graft is tied down, additional sutures at about 3 mm increments are added around the graft to ensure a watertight seal. To detect any potential leak, prior to placement of the chondrocytes, normal saline can be injected under the graft to confirm an adequately sealed cover. At this instant, chondrocytes can be implanted under the watertight sealed periosteal graft, using about one vial per 6-cm-sized defect. After injection of the chondrocytes, fibrin glue is used over the periosteal graft to seal in the implanted cells.

The second generation, and more recent, techniques of ACI all involve a similar first step to obtain a biopsy specimen to be used for autologous chondrocyte expansion. Typically, the biopsy specimens, as has been noted, are collected from the non–weight-bearing area of the medial femoral condyle or from the intercondylar notch. Subsequently, with the second generation ACI techniques, a collagen membrane, as opposed to a periosteal patch, is used to cover the lesion. For the third generation ACI techniques, the cultivated chondrocytes are seeded into a three-dimensional biomaterial scaffold such as with HA, collagen, or an artificial scaffold a few days prior to implantation. Use of the artificial scaffold, refers to the third generation of chondrocyte transplantation techniques that is commonly called the MACI technique. As an illustration, these scaffolds can be protein based, carbohydrate based, or synthetic polymers, which can be woven, spun into nanofibers, or configured as hydrogels.[14] By the time

the scaffolds are loaded with cells, bioreactors are used to provide nutrients and mechanical stimulation to further develop the cultured chondrocytes.[14] In essence, these biocompatible scaffolds allow a more efficient execution of implanting cultured chondrocytes, without the need of a knee arthrotomy, as the use of a matrix no longer requires injection of cells directly into the lesion. Although these later techniques of ACI can be performed all arthroscopically, some locations of defects, such as on the patella, still require an arthrotomy to be implemented for accessibility. After preparing the recipient bed and prior to implantation of the scaffold, a mapper or sizer is used to determine the shape and size of the cartilage defect.[47] As soon as measurements are obtained, the cultured cartilage scaffold is trimmed and tailored to the appropriate size, then implanted into the defect, after removal of solution from the joint, and fixed with fibrin glue.[48] Important to realize, while implanting the scaffold, the cell-seeded side of the implant needs to be placed facing down on the subchondral bone. Under these circumstances, given the efficiency of the subsequent ACI techniques, additional and concurrent interventions can be performed during the same surgical setting.

Postprocedure Healing and Rehabilitation
The postoperative healing, after an ACI technique, proceeds through three phases—proliferation, transition, and remodeling. For this reason, rehabilitation following ACI corresponds with the distinct phases of healing. In the first 6 weeks post procedure, the implanted chondrocytes are undergoing the proliferation phase. To begin with, over 12–18 hours after implantation, cells are allowed to adhere to the subchondral bone. To allow this cell adherence, knee motion is initially restricted for the first 18–24 h. After the short immobilization period, continuous passive motion (CPM) is begun to provide a chondrogenic stimulus. The importance behind use of continuous passive motion has been emphasized by studies showing the synthesis of glycosaminoglycans, chondroitin sulfate, and type II collagen.[48] In addition, use of CPM stimulates the correct spatial distribution of chondrocytes.[38] Along with passive mobilization of the knee, active mobilization of the ipsilateral hip and ankle, with concurrent isometric exercises, is conducted. During the proliferative phase, while soft primitive repair tissue is formed, no weight-bearing is allowed.

The second phase of cartilage healing, known as the transition phase, starts at postprocedure week 7 and lasts for 4–6 months. Depending on the size and location of the lesion treated with ACI, progressive weight-bearing is started with the goal of progressing to full weight-bearing. During this phase, exercises are aimed at achieving full range of motion while restoring full function of the muscles. However, open chain exercises are still avoided during this phase to prevent shear forces across the joint. Throughout this phase of healing, the chondrocytes release matrix into a putty-like consistency.[38] Starting at 6 months and lasting for 12 months, cartilage healing proceeds through the remodeling phase. During this final phase, activities are resumed and progressively proceed toward regular activities by 1 year. At the final phase, the cartilage tissue actively hardens to firm cartilage similar to the adjacent native articular cartilage; yet, the graft continues to mature up to 3 years after ACI.[38]

The gold standard for assessment, post ACI procedure, is arthroscopy. With arthroscopy, the repaired cartilage defect is able to be directly viewed, stiffness of the healed cartilage can be measured by probe indentation, and histomorphologic assessment can be conducted by obtaining a biopsy. Despite this gold standard, MRI is an alternative option that can provide viable information about the treated cartilage defect. In a study by Henderson et al., findings on MRI were able to be followed with second-look arthroscopy and histologic analysis of core biopsies.[49] At 3 months after ACI, MRI demonstrated that 75% of defects had at least 50% defect fill along with 46% having a normal signal and 67% having no significant underlying bone marrow edema.[49] At both 12 and 24 months, the demonstrations on MRI continued to improve to above 95% with defect fill and normal cartilage signal.[49] PostACI assessment continues to be further investigated with studies searching for correlations with functional outcomes in both short-term and long-term follow-up.

Applications of Autologous Chondrocyte Implantation

One of the first studies to evaluate the ACI technique in the United States was performed by Micheli and colleagues on 50 patients in 19 centers across the country.[50] In this study, the mean defect size was 4.2 cm² and 39 of the 50 patients had a prior articular cartilage procedure performed in the knee before receiving an ACI. Regardless of the previous treatment, or the size of the defect, there was no ramification on the results after ACI. At 36 months after ACI, 94% of the patients healed without failure of the graft.[50] Intermediate results, at 2–9 years of follow-up, after ACI were reported on 101 patients.[51] From this cohort, results correlated with location of lesion with good to excellent results in 92% with an isolated femoral

condyle lesion, 67% with multiple lesions, 89% with osteochondritis dissecans, and 65% with a patella lesion. In the final analysis, a learning curve for the ACI procedure was demonstrated by four failures that occurred in the first 23 patients but only three failures that occurred in the last 78 patients.[51] Long-term results, at 5–11 years of follow-up, were reported on 61 patients post ACI procedure.[52] After follow-up of 5–11 years, 51 of the 61 patients had good to excellent results. At the same time, second-look reevaluations of 8 out of the 12 biopsies showed hyaline-like repair tissue at the grafted ACI site.[52] Given these points, a durable outcome, for as long as 11 years after ACI, was reported consistently throughout the years of follow-up in the cohort.[52] From multiple studies, key prognostic factors have been determined to aid in selecting the appropriate candidates for intervention with an ACI technique. Compelling evidence has elucidated the following key factors for ACI: etiology, physiologic age, social factors, patient compliance, timed allowed for recovery, and desired postoperative activity level.[53] With this in mind, complications rates, after ACI, have been reported to be higher with open procedures, with use of a periosteal graft cover, and with first generation ACI techniques. On the other hand, best outcomes after ACI, have been reported with younger patients, with shorter preoperative duration of symptoms, and with fewer prior surgical procedures.[53] In detail, in a study by Knutsen et al., patients younger than 30 years, who underwent an ACI technique for treatment of a cartilage defect, exhibited significantly better Lysholm and Short-Form-36 (SF-36) scores at both 2 and 5 years in comparison to patients older than 30 years who received the same treatment.[54] All things considered, studies on ACI support improved outcomes in the majority of patients and optimal outcomes in patients with positive prognostic factors.

With the succession of different techniques for ACI, studies have been conducted to clarify the clinical outcomes between procedures. In comparison between first and second generation ACI techniques, studies have shown equivalent short-term clinical outcomes as well as similar complications and reoperation rates.[53] In a randomized study by Bartlett et al., 91 patients were randomized to receive either a first generation ACI technique with a type I/type III collagen cover or to receive a third generation ACI technique with a collagen bilayer seeded with chondrocytes.[55] From this study both generations of ACI resulted in clinical improvement at 1 year. After 1 year, arthroscopic assessment and biopsies showed hyaline cartilage in 43.9% of first generation ACI and 36.4% of third generation

ACI; however, there was no difference in reoperation with both groups undergoing additional procedures at 9%.[55] At short-term follow-up, between both generations of ACI, there was no noted significant difference in clinical, arthroscopic, or histologic outcomes.[55] In another randomized study by Zeifang et al., 21 patients with full-thickness cartilage defects at the femoral condyle were randomized to undergo either matrix-associated autologous chondrocyte implantation or the original periosteal flap ACI technique.[56] At both 1 and 2 years of follow-up, there was no significant difference in knee function as assessed by the International Knee Documentation Committee (IKDC) score between the different generations of ACI techniques. In addition, there were no major differences in complications between the treatment groups. As can be seen, short-term results show no significant differences between the different generations of ACI techniques, yet further studies, with longer follow-up, are required to determine the durability between the various techniques of chondrocyte implantation.

The initial ACI technique required an arthrotomy to provide access for injection of the cultured chondrocytes while subsequent ACI techniques are amenable to all arthroscopic procedures by use of a scaffold; given these circumstances, the difference in outcome between open and arthroscopic ACI techniques have been evaluated in several studies. In a systematic review by Harris et al., comparison of open versus arthroscopic ACI resulted in more rapid improvement, fewer complications, and a lower rate of reoperation with the all arthroscopic ACI technique.[53] In a prospective study comparing open and arthroscopic ACI techniques, at 5 years follow-up, results demonstrated significantly improved and better functional outcomes in favor of the all arthroscopic group.[47] Not to mention, up to 19 months after surgery, the arthroscopic ACI group improved and remained stable up to the 5-year follow-up mark, while the open ACI group continued to improve up to 24 months after surgery.[47] Other options to treat cartilage defects, particularly small contained defects, include microfracture or osteochondral grafts, and several studies have compared these techniques to ACI. Important to realize, the summation of studies comparing ACI techniques to microfracture techniques determine better short- and intermediate-term clinical results with ACI implantation.[53] Overtime, clinical outcomes following microfracture tend to plateau or even decline at longer periods of follow-up. In contradistinction, clinical outcomes following ACI techniques tend to remain stable or even continue to improve at longer periods of follow-up.[57] In like matter, in a randomized study by Saris et al., 108 patients with single ICRS grade III/IV cartilage defects of the femoral condyle were randomized to receive microfracture or chondrocyte implantation.[58] At 36 months follow-up, the chondrocyte implantation group resulted in significantly better clinical outcomes while the microfracture group resulted in decline in clinical outcomes.[58] With this in mind, the promising results with ACI techniques led into the evaluation of the cost-effectiveness for treatment of cartilage lesions. Minas and colleagues evaluated the quality of life of 44 patients who had undergone an ACI procedure and calculated the average cost per additional quality-adjusted life year.[59] Up to 24 months post ACI, functional improvements were noted in multiple outcome scores as well as quality of life, as measured by the Short-Form-36 Score. After analysis, the estimated cost per additional quality-adjusted life year was $6701.[59] For these reasons, ACI was determined to be a cost-effective treatment for cartilage lesions of the knee.

Safety of Autologous Chondrocyte Implantation

Given the widespread use of ACI, reports of complications have been collected overtime. With the use of living cultured chondrocytes, one concern is the development of graft hypertrophy. In a systematic review by Harris et al., graft hypertrophy has been noted in 22% after periosteal ACI, 6% after collagen membrane ACI, 4% after Hyalograft C ACI, and 7% after MACI.[53] Arthrofibrosis, especially following open ACI techniques, has been noted to occur in about 2.5% of ACI techniques.[53] After a review of 604 cases, following an ACI procedure, failure or reoperation occurred in 2.8% (17) cases. Important to realize, the rate of failure was noted to increase threefold if a microfracture procedure was performed prior to an ACI technique.[60] Less common complications, following an ACI technique, after review of 13 studies including 917 subjects were reported as three superficial wound infections, one septic arthritis, two reflex sympathetic dystrophies, and two deep venous thromboses.[53] All things considered, the lower rate of complications and lower rate of reoperations have been noted with the all arthroscopic ACI techniques.[53]

STEM CELL

A stem cell is an unspecialized cell with the ability to differentiate into many different types of cells. Not to mention, stem cells are only one generation in maturation from germ layer cells, which is the primary layer of cells

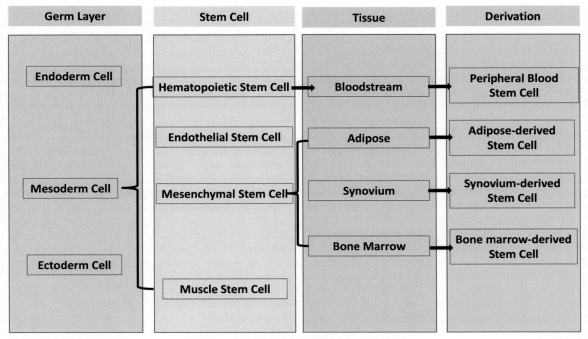

FIG. 4.5 Derivation of Mesenchymal Stem Cells.

that form during embryogenesis (Fig. 4.5).[4] Important to realize, there are four defining qualities and functions of stem cells: (1) proliferation–ability to reproduce; (2) differentiation–ability to mature into different types of cells; (3) mobilization–movement during angiogenesis; and (4) activation–ability to activate and control cells in the surrounding environment through paracrine function.[4] Stem cells, based on these defining qualities, can be considered as embryonic stem cells, adult stem cells, and induced pluripotent stem cells.[11] Embryonic stem cells, derived from the inner cell mass of an embryonic blastocyst, are totipotent with the potential to differentiate into any lineage of cells and the potential for indefinite self-renewal. Adult stem cells, with some level of differentiation, develop into cells that are close in origin. At the same time, these adult stem cells, named by the source of origin, are known, among others as hematopoietic stem cells, MSCs, and endothelial stem cells.[4] Each type of adult stem cell resides within their respective organ system with the function of replacing cells lost through tissue turnover.[11] Induced pluripotent stem cells are derived from a patient's own skin or blood cells through gene transduction using embryonic stem cell transcription factors. After all, MSCs have gained the most attention in orthopaedics due to the direct lineage of tissue in the musculoskeletal system.

In 2006, the International Society for Cellular Therapy provided criteria to define an MSC.[61] Under these circumstances, an MSC is defined as a stem cell with plastic adherence that expresses surface markers of CD105, CD73, and CD90. At the same time, an MSC must also not display surface markers to CD45, CD34, CD14, CD11b, CD79α, CD19, or HLA-DR. Equally important, an MSC, in vitro, must demonstrate the ability to differentiate into definitive cells of the musculoskeletal system. To help identify MSCs, monoclonal antibodies have been developed to the surface markers of CD73, CD105, and CD90.[5] Premier gathering of MSCs was primarily from bone marrow.[11] Given their origin, an MSC may also be called connective tissue progenitor cell or mesenchymal stromal cell. Regardless of nomenclature, an MSC must have the ability to differentiate into the cell lineages of chondrocytes, adipocytes, osteocytes, and myocytes.

Interplay with growth factors and pathways regulates the differentiation of an MSC. Proliferation of MSCs has been found to be primarily under the control of the canonical Wnt/β-Catenin signaling pathway.[62] Under this signaling pathway, a Wnt protein binds to frizzled receptors to inhibit glycogen synthase-kinase-3β (GSK-3β) that in turn allows β-catenin to translocate into the nucleus to induce gene expression and cellular proliferation of MSCs.[62] From this signaling, the Wnt pathway can lead cells toward differentiation of osteogenesis, adipogenesis, or chondrogenesis. Other pathways involved with MSCs include the Sonic Hedgehog pathway that directs cells toward osteogenesis and the TGF-β pathway that directs cells toward chondrogenesis and fibrogenesis.[11] Growth factors found to influence these signaling pathways include FGFs, insulin-like growth factors, granulocyte colony-stimulating factor, and BMPs.[63] In the long run, both growth factors and signaling pathways are synchronized together to determine the fate of an MSC.

Bone marrow was found to be the first source to provide MSCs.[64] However, since bone marrow, multiple sources have been found to contain MSCs.[11] These additional sites that contain MSCs are synovium, amniotic source, peripheral blood, and adipose and allogenic adult tissue. [6,65–67] A unique feature of MSCs, which aids in their isolation, is their ability to adhere to plastic surfaces.[68] Incidentally, the ability to adhere to tissue culture surfaces contributed toward the first isolation of MSCs.[64] With this in mind, marrow-derived MSCs are isolated from aspiration of bone marrow. Adipose-derived MSCs are isolated from the abluminal side of blood vessels in fat. Synovial-derived MSCs are isolated from either synovial tissue or synovial fluid.[4] In the bloodstream, the peripheral blood-derived stem cell (PBSC) can be found as an immature monocyte.[69] The amniotic-derived MSCs is isolated from amniotic fluid or the umbilical cord. Not to mention, the allogenic adult–derived stem cell is isolated from marrow aspirates of volunteer donors.[70] From all sources, MSCs have the ability to become terminally differentiated cells along the lineages of osteocytes, chondrocytes, adipocytes, and myocytes.[71,72] Important to realize, the source of the MSC will influence the differentiation of the cell in favor of the tissue of origin.[5,73] Equally important, MSCs, from different sources, have differences in immunophenotype, cytokine profile, and proteome analysis.[73–75] Despite the origin of MSCs, additional influences have been found to direct the differentiation of MSCs, which includes donor characteristics, isolation methods, and culture conditions.[11] Given these circumstances, the isolation and preparation of MSCs is paramount in providing the optimal quality of stem cells to aid healing in the musculoskeletal system.

Within any given organ, stem cells only comprise a small proportion of the cell concentration. For this reason, any harvest method results in a heterogeneous population of cells that include, among others, inflammatory cells, hematopoietic cells, and endothelial cells. In this case, endothelial cells can inhibit the differentiation of MSCs, thus further highlighting the need to isolate stem cells from other cells of the harvest.[76] Isolation of MSCs takes place by use of monoclonal antibodies to surface makers distinct to MSCs and through use of fluorescence-activated cell sorting.[77] In order to accelerate the isolation method, use of flow cytometry has allowed the process of purifying MSCs to be expedited.[78] After isolation, laboratory culture can be used to increase the population of MSCs. The expansion of MSCs is especially important when certain sources are used because the site of harvest can sway the number of available cells.[4] From in vitro culture, the number of colony-forming units that become apparent can provide an assessment of the amount of cells obtained from the harvest. As an illustration, several studies have demonstrated anywhere from 109 to 664 colony-forming units from 1 mL of bone marrow aspirate.[79] Once the isolated MSCs mature in artificial microenvironments, they can then be used to augment a wide variety of healing in orthopaedic interventions.

Marrow Derived

One of the most commonly used MSCs are bone marrow–derived stem cells. Part of this popularity is due to bone marrow being found as one of the first sources to provide MSCs.[64] Another consideration to this commonality is the accessibility of aspirating bone marrow from sites near to the surgery or from the available iliac crest. When obtaining MSCs from the iliac crest, the posterior iliac crest has been found to outperform the anterior iliac crest.[18] From the posterior iliac crest, the yield of colony-founding MSCs was 1.6 times greater in comparison to the anterior iliac crest. Although the yield was higher from the posterior iliac crest, there were no differences, between the two sites, with regard to viability, phenotype, expansion kinetics, or multilineage differentiation potential of MSCs.[18] Maximizing the yield of the starting population of MSCs, from bone marrow, benefits the subsequent steps of isolation and expansion in culture. Marrow-derived MSCs, from humans, retain the competence to differentiate into tissues of the musculoskeletal system. In vitro, cultured human marrow-derived MSCs, induced with dexamethasone and TGF-β, differentiated into chondrocytes with secretion of aggrecan, proteoglycans, and extracellular matrix containing type II collagen.[80] In the same way, Yoo et al., demonstrated the ability of human bone marrow–derived MSCs (BMSCs) to differentiate into chondrocytes with the expression of type II and type X collagen along with aggrecan, link protein, proteoglycans, biglycan, and decorin.[81] On closer examination, with immunohistochemical staining, antibodies specific for chondroitin 4-sulfate and keratin sulfate were found to be uniformly distributed throughout the terminally differentiated chondrocytes.[81]

In animal models, BMSCs have demonstrated the ability to augment healing of osteochondral defects.[4,11,82] In rabbits, Liu et al., showed that BMSCs embedded in synthetic extracellular matrix, placed into osteochondral defects, resulted in creation of elastic, firm, translucent cartilage with superior integration into the normal cartilage.[82] In a similar fashion, Chong and colleagues also used a rabbit model to demonstrate that the addition of BMSCs following primary Achilles tendon repair improved histological and biomechanical tendon healing.[83] Studies of BMSCs in animal models translated into similar benefits for treatment of cartilage defects in humans.[4,11] Wakitani and colleagues isolated and expanded BMSCs, then embedded these cells in a collagen gel, and transplanted them into the articular cartilage defect in the medial femoral condyle of 12 patients undergoing a high tibial osteotomy.[84] In comparison to the cell-free control group, those patients who received BMSCs showed better arthroscopic and histological scores of white hyaline-like cartilage filling in the chondral defects.[84] Not to mention, in a randomized study by Wong et al., those patients undergoing high tibial osteotomy and receiving marrow-derived MSCs showed significantly better outcome scores and MRI cartilage scores in comparison to those patients who underwent a high tibial osteotomy without additional implantation of MSCs.[85] For the most part, BMSCs are a favored option for MSCs given their accessibility and their ability to multiply in culture without losing the capacity of differentiation.

Adipose Derived

In adipose tissue, the luminal side of the blood vessel serves as a source of adipose-derived MSCs. Along with blood vessels, adipose tissue consists of adipocytes, fibroblasts, vascular smooth muscle cells, endothelial cells, monocytes/macrophages, and lymphocytes. Several studies support adipose-derived MSCs as being more plentiful and more accessible than other sources of MSCs.[4,11] This is supported by the subcutaneous location of adipose and the straightforward isolation of MSCs from adipose. In a study by James et al., 43.2% of the stromal vascular fraction from human lipoaspirate was found to be made up of perivascular stem cells.[77] This concentration translates into per 100 mL of lipoaspirate; 15 million perivascular MSCs can be purified. Important to realize, the proportion and volume of stem cells purified were found to be minimally changed by age, gender, or body mass index of the patient or the

length of storage time between liposuction.[77] Another key finding is that the anatomical site of adipose tissue harvest does not seem to affect the volume of viable MSCs.[86] Surgical technique to harvest adipose tissue uses liposuction, which can be assisted with ultrasound or tumescence. In comparison between the assistance technique for liposuction, tumescence liposuction provides more opportunity for proliferation of harvested MSCs.[87] Once harvested, via liposuction, the adipose tissue is microdissected under sterile conditions to obtain small fat lobules of approximate size $0.5-1\,cm^3$. Without delay, the isolated fat lobules are washed with phosphate-buffered saline then further isolated with use of enzymatic digestion via collagenase, filtered, and centrifuged to remove the remaining erythrocytes. Once independent, the adipose-derived MSCs can be cryopreserved or immediately expanded in vitro on medium. In vitro culture of adipose-derived MSCs can be optimized by use of low-density plating, Dulbecco modified Eagle medium, and low calcium concentration and with antioxidants that includes N-acetyl-L-cysteine and L-ascorbic acid-2-phosphate.[86]

In comparison to other sources of MSCs, adipose-derived MSCs are less immunogenic and less immunosuppressive.[63] In comparison to the more common BMSCs, adipose-derived MSCs are more accessible, are more abundant, and have higher proliferation rates.[86] Although more accessible, adipose-derived MSCs were found to be similar in protein expression and gene expression with BMSCs.[88,89] Specifically, similar gene expression pathways, between BMSCs and adipose-derived MSCs, were found for osteogenic-, chondrogenic-, or lipogenic-like differentiation.[90] With this in mind, the translational application of adipose-derived MSCs has been investigated in animal models. In a rat model, Pecanha et al., demonstrated that adipose-derived stem cell therapy increased and accelerated muscle repair.[63] In a rabbit model, Dragoo et al., evaluated the healing potential of adipose-derived stem cells for full-thickness cartilage defects.[91] From this study, 100% of rabbits, treated with adipose-derived stem cells, healed with hyaline-like cartilage, which revealed a similar collagen type II:I protein ratio to normal articular cartilage.[91] Along with differentiation into cartilage, adipose-derived stem cells have also demonstrated the ability to differentiate into osteocyte-like cells.[90] In a mouse model, Elabd et al., revealed at 4 weeks after implantation that subcutaneously injected adipose-derived stem cells into mice-formed woven bone.[2] Not to mention, the adipose-derived stem cells genetically modified by BMP-2 and applied to a β-tricalcium phosphate carrier were implanted into ulnar bone defects in a canine model to result in increased bone formation.[92] In a prospective cohort study, patients undergoing open-wedge high tibial osteotomy with PRP alone or PRP with adipose-derived MSCs were evaluated with second-look arthroscopy.[93] By all means, on second-look arthroscopy, patients who received adipose-derived MSCs showed significantly greater coverage of cartilage defects. Furthermore, patients who received adipose-derived MSCs demonstrated greater improvements in functional outcomes as measured by the Knee Injury and Osteoarthritis Outcome Score (KOOS) subscales for pain and symptoms and the VAS pain score.[93] With this in mind, patients with knee osteoarthritis received adipose-derived MSCs and then underwent second-look arthroscopy to reveal significantly improved cartilage lesions along with overall improvement in patient satisfaction.[94] After all the animal studies, and limited human studies, of adipose-derived MSCs, further studies are warranted in humans to evaluate the effects of adipose-derived cells for orthopaedic tissue regeneration.

Synovial Derived

The synovium is a thin layer of connective tissue that lines the bursae, joint surface, and tendon sheaths. Two main types of cells are contained within the synovium: type A synoviocytes and type B synoviocytes. Comparatively, type A synoviocytes are macrophages with phagocytic function, while type B synoviocytes are fibroblast-like cells that function to form synovial fluid. In 2001, De Bari and colleagues provided the first evidence of MSCs isolated from adult synovium.[95] From this study, the synovium of adult knee joints was enzymatically treated to release the stem cell population that was culturally expanded and then induced to differentiate into chondrocyte, osteocyte, and adipocyte and myocyte lineages.[95] Another key finding from this study is that donor age, cell passaging, and cryopreservation did not significantly alter the multilineage potential of the synovium-derived stem cells.[95] Under close observation, synovial MSCs have a similar phenotype to type B synoviocytes.[96] Similar to surface markers for other sources of MSCs, synovial MSCs are positive for surface markers of CD44, CD90, and CD105. However, unlike other sources of MSCs, synovial MSCs have a higher expression of CD44, a hyaluronan receptor, which can express uridine diphosphoglucose dehydrogenase that is a vital enzyme involved in hyaluronan synthesis.[96] In comparison to other sources of MSCs, synovium-derived stem cells exhibit higher expansion potential with higher colony-forming efficiency, fold increase, and growth kinetics.[65] In particular, in vitro

chondrogenesis assays showed greater chondrocyte production by synovium-derived cells than other sites of stem cells.[65]

Given these in vitro characteristics, synovial-derived stem cells have been further investigated in animal models. In a rabbit model, Koga and colleagues transplanted undifferentiated synovium-derived MSCs into full-thickness articular cartilage defects of adult rabbits.[97] From this local transplantation, previously undifferentiated synovial MSCs transformed into terminally differentiated chondrocytes. Depending on the local microenvironment, synovial MSCs differentiated into different cells based on the position within the cartilage defect. Under these circumstances, synovial MSCs differentiated into osteocytes in the deeper zone of the cartilage defects and into chondrocytes in the superficial zone of the cartilage defects.[97] In a similar manner, synovial MSCs transplanted into full-thickness articular cartilage defects in a pig model resulted in regeneration of cartilage, as early as 3 months post procedure, as scrutinized on arthroscopic, histologic, and MRI analysis.[98] By the same token, in a bone defect model in rabbits, synovial MSCs with hydroxyapatite were found to accelerate osteoinduction.[99] Synovial-derived MSCs, at the same time, have also demonstrated the ability to terminally differentiate down the myocyte lineage. De Bari et al., implanted adult human synovial membrane–derived MSCs in a mouse model resulting in contribution to skeletal muscle regeneration and persistent functioning of satellite cells.[100] Equally important, healing of tendon to bone was evaluated by Ju and colleagues in a rat Achilles tendon graft model.[101] As demonstrated by Ju et al., synovial MSCs implanted into bone tunnels accelerated early remodeling of tendon to bone healing.[101] In a clinical study, Sekiya et al., transplanted synovial-derived MSCs in patients with a single symptomatic cartilage lesion of the femoral condyle to result in significantly improved MRI score, histologic score, and Lysholm score.[102] Taken together, studies of synovium-derived MSCs show some promising results in animals that are awaiting more equally promising results to be demonstrated in humans.

Peripheral Blood Derived

The peripheral blood–derived stem cell (PBSC) originates from bone marrow and is present in the bloodstream as an immature monocyte. Although present in the bloodstream, PBSCs comprise a low concentration of cells. Often, granulocyte colony-stimulating factor analogues, such as filgrastim, are used to increase the proportion of PBSCs present in the bloodstream.[69,103]

With this in mind, harvesting a high number of PBSCs is possible with a process involving drug stimulation and plasmapheresis.[4] Once isolated, PBSCs, in comparison to MSCs, show that they have the same potential to proliferate. In a study by Huss et al., peripheral blood mononuclear cells were isolated from the heparinized blood of a dog, then cloned in culture with interleukin 6, and found to have MSC characteristic.[104] More commonly, harvested PBSCs are used safely in the field of hematology/oncology for bone marrow transplant.[105] Yet, some favorable results have been authenticated, for use of PBSCs, in orthopaedics.

In a large animal model of mountain sheep, Hopper et al., treated defects in the medial femoral condyle with human peripheral blood–derived MSCs.[106] In this study, the human peripheral blood–derived MSCs were induced under a hypoxic environment to acquire a phenotype of MSCs with upregulation of bmp-2, BMP6, GDF5, and COL1. Without manipulation, the hypoxia-induced peripheral blood–derived MSCs were equally comparable to BMSCs in treatment of osteochondral defects of the knee.[106] As an illustration, a case report of a male athlete with ICRS grade IV chondral lesion of the lateral femoral trochlea was treated with patellofemoral malalignment correction combined with autologous periosteum flap transplantation implanted with peripheral blood–derived MSCs.[107] On second-look arthroscopy, 8 months post procedure, a smooth surface of the lateral femoral trochlea was observed, and the patient was able to return to competitive sports up to the latest follow-up at 7.5 years from surgery.[107] To further demonstrate, in a case series of eight patients with varus deformity of the knee joint, a medial open-wedge high tibial osteotomy was performed with arthroscopic subchondral drilling and followed by postoperative intraarticular injections of peripheral blood stem cells with HA.[108] On follow-up evaluation, second-look arthroscopy showed regeneration of the cartilage and histologic analysis showed significant amounts of proteoglycan and type II collagen.[108] In a randomized study, Saw and colleagues evaluated the histologic and MRI outcomes of patients with chondral lesions treated by arthroscopic subchondral drilling followed by postoperative intraarticular injections of HA with or without peripheral blood stem cells.[109] As evidenced on histologic and radiologic assessment, after second-look arthroscopy, the patients who received an injection of HA plus peripheral blood stem cells showed significant improvement in the quality of articular cartilage repair in comparison to those patients who received an injection of only HA.[109] All things considered, PBSCs show assurance for treatment of chondral lesions; however, further studies are warranted to determine the differential potential and healing potential for other lineages of the musculoskeletal system.

Amniotic Derived

Wharton jelly is the mucoid connective tissue that surrounds the two arteries and one vein of the umbilical cord. Within Wharton jelly, fibroblast-like cells and mesenchymal-like cells can be found and collectively called human umbilical cord perivascular cells (HUCPV).[110] Other sources of amniotic-derived stem cells, in addition to the umbilical cord, are amniotic fluid and placenta tissue.[111] From these amniotic sources, these mesenchymal cells express surface markers CD44 and CD105 of stem cells and lack surface markers CD34 and CD45 of hematopoietic cells. Evaluation of the mesenchymal cells, isolated from amniotic sources, exhibit multilineage potential with the ability to differentiate into cells of the adipogenic, chondrogenic, and osteogenic lineages.[112] Under closer inspection, with gene expression analysis, amniotic-derived MSC have been found to express genes of the Wnt pathway, which is a known pathway for proliferation of MSCs.[113,114] Other genes, similarly expressed in BMSCs, were also found to be highly expressed in umbilical-derived stem cells such as vimentin, osteonectin, and collagens.[114] In comparison to BMSCs, amniotic-derived MSCs show a higher proliferative potential and show a higher expressed level of CD146, which is a marker of MSCs.[110] In particular, amniotic-derived MSCs proceed more quickly into terminal differentiation of the osteogenic lineage than marrow-derived MSCs.[113] Not to mention, human amniotic-derived stem cells have also demonstrated nontumorigenicity and nonimmunogenicity, given the low levels of major histocompatibility complex, thus allowing tolerance in transplantation to other humans.[115,116]

On a collagen scaffold, in the presence of a chondrogenic medium, amniotic-derived stem cells establish enhanced chondrogenesis in comparison to BMSCs.[117] In a similar fashion, Nogami et al., demonstrated the ability of isolated human amniotic MSCs, in chondrogenic medium containing TGF-β and BMP-2, to undergo chondrogenesis.[116] In an animal model, human placenta-derived MSCs, grown on silk fibroin biomaterial, were implanted into articular cartilage defects in adult rabbits to result in newly formed hyaline cartilage that filled in the articular defects.[111] On osteochondral explants, from adult arthritic knee tissue resected during total knee arthroplasty, human mesenchymal chondroprogenitor cells, derived from embryonic stem cells, were found to be capable of integrating into the partial-thickness defects of the ex vivo articular cartilage.[118] For the most part, potential from amniotic-derived stem cells has been demonstrated in preclinical studies, and future clinical studies will be needed to further verify the validity of amniotic-derived MSCs as efficacious orthobiologics.

Allogenic Adult Derived

From the marrow aspirates of donors, human MSCs have been isolated and expanded in colonies to retain their multilineage potential. In this case, the MSCs, derived from adult donors, can be used in allogenic transplantation to augment healing in orthopaedic conditions. Once isolated, the allogenic adult–derived MSCs can be induced to terminally differentiate into lineages of adipocytes, chondrocytes, or osteocytes.[70] In a rabbit model, Tay et al., created full-thickness articular cartilage defects on the medial femoral condyle of rabbits and then treated these injuries with either allogenic MSCs or ACI.[119] In comparison, allogenic MSCs, embedded in alginate, showed similar cartilage regenerative profiles and outcome scores as the group of rabbits that received treatment with ACI.[119] To evaluate the immune response of allogenic MSCs, Arinzeh et al., implanted adult human–derived allogenic MSCs into bone defects of the femoral diaphysis in dogs without the use of immunosuppressive therapy.[120] At any time point, after implantation of the allogenic MSCs, no adverse host response was detected with histology showing no lymphocytic infiltration and serum showing no antibodies against the allogeneic cells. At the same time, the allogenic-derived MSCs contributed toward callus formation and accelerated healing of the bone defect.[120] Given these findings in animal models, allogenic-derived MSCs demonstrate safety, with no immune response elicited, and demonstrate efficacy, with accelerated healing attained. The lack of donor morbidity, from allogenic-derived MSCs, is a favorable feature in comparison to harvest sites of other stem cells, and future clinical studies are warranted to further validate the effectiveness of donor stem cells in enhancing healing for orthopaedic conditions.

Future Directions of Stem Cells in Orthopaedics

Future studies on MSCs as biologics to augment healing in orthopaedics is warranted. In the first place, the exact mechanism and pathways of MSCs is poorly understood, especially in the natural environment. Assays to establish the function and maturation of MSCs require further refinement; particularly in preserving stem cell–like properties through clonal expansion. Once the laboratory process is polished, the most appropriate way to deliver these stem cells into patients' needs to be distinguished. Interactions between stem cells and potential carriers, such as patches, scaffolds, and hydrogels may serve as a source of transplantation into the target tissue. After delivery, the clinical studies will require appropriate controls for the evaluation of stem cells. In the long-term, proof of safety from stem cells will be provided by long-term follow-up of clinical studies. The remaining directions will only be possible through collaboration with academia, industry, and regulatory bodies to establish a safe and effective stem cell treatment for patients.

REFERENCES

1. Alberts B. *Molecular Biology of the Cell.* 6th ed. New York, NY: Garland Science, Taylor and Francis Group; 2015.
2. Elabd C, Chiellini C, Massoudi A, et al. Human adipose tissue-derived multipotent stem cells differentiate in vitro and in vivo into osteocyte-like cells. *Biochem Biophys Res Commun.* 2007;361(2):342–348.
3. Harford JS, Dekker TJ, Adams SB. Bone marrow aspirate concentrate for bone healing in foot and ankle surgery. *Foot Ankle Clin.* 2016;21(4):839–845.
4. Anz AW, Hackel JG, Nilssen EC, Andrews JR. Application of biologics in the treatment of the rotator cuff, meniscus, cartilage, and osteoarthritis. *J Am Acad Orthop Surg.* 2014;22(2):68–79.
5. Holton J, Imam M, Ward J, Snow M. The basic science of bone marrow aspirate concentrate in chondral injuries. *Orthop Rev (Pavia).* 2016;8(3):6659.
6. Delorme B, Charbord P. Culture and characterization of human bone marrow mesenchymal stem cells. *Methods Mol Med.* 2007;140:67–81.
7. Bain BJ. The bone marrow aspirate of healthy subjects. *Br J Haematol.* 1996;94(1):206–209.
8. Cassano JM, Kennedy JG, Ross KA, Fraser EJ, Goodale MB, Fortier LA. Bone marrow concentrate and platelet-rich plasma differ in cell distribution and interleukin 1 receptor antagonist protein concentration. *Knee Surg Sports Traumatol Arthrosc.* 2018;26(1):333–342.
9. Hernigou P, Poignard A, Manicom O, Mathieu G, Rouard H. The use of percutaneous autologous bone marrow transplantation in nonunion and avascular necrosis of bone. *J Bone Joint Surg Br.* 2005;87(7):896–902.
10. Connolly JF, Guse R, Tiedeman J, Dehne R. Autologous marrow injection for delayed unions of the tibia: a preliminary report. *J Orthop Trauma.* 1989;3(4):276–282.
11. LaPrade RF, Dragoo JL, Koh JL, Murray IR, Geeslin AG, Chu CR. AAOS research symposium updates and consensus: biologic treatment of orthopaedic injuries. *J Am Acad Orthop Surg.* 2016;24(7):e62–e78.

12. Hernigou P, Poignard A, Beaujean F, Rouard H. Percutaneous autologous bone-marrow grafting for nonunions. Influence of the number and concentration of progenitor cells. *J Bone Joint Surg Am.* 2005;87(7):1430–1437.

13. Connolly J, Guse R, Lippiello L, Dehne R. Development of an osteogenic bone-marrow preparation. *J Bone Joint Surg Am.* 1989;71(5):684–691.

14. Tuan RS, Chen AF, Klatt BA. Cartilage regeneration. *J Am Acad Orthop Surg.* 2013;21(5):303–311.

15. Sakou T. Bone morphogenetic proteins: from basic studies to clinical approaches. *Bone.* 1998;22(6):591–603.

16. McLain RF, Fleming JE, Boehm CA, Muschler GF. Aspiration of osteoprogenitor cells for augmenting spinal fusion: comparison of progenitor cell concentrations from the vertebral body and iliac crest. *J Bone Joint Surg Am.* 2005;87(12):2655–2661.

17. Hyer CF, Berlet GC, Bussewitz BW, Hankins T, Ziegler HL, Philbin TM. Quantitative assessment of the yield of osteoblastic connective tissue progenitors in bone marrow aspirate from the iliac crest, tibia, and calcaneus. *J Bone Joint Surg Am.* 2013;95(14):1312–1316.

18. Pierini M, Di Bella C, Dozza B, et al. The posterior iliac crest outperforms the anterior iliac crest when obtaining mesenchymal stem cells from bone marrow. *J Bone Joint Surg Am.* 2013;95(12):1101–1107.

19. Marx RE, Tursun R. A qualitative and quantitative analysis of autologous human multipotent adult stem cells derived from three anatomic areas by marrow aspiration: tibia, anterior ilium, and posterior ilium. *Int J Oral Maxillofac Implants.* 2013;28(5):e290–e294.

20. Peters AE, Watts AE. Biopsy needle advancement during bone marrow aspiration increases mesenchymal stem cell concentration. *Front Vet Sci.* 2016;3:23.

21. Hernigou P, Homma Y, Flouzat Lachaniette CH, et al. Benefits of small volume and small syringe for bone marrow aspirations of mesenchymal stem cells. *Int Orthop.* 2013;37(11):2279–2287.

22. Batinic D, Marusic M, Pavletic Z, et al. Relationship between differing volumes of bone marrow aspirates and their cellular composition. *Bone Marrow Transpl.* 1990;6(2):103–107.

23. Muschler GF, Boehm C, Easley K. Aspiration to obtain osteoblast progenitor cells from human bone marrow: the influence of aspiration volume. *J Bone Joint Surg Am.* 1997;79(11):1699–1709.

24. Bacigalupo A, Tong J, Podesta M, et al. Bone marrow harvest for marrow transplantation: effect of multiple small (2 ml) or large (20 ml) aspirates. *Bone Marrow Transpl.* 1992;9(6):467–470.

25. Hegde V, Shonuga O, Ellis S, et al. A prospective comparison of 3 approved systems for autologous bone marrow concentration demonstrated nonequivalency in progenitor cell number and concentration. *J Orthop Trauma.* 2014;28(10):591–598.

26. Homma Y, Zimmermann G, Hernigou P. Cellular therapies for the treatment of non-union: the past, present and future. *Injury.* 2013;44(suppl 1):S46–S49.

27. Gianakos A, Ni A, Zambrana L, Kennedy JG, Lane JM. Bone marrow aspirate concentrate in animal long bone healing: an analysis of basic science evidence. *J Orthop Trauma.* 2016;30(1):1–9.

28. Chahla J, Dean CS, Moatshe G, Pascual-Garrido C, Serra Cruz R, LaPrade RF. Concentrated bone marrow aspirate for the treatment of chondral injuries and osteoarthritis of the knee: a systematic review of outcomes. *Orthop J Sports Med.* 2016;4(1):2325967115625481.

29. Sampson S, Botto-van Bemden A, Aufiero D. Autologous bone marrow concentrate: review and application of a novel intra-articular orthobiologic for cartilage disease. *Phys Sportsmed.* 2013;41(3):7–18.

30. Saw KY, Hussin P, Loke SC, et al. Articular cartilage regeneration with autologous marrow aspirate and hyaluronic Acid: an experimental study in a goat model. *Arthroscopy.* 2009;25(12):1391–1400.

31. Fortier LA, Potter HG, Rickey EJ, et al. Concentrated bone marrow aspirate improves full-thickness cartilage repair compared with microfracture in the equine model. *J Bone Joint Surg Am.* 2010;92(10):1927–1937.

32. Gobbi A, Chaurasia S, Karnatzikos G, Nakamura N. Matrix-induced autologous chondrocyte implantation versus multipotent stem cells for the treatment of large patellofemoral chondral lesions: a nonrandomized prospective trial. *Cartilage.* 2015;6(2):82–97.

33. Dean CS, Liechti DJ, Chahla J, Moatshe G, LaPrade RF. Clinical outcomes of high tibial osteotomy for knee instability: a systematic review. *Orthop J Sports Med.* 2016;4(3):2325967116633419.

34. Hendrich C, Franz E, Waertel G, Krebs R, Jager M. Safety of autologous bone marrow aspiration concentrate transplantation: initial experiences in 101 patients. *Orthop Rev (Pavia).* 2009;1(2):e32.

35. Hernigou P, Homma Y, Flouzat-Lachaniette CH, Poignard A, Chevallier N, Rouard H. Cancer risk is not increased in patients treated for orthopaedic diseases with autologous bone marrow cell concentrate. *J Bone Joint Surg Am.* 2013;95(24):2215–2221.

36. Kim JD, Lee GW, Jung GH, et al. Clinical outcome of autologous bone marrow aspirates concentrate (BMAC) injection in degenerative arthritis of the knee. *Eur J Orthop Surg Traumatol.* 2014;24(8):1505–1511.

37. Centeno C, Pitts J, Al-Sayegh H, Freeman M. Efficacy of autologous bone marrow concentrate for knee osteoarthritis with and without adipose graft. *Biomed Res Int.* 2014;2014:370621.

38. Jones DG, Peterson L. Autologous chondrocyte implantation. *J Bone Joint Surg Am.* 2006;88(11):2502–2520.

39. Oddy MJ, Jones MJ, Pendegrass CJ, Pilling JR, Wimhurst JA. Assessment of reproducibility and accuracy in templating hybrid total hip arthroplasty using digital radiographs. *J Bone Joint Surg Br.* 2006;88(5):581–585.

40. Cameron ML, Briggs KK, Steadman JR. Reproducibility and reliability of the outerbridge classification for grading chondral lesions of the knee arthroscopically. *Am J Sports Med.* 2003;31(1):83–86.

41. Mainil-Varlet P, Aigner T, Brittberg M, et al. Histological assessment of cartilage repair: a report by the histology endpoint committee of the international cartilage repair society (ICRS). *J Bone Joint Surg Am*. 2003;85-A(suppl 2):45–57.

42. Curl WW, Krome J, Gordon ES, Rushing J, Smith BP, Poehling GG. Cartilage injuries: a review of 31,516 knee arthroscopies. *Arthroscopy*. 1997;13(4):456–460.

43. Hjelle K, Solheim E, Strand T, Muri R, Brittberg M. Articular cartilage defects in 1,000 knee arthroscopies. *Arthroscopy*. 2002;18(7):730–734.

44. Steadman JR, Rodkey WG, Briggs KK, Rodrigo JJ. [The microfracture technic in the management of complete cartilage defects in the knee joint]. *Orthopade*. 1999;28(1):26–32.

45. Grande DA, Pitman MI, Peterson L, Menche D, Klein M. The repair of experimentally produced defects in rabbit articular cartilage by autologous chondrocyte transplantation. *J Orthop Res*. 1989;7(2):208–218.

46. Brittberg M, Lindahl A, Nilsson A, Ohlsson C, Isaksson O, Peterson L. Treatment of deep cartilage defects in the knee with autologous chondrocyte transplantation. *N Engl J Med*. 1994;331(14):889–895.

47. Ferruzzi A, Buda R, Faldini C, et al. Autologous chondrocyte implantation in the knee joint: open compared with arthroscopic technique. Comparison at a minimum follow-up of five years. *J Bone Joint Surg Am*. 2008;90(suppl 4):90–101.

48. Jacobi M, Villa V, Magnussen RA, Neyret P. MACI - a new era? *Sports Med Arthrosc Rehabil Ther Technol*. 2011;3(1):10.

49. Henderson I, Francisco R, Oakes B, Cameron J. Autologous chondrocyte implantation for treatment of focal chondral defects of the knee–a clinical, arthroscopic, MRI and histologic evaluation at 2 years. *Knee*. 2005;12(3):209–216.

50. Micheli LJ, Browne JE, Erggelet C, et al. Autologous chondrocyte implantation of the knee: multicenter experience and minimum 3-year follow-up. *Clin J Sport Med*. 2001;11(4):223–228.

51. Peterson L, Minas T, Brittberg M, Nilsson A, Sjogren-Jansson E, Lindahl A. Two- to 9-year outcome after autologous chondrocyte transplantation of the knee. *Clin Orthop Relat Res*. 2000;(374):212–234.

52. Peterson L, Brittberg M, Kiviranta I, Akerlund EL, Lindahl A. Autologous chondrocyte transplantation. Biomechanics and long-term durability. *Am J Sports Med*. 2002;30(1):2–12.

53. Harris JD, Siston RA, Pan X, Flanigan DC. Autologous chondrocyte implantation: a systematic review. *J Bone Joint Surg Am*. 2010;92(12):2220–2233.

54. Knutsen G, Engebretsen L, Ludvigsen TC, et al. Autologous chondrocyte implantation compared with microfracture in the knee. A randomized trial. *J Bone Joint Surg Am*. 2004;86-A(3):455–464.

55. Bartlett W, Skinner JA, Gooding CR, et al. Autologous chondrocyte implantation versus matrix-induced autologous chondrocyte implantation for osteochondral defects of the knee: a prospective, randomised study. *J Bone Joint Surg Br*. 2005;87(5):640–645.

56. Zeifang F, Oberle D, Nierhoff C, Richter W, Moradi B, Schmitt H. Autologous chondrocyte implantation using the original periosteum-cover technique versus matrix-associated autologous chondrocyte implantation: a randomized clinical trial. *Am J Sports Med*. 2010;38(5):924–933.

57. Harrison AK, Flatow EL. Arthroscopic decompression with acromioplasty and structured exercise was no more effective and was more expensive than exercise alone. *J Bone Joint Surg Am*. 2010;92(10):1999.

58. Saris DB, Vanlauwe J, Victor J, et al. Treatment of symptomatic cartilage defects of the knee: characterized chondrocyte implantation results in better clinical outcome at 36 months in a randomized trial compared to microfracture. *Am J Sports Med*. 2009;37(suppl 1):10S–19S.

59. Minas T. Chondrocyte implantation in the repair of chondral lesions of the knee: economics and quality of life. *Am J Orthop (Belle Mead NJ)*. 1998;27(11):739–744.

60. Minas T, Gomoll AH, Rosenberger R, Royce RO, Bryant T. Increased failure rate of autologous chondrocyte implantation after previous treatment with marrow stimulation techniques. *Am J Sports Med*. 2009;37(5):902–908.

61. Dominici M, Le Blanc K, Mueller I, et al. Minimal criteria for defining multipotent mesenchymal stromal cells. The International Society for Cellular Therapy position statement. *Cytotherapy*. 2006;8(4):315–317.

62. Etheridge SL, Spencer GJ, Heath DJ, Genever PG. Expression profiling and functional analysis of wnt signaling mechanisms in mesenchymal stem cells. *Stem Cells*. 2004;22(5):849–860.

63. Pecanha R, Bagno LL, Ribeiro MB, et al. Adipose-derived stem-cell treatment of skeletal muscle injury. *J Bone Joint Surg Am*. 2012;94(7):609–617.

64. Hung SC, Chen NJ, Hsieh SL, Li H, Ma HL, Lo WH. Isolation and characterization of size-sieved stem cells from human bone marrow. *Stem Cells*. 2002;20(3):249–258.

65. Yoshimura H, Muneta T, Nimura A, Yokoyama A, Koga H, Sekiya I. Comparison of rat mesenchymal stem cells derived from bone marrow, synovium, periosteum, adipose tissue, and muscle. *Cell Tissue Res*. 2007;327(3):449–462.

66. Wagner W, Wein F, Seckinger A, et al. Comparative characteristics of mesenchymal stem cells from human bone marrow, adipose tissue, and umbilical cord blood. *Exp Hematol*. 2005;33(11):1402–1416.

67. Bianco P, Riminucci M, Gronthos S, Robey PG. Bone marrow stromal stem cells: nature, biology, and potential applications. *Stem Cells*. 2001;19(3):180–192.

68. Kassem M, Kristiansen M, Abdallah BM. Mesenchymal stem cells: cell biology and potential use in therapy. *Basic Clin Pharmacol Toxicol*. 2004;95(5):209–214.

69. Cesselli D, Beltrami AP, Rigo S, et al. Multipotent progenitor cells are present in human peripheral blood. *Circ Res*. 2009;104(10):1225–1234.

70. Pittenger MF, Mackay AM, Beck SC, et al. Multilineage potential of adult human mesenchymal stem cells. *Science*. 1999;284(5411):143–147.

71. De Bari C, Dell'Accio F, Vanlauwe J, et al. Mesenchymal multipotency of adult human periosteal cells demonstrated by single-cell lineage analysis. *Arthritis Rheum*. 2006;54(4):1209–1221.

72. Zuk PA, Zhu M, Ashjian P, et al. Human adipose tissue is a source of multipotent stem cells. *Mol Biol Cell*. 2002;13(12):4279–4295.

73. Katz AJ, Tholpady A, Tholpady SS, Shang H, Ogle RC. Cell surface and transcriptional characterization of human adipose-derived adherent stromal (hADAS) cells. *Stem Cells*. 2005;23(3):412–423.

74. Mitchell JB, McIntosh K, Zvonic S, et al. Immunophenotype of human adipose-derived cells: temporal changes in stromal-associated and stem cell-associated markers. *Stem Cells*. 2006;24(2):376–385.

75. Kilroy GE, Foster SJ, Wu X, et al. Cytokine profile of human adipose-derived stem cells: expression of angiogenic, hematopoietic, and pro-inflammatory factors. *J Cell Physiol*. 2007;212(3):702–709.

76. Meury T, Verrier S, Alini M. Human endothelial cells inhibit BMSC differentiation into mature osteoblasts in vitro by interfering with osterix expression. *J Cell Biochem*. 2006;98(4):992–1006.

77. James AW, Zara JN, Corselli M, et al. An abundant perivascular source of stem cells for bone tissue engineering. *Stem Cells Transl Med*. 2012;1(9):673–684.

78. Corselli M, Crisan M, Murray IR, et al. Identification of perivascular mesenchymal stromal/stem cells by flow cytometry. *Cytom a*. 2013;83(8):714–720.

79. Murphy MB, Moncivais K, Caplan AI. Mesenchymal stem cells: environmentally responsive therapeutics for regenerative medicine. *Exp Mol Med*. 2013;45:e54.

80. Mackay AM, Beck SC, Murphy JM, Barry FP, Chichester CO, Pittenger MF. Chondrogenic differentiation of cultured human mesenchymal stem cells from marrow. *Tissue Eng*. 1998;4(4):415–428.

81. Yoo JU, Barthel TS, Nishimura K, et al. The chondrogenic potential of human bone-marrow-derived mesenchymal progenitor cells. *J Bone Joint Surg Am*. 1998;80(12):1745–1757.

82. Liu Y, Shu XZ, Prestwich GD. Osteochondral defect repair with autologous bone marrow-derived mesenchymal stem cells in an injectable, in situ, cross-linked synthetic extracellular matrix. *Tissue Eng*. 2006;12(12):3405–3416.

83. Chong AK, Ang AD, Goh JC, et al. Bone marrow-derived mesenchymal stem cells influence early tendon-healing in a rabbit achilles tendon model. *J Bone Joint Surg Am*. 2007;89(1):74–81.

84. Wakitani S, Imoto K, Yamamoto T, Saito M, Murata N, Yoneda M. Human autologous culture expanded bone marrow mesenchymal cell transplantation for repair of cartilage defects in osteoarthritic knees. *Osteoarthr Cartil*. 2002;10(3):199–206.

85. Wong KL, Lee KB, Tai BC, Law P, Lee EH, Hui JH. Injectable cultured bone marrow-derived mesenchymal stem cells in varus knees with cartilage defects undergoing high tibial osteotomy: a prospective, randomized controlled clinical trial with 2 years' follow-up. *Arthroscopy*. 2013;29(12):2020–2028.

86. Schaffler A, Buchler C. Concise review: adipose tissue-derived stromal cells–basic and clinical implications for novel cell-based therapies. *Stem Cells*. 2007;25(4):818–827.

87. Oedayrajsingh-Varma MJ, van Ham SM, Knippenberg M, et al. Adipose tissue-derived mesenchymal stem cell yield and growth characteristics are affected by the tissue-harvesting procedure. *Cytotherapy*. 2006;8(2):166–177.

88. Gronthos S, Franklin DM, Leddy HA, Robey PG, Storms RW, Gimble JM. Surface protein characterization of human adipose tissue-derived stromal cells. *J Cell Physiol*. 2001;189(1):54–63.

89. Liu TM, Martina M, Hutmacher DW, Hui JH, Lee EH, Lim B. Identification of common pathways mediating differentiation of bone marrow- and adipose tissue-derived human mesenchymal stem cells into three mesenchymal lineages. *Stem Cells*. 2007;25(3):750–760.

90. Tapp H, Hanley Jr EN, Patt JC, Gruber HE. Adipose-derived stem cells: characterization and current application in orthopaedic tissue repair. *Exp Biol Med (Maywood)*. 2009;234(1):1–9.

91. Dragoo JL, Carlson G, McCormick F, et al. Healing full-thickness cartilage defects using adipose-derived stem cells. *Tissue Eng*. 2007;13(7):1615–1621.

92. Li H, Dai K, Tang T, Zhang X, Yan M, Lou J. Bone regeneration by implantation of adipose-derived stromal cells expressing BMP-2. *Biochem Biophys Res Commun*. 2007;356(4):836–842.

93. Koh YG, Kwon OR, Kim YS, Choi YJ. Comparative outcomes of open-wedge high tibial osteotomy with platelet-rich plasma alone or in combination with mesenchymal stem cell treatment: a prospective study. *Arthroscopy*. 2014;30(11):1453–1460.

94. Koh YG, Choi YJ, Kwon OR, Kim YS. Second-look arthroscopic evaluation of cartilage lesions after mesenchymal stem cell implantation in osteoarthritic knees. *Am J Sports Med*. 2014;42(7):1628–1637.

95. De Bari C, Dell'Accio F, Tylzanowski P, Luyten FP. Multipotent mesenchymal stem cells from adult human synovial membrane. *Arthritis Rheum*. 2001;44(8):1928–1942.

96. Atesok K, Doral MN, Bilge O, Sekiya I. Synovial stem cells in musculoskeletal regeneration. *J Am Acad Orthop Surg*. 2013;21(4):258–259.

97. Koga H, Muneta T, Ju YJ, et al. Synovial stem cells are regionally specified according to local microenvironments after implantation for cartilage regeneration. *Stem Cells*. 2007;25(3):689–696.

98. Nakamura T, Sekiya I, Muneta T, et al. Arthroscopic, histological and MRI analyses of cartilage repair after a minimally invasive method of transplantation of allogeneic synovial mesenchymal stromal cells into cartilage defects in pigs. *Cytotherapy*. 2012;14(3):327–338.

99. Matsusaki M, Kadowaki K, Tateishi K, et al. Scaffold-free tissue-engineered construct-hydroxyapatite composites generated by an alternate soaking process: potential for repair of bone defects. *Tissue Eng A.* 2009;15(1):55–63.

100. De Bari C, Dell'Accio F, Vandenabeele F, Vermeesch JR, Raymackers JM, Luyten FP. Skeletal muscle repair by adult human mesenchymal stem cells from synovial membrane. *J Cell Biol.* 2003;160(6):909–918.

101. Ju YJ, Muneta T, Yoshimura H, Koga H, Sekiya I. Synovial mesenchymal stem cells accelerate early remodeling of tendon-bone healing. *Cell Tissue Res.* 2008;332(3):469–478.

102. Sekiya I, Muneta T, Horie M, Koga H. Arthroscopic transplantation of synovial stem cells improves clinical outcomes in knees with cartilage defects. *Clin Orthop Relat Res.* 2015;473(7):2316–2326.

103. Bensinger W, Singer J, Appelbaum F, et al. Autologous transplantation with peripheral blood mononuclear cells collected after administration of recombinant granulocyte stimulating factor. *Blood.* 1993;81(11):3158–3163.

104. Huss R, Lange C, Weissinger EM, Kolb HJ, Thalmeier K. Evidence of peripheral blood-derived, plastic-adherent CD34(-/low) hematopoietic stem cell clones with mesenchymal stem cell characteristics. *Stem Cells.* 2000;18(4):252–260.

105. Holig K, Kramer M, Kroschinsky F, et al. Safety and efficacy of hematopoietic stem cell collection from mobilized peripheral blood in unrelated volunteers: 12 years of single-center experience in 3928 donors. *Blood.* 2009;114(18):3757–3763.

106. Hopper N, Henson F, Brooks R, Ali E, Rushton N, Wardale J. Peripheral blood derived mononuclear cells enhance osteoarthritic human chondrocyte migration. *Arthritis Res Ther.* 2015;17:199.

107. Fu WL, Ao YF, Ke XY, et al. Repair of large full-thickness cartilage defect by activating endogenous peripheral blood stem cells and autologous periosteum flap transplantation combined with patellofemoral realignment. *Knee.* 2014;21(2):609–612.

108. Saw KY, Anz A, Jee CS, Ng RC, Mohtarrudin N, Ragavanaidu K. High tibial osteotomy in combination with chondrogenesis after stem cell therapy: a histologic report of 8 cases. *Arthroscopy.* 2015;31(10):1909–1920.

109. Saw KY, Anz A, Siew-Yoke Jee C, et al. Articular cartilage regeneration with autologous peripheral blood stem cells versus hyaluronic acid: a randomized controlled trial. *Arthroscopy.* 2013;29(4):684–694.

110. Sarugaser R, Lickorish D, Baksh D, Hosseini MM, Davies JE. Human umbilical cord perivascular (HUCPV) cells: a source of mesenchymal progenitors. *Stem Cells.* 2005;23(2):220–229.

111. Li F, Chen YZ, Miao ZN, Zheng SY, Jin J. Human placenta-derived mesenchymal stem cells with silk fibroin biomaterial in the repair of articular cartilage defects. *Cell Reprogr.* 2012;14(4):334–341.

112. Wang HS, Hung SC, Peng ST, et al. Mesenchymal stem cells in the Wharton's jelly of the human umbilical cord. *Stem Cells.* 2004;22(7):1330–1337.

113. Baksh D, Yao R, Tuan RS. Comparison of proliferative and multilineage differentiation potential of human mesenchymal stem cells derived from umbilical cord and bone marrow. *Stem Cells.* 2007;25(6):1384–1392.

114. Panepucci RA, Siufi JL, Silva Jr WA, et al. Comparison of gene expression of umbilical cord vein and bone marrow-derived mesenchymal stem cells. *Stem Cells.* 2004;22(7):1263–1278.

115. Gauthaman K, Fong CY, Suganya CA, et al. Extra-embryonic human Wharton's jelly stem cells do not induce tumorigenesis, unlike human embryonic stem cells. *Reprod Biomed Online.* 2012;24(2):235–246.

116. Nogami M, Tsuno H, Koike C, et al. Isolation and characterization of human amniotic mesenchymal stem cells and their chondrogenic differentiation. *Transplantation.* 2012;93(12):1221–1228.

117. Fong CY, Subramanian A, Gauthaman K, et al. Human umbilical cord Wharton's jelly stem cells undergo enhanced chondrogenic differentiation when grown on nanofibrous scaffolds and in a sequential two-stage culture medium environment. *Stem Cell Rev.* 2012;8(1):195–209.

118. Olee T, Grogan SP, Lotz MK, Colwell Jr CW, D'Lima DD, Snyder EY. Repair of cartilage defects in arthritic tissue with differentiated human embryonic stem cells. *Tissue Eng A.* 2014;20(3–4):683–692.

119. Tay LX, Ahmad RE, Dashtdar H, et al. Treatment outcomes of alginate-embedded allogenic mesenchymal stem cells versus autologous chondrocytes for the repair of focal articular cartilage defects in a rabbit model. *Am J Sports Med.* 2012;40(1):83–90.

120. Arinzeh TL, Peter SJ, Archambault MP, et al. Allogeneic mesenchymal stem cells regenerate bone in a critical-sized canine segmental defect. *J Bone Joint Surg Am.* 2003;85-A(10):1927–1935.

CHAPTER 5

Allograft Tissue Safety and Technology

MARK A. MOORE, PHD • BRIAN SAMSELL, BS • JULIE MCLEAN, PHD

INTRODUCTION

Biologic tissues are among the many clinical options available to orthopedic surgeons, with over 1 million annual implants of human allografts alone.[1] Such biologic tissues may be considered structural, for example, tendons or cortical bone struts, or nonstructural, such as ground demineralized bone matrices (DBMs) or amniotic membranes. Their intended use may mimic their original anatomical function, such as using a patellar ligament for anterior cruciate ligament (ACL) reconstruction or a cortical bone segment to repair a long-bone fracture. In other circumstances, their use may differ from original anatomy, such as using a dermal layer for rotator cuff repair or a ground amniotic membrane combined with demineralized cortical bone for a spine fusion procedure. This chapter focuses on the intent and science of various means of processing human allograft tissues to ensure safety and clinical use.

Although xenografts, derived from nonhuman sources, have found clinical use in a variety of surgical disciplines, including the use of porcine heart valves for heart valve replacement surgery[2] and ground bovine bone for dental procedures,[3,4] their use in orthopedic surgery has met with more limited use and success. In particular, porcine-derived small intestinal submucosa did not perform well as a tissue augmentation material,[5,6] and bovine tendons are not commonly used[7]; thus, xenografts will not be discussed in this chapter.

Although autografts, taken directly from the patient, are widely used[8,9] for procedures such as ACL reconstruction or spinal implant of an iliac crest segment, these grafts are not subject to any significant processing other than some cleaning, shaping, or suture attachment before intrasurgery transplantation and therefore are also not covered in this chapter. Other autograft materials, such as those used for autologous cartilage implantation[10] or blood-derived preparations such as platelet-rich plasma,[11,12] are described elsewhere in this book.

Before being used by the orthopedic surgeon, allografts are commonly processed through physical, chemical, or biochemical means. Such processing steps are typically performed to accomplish one or more objectives such as:

- to reduce risk of disease transmission (e.g., through various disinfection or sterilization steps);
- to reduce immunogenic response (e.g., through decellularization);
- to reduce barriers to optimal physiological activity (e.g., by demineralizing cortical bone to enhance bioavailability of growth factors);
- to physically convert grafts into more usable forms (e.g., shaping a bone graft for placement as an intervertebral body spacer);
- to combine grafts with synthetics to enhance ease of use (e.g., by combining ground demineralized bone with a carrier to produce a putty-like material);
- to preserve tissue to increase shelf life or simplify storage (e.g., lyophilization of ground bone that enables retention at ambient temperatures).

With the focus here on human allografts, a brief historical and regulatory perspective is provided as background, followed by sections on reduction of disease transmission, enhancing fusion potential of bone void fillers, lowering immunogenic response by decellularization, preservation methods, and future directions.

BACKGROUND

Human allografts have been used in orthopedic surgery for many decades. In the 19th century William Macewen[13] described the successful use of allogeneic cortical bone fragments to graft a replacement for a missing humeral mid-shaft. Over 100 years ago, Fred Albee published a long list of surgical uses of bone allografts including applications and stated, "*[I have] been able during the past 2 years to avoid entirely the use of metal … for internal bone fixation purposes … made possible, largely, by utilizing the best of well known mechanical devices hitherto rarely, if at all, used in surgery, such as bone inlays, wedges, dowels, tongue and groove joints, mortised and dovetailed joints.*"[14]

Through the 20th century bone grafts continued to be used, and tendon allografts started gaining widespread acceptance by the 1980s.[15–17] During

Biologics in Orthopaedic Surgery. https://doi.org/10.1016/B978-0-323-55140-3.00005-9

the mid- to late-20th century, most "bone banks" for allografts were hospital-based with tissue derived from deceased or amputated patients.[18] These tissues often underwent only minimal chemical processing, such as antibiotic or disinfectant soaks. In addition, any physical alteration of these tissues was typically performed by the surgical team at the time of implantation and included bone shaping or grinding or tendon trimming or suturing. In answer to the need for better defined methods for ensuring graft safety and consistency, as well as appropriate respect for the tissue donors and their families, more formal systems began to be established by the Navy Tissue Bank in Bethesda, MD.[17-19]

Tissue Bank Standards and Regulation

In the latter half of the 20th century, the methodologies and practices developed by the Navy Tissue Bank were increasingly adopted by other organizations. In 1976 the American Association of Tissue Banks (AATB) was formed, and in 1984 it issued the first set of tissue-processing standards, which established guidelines such as acceptable time from death to recovery, storage conditions for tissues, microbial testing requirements, definitions of demineralization, freeze-drying, and so forth. A certification program was also established to assure the surgical community that qualified tissue banks met AATB standards.

Similarly, around the turn of the 21st century, the US Food and Drug Administration (FDA) developed the classification of Human Cell and Tissue Products (HCT/Ps) as a separate regulatory classification into which most human tissue transplants fell. This classification applies to most human tissue transplants. It differs from a medical device classification, in which, to qualify as an HCT/P, the tissue needs to meet standards of not exceeding "minimal manipulation" such that the "original relevant characteristics" are not altered, and also "homologous use" meaning the tissue is used clinically in a similar manner to that intended in the body of origin.[20,21] A clear example of a tissue meeting these requirements would be a hamstring tendon that is recovered intact, disinfected, sterilized, and then used for tendon replacement. Conversely, although bone void filler putty containing DBM would be considered for homologous use, it may be considered more than minimally manipulated because of the addition of a synthetic carrier and thus be classified as a medical device requiring FDA clearance before distribution. In further example, a disinfected and freeze-dried cortical bone segment used as an intervertebral body spacer is considered both minimally manipulated and intended for homologous use. As processors continue to become

more innovative in the use and treatment of human tissues, these definitions will undoubtedly be tested and clarified.

In adding further regulatory safeguards especially with respect to the risk of disease transmission, FDA issued the "Interim Rule" in 1993 to "require certain infectious disease testing, donor screening, and record-keeping facilities to help prevent the transmission of AIDS and hepatitis through human tissue used in transplantation."[22] In general, methods to reduce risk of disease transmission, such as antibiotic soaks, peroxide disinfection, and sterilization using radiation methods, are considered to be no more than minimal manipulation. Further on the regulatory front, in 2005, FDA established,[20,21] in conjunction with tissue bank input, a standard of good tissue practices to "create a unified registration and listing system for establishments that manufacture HCT/Ps and to establish donor eligibility, current good tissue practice, and other procedures to prevent the introduction, transmission, and spread of communicable disease."

In summary, the US system of AATB Standards and FDA regulations and inspections provide many safeguards for the provision of effective transplantable allograft tissues.

REDUCING RISK OF DISEASE TRANSMISSION IN TRANSPLANTED ALLOGRAFTS

Human tissue carries an inherent, yet minimal, risk of disease transmission, which has been made essentially negligible through advancements in cleaning and processing methodologies. A 2005 survey from AATB estimated an overall allograft-associated infection rate of 0.014%.[23] It is important to note that this survey preceded widespread implementation of more advanced methods aimed at reducing the risk of disease transmission, including FDA-mandated and sensitive nucleic acid testing (NAT) for certain viruses as well as routine terminal sterilization. Although well-documented cases of disease transmission have occurred,[24-26] modern tissue bank practices and processes have successfully diminished incidences over the last few decades. In a case beginning in 1985, four organs and 54 allograft tissues were distributed from an HIV-infected donor who had a favorable screening history and negative serology test.[25] All four organ recipients and the three recipients who received fresh frozen bone tissue tested positive for HIV. Investigators suspected that the transmissions occurred because the seronegative donor had very recently become infected and, being in the "window" period, had not yet developed an HIV-1 antibody detectable by the tests in use at the time. In 2002 another case surfaced where 40 recipients received organs and tissues from a donor infected with hepatitis C virus (HCV), and 8 consequently developed HCV infections.[26] As with the earlier HIV transmission case, the donor was seronegative for HCV, and NAT had not been performed. Subsequent NAT of stored serum from the donor detected the virus, which highlighted the importance of using more sensitive testing before releasing donor tissue. NAT for HIV and HCV is now required by FDA after being added as a requirement by AATB in 2005.[27] There have also been reported cases of transmission of tuberculosis, various *Clostridium species*, Group A *Streptococci*, and rabies.[28] Overall, the relative risk of disease transmission is small considering the millions of allografts transplanted; however, the possibility of transmission makes avoidance, control, and reduction of microbial and viral bioburden integral to tissue-processing practices.

Reducing Risk of Disease Transmission: Approach

Allograft tissue providers reduce risk of disease transmission by three primary means:

1. minimizing occurrence of processing donor tissue with unacceptable bioburden;
2. controlling environment and tissue-handling practices to avoid contamination; and
3. reducing any remaining bioburden through disinfection and sterilization techniques.

In the first category, the occurrence of recovering or processing tissue that is contaminated can be minimized through stringent bioburden tests, including anaerobic and aerobic culture tests for bacteria and fungi, as well as serological testing and NAT to detect specific viruses. Specific tests are required by FDA and also to meet AATB standards. Note that proper infectious disease tests must be validated for use specifically with cadaveric specimens.[21] A detailed donor-screening process is also critical for minimizing bioburden; medical records and social history, such as travel, tattoos, high-risk sexual behavior, illicit drug use, and incarceration, as well as physical examination, help assess donor eligibility.[28]

In the second category, bioburden loads can be controlled by using aseptic handling techniques during recovery and processing to prevent contamination of the tissue by pathogens. However, it is important to note that using aseptic conditions by themselves can only prevent additional contamination but will not reduce or eliminate any existing bioburden. For

the third risk-reduction category, processing methods designed to reduce any remaining bioburden are addressed in the following sections.

Bioburden Reduction Methods

Bioburden loads can be reduced by cleaning and disinfecting the tissue. These steps vary by tissue type and may include:

- debridement;
- low doses of preirradiation (irradiation before other chemical processing steps);
- physical methods such as lavage, pulsatile fluid flow, centrifuge, fluid bath rotation, and sonication;
- enzymatic digestion of cellular material;
- penetrating agents such as supercritical CO_2 in combination with chemical activators;
- milder chemicals including alcohol, detergents, and antibiotics;
- more aggressive chemicals such as NaOH, acetone, and peroxide.

Cleaning processes can remove bone marrow elements, lipids, and low-molecular-weight proteins, thus reducing any graft immunogenic potential as well as bacterial, viral, and fungal contamination.[29] More aggressive agents that may be commonly used to disinfect bone, such as hydrogen peroxide, are not typically used for soft tissue grafts. At least one process that includes the use of hydrogen peroxide on tendons was correlated with a significant increase in risk for revision ACL repair.[30] In this case, however, the contribution of the hydrogen peroxide to apparent graft weakening is unclear because the process also includes pulsatile fluid flow. Cellular remnants and, presumably, associated infectious agents may also be removed through tissue decellularization methods, which will also be discussed in a later section. These methods include the use of chemicals such as nondenaturing anionic detergent, recombinant endonuclease, sodium dodecyl sulfate, sodium hydroxide, sodium peroxide, sodium chloride, and antibiotics.[31-34]

Assurance of Tissue Sterility

After processing to reduce or eliminate bioburden, the tissue is typically either tested for sterility or subjected to a terminal sterilization step. Testing for sterility usually involves sampling a portion of the tissue or processing solutions according to United States Pharmacopeia <71> sterility test guidelines before packaging. It is important to note that the United States Pharmacopeia <71> label does not necessarily indicate that the tissue product is sterile but rather that a sample of the product batch was culture negative thus passing the test for sterility.[35,36] As an alternative to testing for sterility, the tissue may be processed, packaged, and then subjected to sterilization after placement in its final package thus at the terminus of the process. In this case of terminal sterilization the chosen method must effectively penetrate the packaging; such options will be discussed in subsequent sections.

In terms of measuring sterility, an absolute assurance of sterility is not probabilistically feasible, but there is a measure known as sterility assurance level, commonly referred to as SAL. This designation indicates the degree, or level, of assurance of sterility achieved through a validated sterilization process. The two most common SALs for allografts are 10^{-3} and 10^{-6}. A product labeled with an SAL of 10^{-3} indicates that there is a 1 in 1,000 chance of a single viable microbe present in the tissue, whereas an SAL of 10^{-6} indicates a greater degree of sterility with a 1 in 1,000,000 chance of the same. An SAL of 10^{-6} is the required level of sterilization by the Center for Disease Control and Prevention for medical instruments that breach the skin[37] and is thus often referred to as a medical device level of sterility. This level of sterility can only be achieved through terminal sterilization, though some terminally sterilized tissue products still retain an SAL of only 10^{-3}.[38]

Note that SAL is only a measure of microbial sterility and is unrelated to viruses, although the methods used to achieve an acceptable SAL may be effective at lowering viral risk. As mentioned previously, tissue processors use strict donor-screening and viral test methods to prevent viral transmission. Furthermore, several processing methods have been demonstrated to result in significant viral inactivation. For example, low-dose gamma irradiation was demonstrated to inactivate a broad spectrum of viruses, including HIV and enveloped, nonenveloped, DNA, and RNA viruses.[39] Another processing method uses vacuum and oscillating pressure combined with chemical agents to inactivate pathogens.[40] The use of a terminal sterilization process with the ability to inactivate a wide range of virus types is particularly advantageous as new viruses (e.g., Zika, severe acute respiratory syndrome, and so forth) emerge for which validated blood tests may not yet exist.

Terminal Sterilization

Reported methods to terminally sterilize allografts in their final packaging include plasma H_2O_2, ethylene oxide (EO), supercritical CO_2, electron beam irradiation, and gamma irradiation, all with benefits and risks. Plasma H_2O_2 has the disadvantage of removing osteoinductive potential from DBM[41] and may damage soft tissues. Although EO is commonly used to sterilize medical instruments, it has been reported to cause persistent synovial effusions and inflammatory responses in EO-treated allografts.[42] Both supercritical CO_2 and electron beam irradiation have been reported capable of safely providing terminal sterilization without significantly damaging tissue.[43,44] However, these processes are relatively unproven clinically and account for a small percentage of sterilized tissue. The most frequently used method of terminal sterilization is gamma irradiation.[45]

Gamma Irradiation

Gamma irradiation is the most common sterilization treatment method used on allografts and is also used in a majority of processed tendons whether for terminal sterilization or as an intermediate step.[45] Although there have been reports of negative outcomes with gamma-irradiated allografts,[46,47] the tissues studied were either first treated with harsh chemical pretreatments or by applying irradiation at higher, less desirable temperatures.[46-48] Other studies have demonstrated that the use of irradiated grafts did not negatively affect clinical efficacy.[30,49-51]

In interpreting these inconsistent results, it is important to note four key variables that allow a reader to more accurately evaluate the method used for applying gamma irradiation and the potential impact on clinical outcomes. These four key variables[48] include:
- target dose
- dose range.
- temperature at irradiation
- tissue treatment before irradiation

Target dose refers to the intended dose delivered to the tissue, although tissues actually receive a range of dosages due to the nature of irradiation. A dose range is a more precise description because it conveys both the minimum and maximum amount of radiation exposure a graft has received. A narrow dose range indicates a higher degree of control. Bone allografts irradiated with approximately 25 kGy (or 2.5 Mrad) have shown similar clinical results to nonirradiated bone, but irradiation dosages greater than this may negatively impact biomechanical properties,[52,53] although the clinical significance is unclear. Soft tissue allografts are reported to perform well when treated at <20 kGy (2.0 Mrad).[30,54]

The irradiation of allografts at low temperatures, e.g., on dry ice, has also been shown to effectively mitigate potential damage to the graft by minimizing the generation of free radicals.[55,56] If the temperature of irradiation is not provided in a study, it may indicate that the grafts were irradiated at ambient temperature and more prone to damage. Thus, the temperature of irradiation should always be taken into account when analyzing the results of a study. Some studies[47] report results that come from grafts irradiated at ambient temperature; it is important to note that these outcomes cannot be accurately applied to grafts more carefully irradiated at ultra-low temperatures. In support, after reviewing 5968 cases of ACL repair, Tejwani et al.[30] did not find an increased risk of revision surgery with the use of two proprietary process that use low-dose (<1.8 Mrad) gamma irradiation applied at a low temperature. This outcome, along with the findings of other studies,[50,51,57] support the clinical efficacy of low-temperature irradiated sterile tendons.

In summary, advanced tissue recovery and processing methods include steps to ensure bioburden prevention, control, and reduction. However, methods used by tissue processors vary at each step resulting in differences among available allografts. Tissue may either be offered aseptically or with a terminal sterilization step to reach an SAL of 10^{-3} or 10^{-6}. The type of terminal sterilization used also differs and can impact the clinical performance of the allograft tissue. Low-dose gamma irradiation at a low temperature is still the most common method with well-documented success,[50,51,57] but bench-top studies have shown encouraging early results for supercritical CO_2 and electron beam irradiation.[43,44,58,59]

ENHANCING FUSION POTENTIAL OF ALLOGRAFT BONE VOID FILLERS

Bone allografts have long been used to provide structural support and to fill voids. Traditionally, these grafts have been processed as previously described to reduce risk of disease transmission and also to meet specific surgical dimensional needs through cutting, machining, and grinding. Traditional allografts, such as cortical struts, ground cortical bone, cancellous cubes, femoral heads, and shaped interbody spacers, have played, and continue to play, a prominent role in orthopedic surgery. In addition, as reviewed in this chapter, when accelerated fusion is an objective, the orthopedic surgeon now also has a wide array of more advanced options to facilitate new bone growth.

The breakthrough in this field came with the discovery that certain extractable bone elements could promote bone growth[60-64] and, subsequently, when Marshall Urist and colleagues isolated the proteinaceous factors that were found to stimulate or induce new bone formation.[65-67] This family of osteoinductive proteins was named bone morphogenic proteins (BMPs).

We now recognize that three key properties are required for new bone formation and growth: (1) osteoconductivity (scaffolding), (2) osteoinductivity (signals such as BMPs), and (3) osteogenicity (cells). In order, new bone must have a scaffold to grow, referred to as an osteoconductive matrix. Then cytokine signals are required to induce precursor cells to either differentiate toward the osteoblastic lineage or for cells to further express the osteoblastic phenotype of bone formation; these factors are thus considered osteoinductive. Finally, new bone growth requires the presence of bone-forming cells such as osteoblasts or precursors to produce an extracellular, mineralizing matrix, and this cellular component is referred to as osteogenic. Different bone-grafting options may provide one, two, or all three of these properties. For example, a processed cancellous cube is still considered an osteoconductive scaffold capable of supporting new bone growth by interacting with host bone and signals despite potentially having neither significant osteoinductive capacity, being low in native growth factors, nor any osteogenic potential, being devitalized. In another example, a recombinant form of one commercially available specific human growth factor, BMP-2, would be considered as an osteoinductive signal[68] but would require the additional presence of osteogenic and osteoconductive components to drive bone formation. Furthermore, an autograft bone and marrow mixture derived from the patient may theoretically provide all three components necessary for new bone formation, but the quantity and quality of grafting material may depend on the surgical site, health, and age of the patient. As an alternative, viable cellular allografts can theoretically provide all three components, and these will be described further in the following sections.

Beyond simply filling bone voids, allografts can also be processed in different manners to enhance fusion potential. The most prevalent processing method involves taking advantage of the pervasiveness of native BMPs found in cortical bone. Through careful demineralization, these factors can become bioavailable in the resultant DBM. Typically, a dilute hydrochloric acid solution is used to dissolve some of the bone's mineral phase (apatitic calcium phosphate), thus exposing these growth factors. In fact, this process mimics the natural action of osteoclasts in bone remodeling as they create a localized acidic environment which similarly dissolves the mineral phase, releasing BMPs to signal cells to lay down new bone.[69-72] If undertreated, hypodemineralization would result in osteoinductive factors still being trapped in the bone matrix and unavailable for rapid signaling, whereas hyperdemineralization may lead to those factors either being eluted out of the matrix during demineralization or overly acid-exposed and denatured, thus yielding a nonosteoinductive material.

At least one study demonstrates this relationship by correlation of the residual calcium levels, as a measure of demineralization, to new bone formation using a rodent bone growth model.[73] The authors support the premise that overdemineralization or underdemineralization lowers the osteoinductive potential of DBMs, indicating that there is an optimal range in the middle. Thus given the presence of bioavailable growth factors within a human bony matrix, properly demineralized DBMs are considered both osteoinductive and osteoconductive, still relying on the patient's own cells for the osteogenic component. To improve handling, many DBM formulations also use a carrier such as glycerol, hyaluronic acid, starch, and so forth. An extensive study of the impact of these carriers on long-term clinical outcomes is generally lacking, although clinical evidence supports glycerol and hyaluronic acid as DBM carriers.[74-76]

More recently, cellular bone allografts have emerged as a new option.[77] These grafts are formulated to provide all three elements of bone formation. The osteoconductive component is bone in the form of chips, fibers, or particulates. The osteogenic component is comprised of cells either adhering to the bone component or added from another source, for example, adipose-derived cells or amniotic tissue. The osteoinductive component may be DBM derived from the same donor or may rely on endogenous trophic factors inherent to the cellular component. Most current cellular bone void filler approaches rely on inclusion of mesenchymal stem cells, assuming that they will produce factors conducive to the healing process and that they will differentiate down the osteoblastic lineage to initiate bone formation. The impact of the patient's local environment on the differentiation pathway and timing is not well understood. This question becomes increasingly complex when the cell component derives from a nonbone source such as placenta or adipose tissue. Alternatively, cellular bone void fillers can include living cells that are integral to the donor bone and thus, being "bone cells," are already committed to the osteoblastic lineage. Longer term, controlled clinical data would be beneficial in helping support providing the orthopedist with a single grafting material with all three components of bone formation.

LOWERING ALLOGRAFT IMMUNOGENIC POTENTIAL: DECELLULARIZATION

Most allografts are generally considered nonimmunogenic either due to the nature of human tissue being transplanted into humans, as a consequence of cleaning processes that remove cellular material such as bone marrow elements,[29] or through preservation processes, including freezing and freeze-drying.[78] However, depending on the tissue type and intended clinical application, unprocessed allograft tissue can pose issues with immunogenicity,[18,78] which need to be minimized for an allograft to be optimally biocompatible upon implantation.[79] Furthermore, different types of tissue exhibit varying degrees of immunogenicity, as measured by antigenicity. Skin is generally more immunogenic[80] than bone and tendon tissues, which exhibit lower immunogenicity[81] that can generally be resolved through the typical allograft-cleaning processes. More immunogenic tissues may need alternative processes to lower antigenicity. One method treats tissue with glutaraldehyde, an aldehyde fixative, to greatly reduce immunogenicity by cross-linking antigens.[82] However, glutaraldehyde has been associated with allergic reactions and may have contributed to the extremely high ACL failure rates reported in one study.[83] Another method, frequently applied to dermal tissue, uses decellularization to reduce potential immunogenicity and is intended to yield a biocompatible scaffold as a favorable environment for host recellularization and remodeling.[84] Although there are several different decellularization methods in use, the common goal is to eliminate cellular remnants that could cause an immune response while preserving the tissue architecture and maintaining the mechanical properties of the scaffold.[85,86] Once the dermal tissue is decellularized, this scaffold can be used in orthopedic procedures, such as superior capsule shoulder reconstruction, Achilles tendon repair, and others.[87-91]

As noted previously, decellularization processes can include both chemical and mechanical extraction methods.[92] More specifically, decellularization techniques are reported to use anionic agents (e.g., sodium dodecyl sulfate, sodium chloride), alkali compounds (e.g., sodium hydroxide), and oxidizing agents (e.g., hydrogen peroxide) to solubilize cellular remnants before removal.[31-34] However, the type of chemicals used and the duration of the decellularization process can affect the strength of the graft by removing collagen and glycosaminoglycans in addition to the immunogenic components,[33] making the differences among decellularization processes worthy of consideration.

The amount of cellular remnants remaining after decellularization may be indicated using residual DNA content; a lower DNA content would theoretically indicate a cleaner matrix and more favorable host response.[33] The residual DNA content of grafts varies widely. Published reports include ranges from less than 25 to greater than 250-ng DNA/mg dry weight for acellular dermal matrix (ADM) tissues.[32,93,94] As residual DNA levels may correlate with host response, it is not surprising that different ADMs incorporate at different rates,[33] as specifically noted when an ADM with lower residual DNA content was found to more rapidly integrate and recellularize in a comparative animal model.[32,95,96]

Recellularization

Once an ADM has been implanted, host cells may begin repopulating the scaffold and initiating incorporation of the graft. This process starts with the migration of inflammatory host cells, followed by matrix remodeling, and then finally revascularization, leading to recellularization.[96] Although the exact mechanism of host integration is not fully understood, differences in incorporation rates likely begin at the initiation of the process. The initial inflammatory host response is mediated by macrophages and monocytes, which must achieve a careful balance between wound healing and tissue destruction.[97] Macrophages regulate the expression of interleukin-1b,[98] a cytokine which contributes to the wound-healing process by controlling fibroblast activation.[97] The M1 macrophage phenotype is more associated with an inflammatory response, whereas the M2 macrophage phenotype is associated with tissue repair and constructive tissue remodeling.[99,100] Agrawal et al.[95] investigated the mechanism of incorporation by examining the effect of macrophage phenotype expression on matrix remodeling using three different human ADMs and one synthetic/bovine ADM. The ADM products displayed differing patterns and timing of macrophage infiltration, leading the authors to conclude that this variability was due to the distinct decellularization processes used for each of the ADM products. Capito et al.[96] also concluded that different decellularization processes may have accounted for the varying degrees of cellular and vascular ingrowth shown by the four different materials in this study.

As discussed in this chapter, decellularization can be beneficial for further reducing immunogenicity of certain tissue types. Different methods can result in different rates of recellularization, which may impact incorporation rates and ultimate tissue remodeling.

ALLOGRAFT PRESERVATION AND STORAGE METHODS

Unlike organs and composite tissue allotransplants, which are typically transplanted within hours after the donor's death, allografts may be stored from weeks to years before use. Consequently, these grafts must be processed in ways that maintain their safety and clinical efficacy for an extended period of time. In addition to the processing and sterilization methods described previously, another factor which can impact the use and clinical effectiveness of allografts is the manner in which they are preserved, stored, and handled before use. Currently, allograft preservation typically includes using storage media, cryopreservation, or freeze-drying to store grafts in ambient, refrigerated, or frozen states. The storage temperature determines requirements for shipping, on-site storage, and presurgery preparation. There are several main considerations concerning the preservation and storage of allograft tissues: (1) cell viability if applicable, (2) maintaining the structural integrity and native properties of the bone or extracellular matrix, and (3) convenient storage and use. This section reviews the main types of preservation and storage, as well as their advantages and disadvantages. It is arranged by storage temperature, followed by preservation methods, if applicable. The methods are also summarized in Table 5.1.

Refrigeration

The simplest type of preservation is to store aseptically recovered tissues by refrigeration; however, the simplicity of the preservation belies the complex logistics involved when using so-called "fresh" tissues. Currently, fresh grafts have a very limited shelf life between release and expiration in which they can be implanted. The most commonly used fresh tissues in orthopedic surgery are osteochondral allografts used for cartilage restoration in the knee, shoulder, and talus.[101-104] The advantage of this preservation type is that it can maintain viable cells. In the case of osteochondral grafts, this includes viable chondrocytes that may help restore the recipient's articular surfaces. These living cells are immunoprivileged and do not require immunosuppressants, making this graft type advantageous because the donor cells can contribute to generating collagenous extracellular matrix.[105] To maintain viable cells, the tissue processor will aseptically recover the tissue, take cultures, debride and disinfect, size, and treat with antibiotics. The tissue processor will avoid using methods which remove cellular material either deliberately, as

TABLE 5.1
Allograft Preservation and Storage Methods

Preservation Method		Storage Temperature	Advantages	Potential Disadvantages
Fresh		Refrigerated at 1–10°C	• Viable cells	• Complex logistics • Limited shelf life
Frozen		Frozen at −40 to −80°C	• Fully hydrated • Long shelf life	• Thaw time • Need validated and monitored freezer for storage • Shipping costs
Cryopreserved		Liquid nitrogen (LN2) or −80°C	• Cell viability • Maintains biomechanical properties • Long shelf life	• Need validated and monitored freezer or LN2 tanks to store on site • Shipping costs
Freeze-dried		Ambient temperature	• Easy storage • Long shelf life	• Altered biomechanical properties • Long rehydration time
Preservant treated	Glycerol	Ambient temperature	• Fully hydrated • Easy storage • Long shelf life • More options in operating room • Maintains biomechanical properties	• Reaction to preservation solutions in susceptible patients
	Ethanol	Ambient temperature	• Easy storage • Long shelf life • More options in operating room	• Reaction to preservation solutions in susceptible patients • Potential tissue alterations if solution is dehydrating

those used in decellularization processes previously discussed, or incidentally, as a result of some type of chemical or physical cleaning processes.[105] Once processed, the allograft is packaged and stored at 1–10°C in quarantine until the bacterial, fungal, and viral tests results are obtained. Storage time is a critical factor for these grafts as studies have shown that cell viability decreases with time.[104] Storage media can also impact cell viability, and this is an area of ongoing research and development.[106–109]

If the graft is cleared for distribution, the current graft expiration times are generally fewer than 60 days, including the quarantine period. Because surgery cannot be reasonably scheduled until a suitable match is found, this short window of availability contributes to the logistical complexity involved with using fresh allografts. Despite these challenges, fresh osteochondral allografts are becoming more popular.[101] Although fresh tissues have advantages in some particular circumstances, current time constraints can make their use challenging for surgeons, patients, hospitals, and tissue processors alike.

Frozen and Cryopreserved Allografts

Unlike fresh, refrigerated tissues, some frozen allografts may be stored for years before implantation. Freezing, without using special cryopreservation methods and solutions, can cause the formation of ice crystals within the cells or extracellular matrix, resulting in lysis. Therefore, this type of preservation is used for allografts in which maintenance of viability is not an objective, such as in structural bone allografts, tendons, and acellular dermis. For frozen grafts not processed with cryopreservants, the process generally includes pathogen testing, debridement, cleaning, and disinfecting to remove remnant cells, marrow, lipids, and bioburden before being frozen and stored. For tissues that do contain living cells, for example, cellular bone void fillers or osteochondral grafts, cryopreservation solutions are used. Cryopreservation can extend the storage time for tissues that require viable cells, avoiding the logistical, time-sensitive issues noted for fresh refrigerated allografts.

Cryopreservation methods include controlling the rate of the freezing process and reducing the formation of ice crystals by removing water from the cells and replacing it with a cryopreservant. Common cryopreservants include glycerol and dimethyl sulfoxide.[110] Tissues are processed, treated with cryopreservant, and slowly cooled to cryogenic temperatures.[111] Cryopreserved allografts are then either stored in ultra-low-temperature freezers or using liquid nitrogen to maintain temperature below the transition phase of ice to an amorphous glass, which will prevent the reformation of ice crystals and can maintain the state of tissues for several years.[112] This preservation method allows for longer storage time for allografts which require viable cells, such as cellular bone void fillers and osteochondral grafts, avoiding the complex timing logistics seen with fresh allografts. However, the tissues must remain frozen until use and therefore require special shipping conditions, as well as on-site storage in a validated freezer that is monitored 24/7 for temperature.[113] Frozen tissue may also require a lengthy thawing time depending on the tissue type, and once the allograft has been thawed, the allograft must be used or discarded. Although freezing is an effective form of allograft preservation, its specialized shipping and storage requirements have motivated the development of alternate methods.

Ambient Temperature
Freeze-dried
To avoid the shipping and storage limitations associated with frozen tissues, another preservation option is freeze-drying, also known as lyophilization, which can be used for ligaments, bone, and dermis. After the tissue has been cleaned and processed, freeze-drying is achieved by using specialized equipment to reduce the residual moisture to a level that maintains tissue quality, which may vary depending on the tissue type. The lyophilization process must be validated and monitored, and the storage conditions must maintain the appropriate moisture level.[114] An advantage of freeze-drying is that the allograft can typically be stored for years at ambient temperature and then rehydrated when needed. With ambient temperature storage, there is no need for a special freezer or specialized shipping conditions. However, the rehydration time can be lengthy, and some grafts may never fully rehydrate. Even full hydration may not be able to restore the tissue's native properties and may leave tissues in a fragile state, making them susceptible to damage during implantation. For example, some studies have found that freeze-dried bone may exhibit brittleness and weakness compared with frozen or glycerol-preserved bone, which could be especially problematic for a weight-bearing graft.[115-117]

In addition, preclinical and clinical reports[118-120] have raised concerns about immunologic response to freeze-dried bone and tendons. In spite of these potential limitations, freeze-dried allografts, especially ground bone void fillers, are widely used and clinically successful.[121-124]

Media-derived preservation
To provide the convenience of ambient storage while avoiding potential tissue alterations inherent with freeze-drying, some tissue processors have developed solution-based methods of ambient preservation. Currently, there are two main preservants used for allografts, namely solutions containing ethanol or glycerol, although saline solution is used for some bone grafts. Ethanol storage is a traditional and economical method used to preserve tissues. Ecologists and natural history museums have been using this method to preserve intact specimens for many decades. It is also used in forensic science to preserve DNA samples. Ethanol preserves tissue by driving water out of tissue and cells, essentially dehydrating the tissue.[125] The other most common ambient temperature storage method is to treat the tissue with glycerol, which acts as a humectant to protect the tissues, keeping them fully hydrated. Glycerol is a nontoxic, biodegradable liquid that the FDA classifies as "generally recognized as safe."[126] It is a common ingredient in over 1500 food, cosmetic, and pharmaceutical products[127] and has been widely used in DBM allografts for spinal applications since 1991. By holding in moisture, glycerol allows allografts to be stored at ambient temperature without drying out. Ethanol storage is most commonly used on ADM allografts, whereas glycerol storage can be effectively used for bone as well as ADMs. In clinical studies comparing glycerol-preserved bone to either freeze-dried or frozen bone, the authors found that glycerol-preserved bone performed as well as freeze-dried and frozen bone while having a shorter preparation time.[117,128]

Both glycerol and alcohol preservation methods endow tissues with desirable storage characteristics, eliminating the need for the lengthy thawing and rehydration times that accompany frozen or freeze-dried allografts. The advantages include ease of shipping and storage, as well as increased flexibility for the operating room staff. Unlike frozen tissues that may need thawing to begin well in advance of a scheduled surgery, a surgeon can decide whether or not to use a glycerol- or alcohol-preserved allograft once surgery has already begun, allowing the surgeon the option to make real-time decisions based on the state of the patient. Given the proven clinical effectiveness and convenience of ambient-stored allografts, it is likely that tissue banks will seek to develop and improve these storage methods for a wider variety of tissues.

FUTURE DIRECTIONS

Human allograft tissues have played an increasing role in orthopedic practice, and their use is likely to continue and increase. Although future development of more human-like synthetics and xenografts may lead to a decline in the use of some traditional human tissues, the natural matrix structure and human cellular content available with allografts is hard to replicate. Limitations and considerations noted previously point to areas of improvement and are subjects of active research within industry and academia, which include:

- increased cell viability and viability time in osteochondral grafts;
- increasing type of tissues preserved for ambient temperature storage;
- development of more time-efficient and less aggressive disinfection and sterilization technologies;
- rapid test methods to detect microbes and viruses before donor tissue is even recovered;
- use of late clinical stage antibiotics and antiviral agents to further assure allograft safety;
- preconditioning of implanted cells or genetic transfection of transplanted cells to overexpress key factors such as BMPs or insulin-like growth factor;
- nontoxic, slowly degradable cross-linking methods to allow tissues to have favorable initial biomechanical properties and low immunogenicity but also to eventually remodel;
- modifications of allografts to promote recruitment of key cell types based on the clinical application;
- seeding autologous cells in situ on allogeneic scaffolds;
- isolating key proteins from allografts as a chemotactic coating in combination with synthetic implants;
- modifications to allow injection and deployment of structural and nonstructural grafts in minimally invasive procedures;
- use of human-derived cells, perhaps genetically altered, for direct injection at clinical site or provided systemically;
- use of allograft-sourced induced pluripotent stem cells as a source of personalized medicine treatments (e.g., induce cells along a lineage specific to treat a patient's unique condition);
- expandable allografts for geometrically challenging bone void filling applications.

The use of allografts moving forward should likely not only include basic anatomic grafts but also dramatically modified human components provided as injectables, coatings, cellular therapies, and in combination with other materials.

SUMMARY

Allografts are widely used in orthopedic practice. Historically, tissues were typically provided as simple intact anatomical grafts, such as tendons, long bones, skin, and so forth. As introduced in this chapter, technologies to process allografts include physical shaping, demineralization, decellularization, and preservation methodologies. These processes, which tend to alter or deconstruct the grafts or change their physical state, are designed to yield tissues that are clinically effective while advanced disinfection and sterilization technologies assure safety. Looking forward, human tissues should serve a very useful role still as intact structures, partially deconstructed, or altered grafts. However, advances will increasingly propel the use of tissue as reconstructed or more biologically integrative constructs using protein isolation and reconstitution methods, genetic alterations, in situ cell seeding, and other advances.

DISCLOSURE STATEMENT

Dr. Moore, Mr. Samsell, and Dr. McLean are employees of LifeNet Health, a nonprofit organization.

REFERENCES

1. Tomford WW, Ortiz-Cruz EJ. The use of allografts in orthopedics. In: Warwick RM, Brubaker SA, eds. *Tissue and Cell Clinical Use: An Essential Guide*. Wiley-Blackwell; 2012:152–169.
2. Manji RA, Menkis AH, Ekser B, Cooper DK. Porcine bioprosthetic heart valves: the next generation. *Am Heart J*. 2012;164(2):177–185.
3. Hammerle CH, Jung RE, Yaman D, Lang NP. Ridge augmentation by applying bioresorbable membranes and deproteinized bovine bone mineral: a report of twelve consecutive cases. *Clin Oral Implants Res*. 2008;19(1):19–25.
4. Rodella LF, Favero G, Labanca M. Biomaterials in maxillofacial surgery: membranes and grafts. *Int J Biomed Sci*. 2011;7(2):81–88.

5. Iannotti JP, Codsi MJ, Kwon YW, Derwin K, Ciccone J, Brems JJ. Porcine small intestine submucosa augmentation of surgical repair of chronic two-tendon rotator cuff tears. A randomized, controlled trial. *J Bone Joint Surg Am.* 2006;88(6):1238–1244.

6. Zheng MH, Chen J, Kirilak Y, Willers C, Xu J, Wood D. Porcine small intestine submucosa (SIS) is not an acellular collagenous matrix and contains porcine DNA: possible implications in human implantation. *J Biomed Mater Res B Appl Biomater.* 2005;73(1):61–67.

7. Colaço HB, Shah Z, Back D, Davies A, Ajuied A. (iv) Xenograft in orthopaedics. *Orthop Trauma.* 2015;29(4):253–260.

8. Chang SK, Egami DK, Shaieb MD, Kan DM, Richardson AB. Anterior cruciate ligament reconstruction: allograft versus autograft. *Arthroscopy.* 2003;19(5):453–462.

9. Hu J, Qu J, Xu D, Zhou J, Lu H. Allograft versus autograft for anterior cruciate ligament reconstruction: an up-to-date meta-analysis of prospective studies. *Int Orthop.* 2013;37(2):311–320.

10. Clar C, Cummins E, McIntyre L, et al. Clinical and cost-effectiveness of autologous chondrocyte implantation for cartilage defects in knee joints: systematic review and economic evaluation. *Health Technol Assess.* 2005;9(47):1–82.

11. Arnoczky SP, Delos D, Rodeo SA. What is platelet-rich plasma? *Oper Tech Sports Med.* 2011;19(3):142–148.

12. Cole BJ, Seroyer ST, Filardo G, Bajaj S, Fortier LA. Platelet-rich plasma: where are we now and where are we going? *Sports Health.* 2010;2(3):203–210.

13. Macewen W. Observations concerning transplantation of bone, illustrated by a case of interhuman osseous transplantation, whereby two-thirds of the shaft of a humerus was restored. *Proc Roy Soc Lond.* 1881;32:232–247.

14. Albee FH. *Bone-Graft Surgery.* Philadelphia: W. B. Saunders Company; 1915.

15. Gitelis SaC BJ. The use of allografts in orthopaedic surgery. *AAOS Instr Course Lect.* 2002;51:507–520.

16. Davarinos N, O'Neill BJ, Curtin W. A brief history of anterior cruciate ligament reconstruction. *Adv Orthop Surg.* 2014;2014:1–6.

17. Anderson MW, Bottenfield S. Tissue banking- past, present, and future. In: Youngner SJ, Anderson MW, Schapiro R, eds. *Transplanting Human Tissue: Ethics, Policy and Practice.* Oxford, New York: Oxford University Press; 2004:14–35.

18. Nather A, Zheng S. Evolution of allograft transplantation. In: Nather A, Yusof N, Hilmy N, eds. *Allograft Procurement, Processing and Transplantation: A Comprehensive Guide for Tissue Banks.* World Scientific Publishing Co; 2017:3–28.

19. Strong DM. The US Navy tissue bank: 50 Years on the cutting edge. *Cell Tissue Bank.* 2000;1(1):9–16.

20. Food and Drug Administration. *Part 127 of Code of Federal Regulations Title 21- Human Cells, Tissues, and Cellular and Tissue-Based Products;* 2016.

21. Food and Drug Administration (FDA). *Guidance for Industry: Regulation of Human Cells, Tissues, and Cellular and Tissue-Based Products (HCT/Ps);* 2007:1–15.

22. Federal Register. *Interim Rule.* 1993;58(238):65514–65521.

23. American Association of Tissue Banks. *AATB "Allograft-associated Infections" Survey Report;* 2005.

24. Centers for Disease Control, Prevention (CDC). Update: unexplained deaths following knee surgery–Minnesota. *MMWR Morb Mortal Wkly Rep 2001.* 2001;50(48):1080.

25. Simonds RJ, Holmberg SD, Hurwitz RL, et al. Transmission of human immunodeficiency virus type 1 from a seronegative organ and tissue donor. *N Engl J Med.* 1992;326(11):726–732.

26. Tugwell BD, Patel PR, Williams IT, et al. Transmission of hepatitis C virus to several organ and tissue recipients from an antibody-negative donor. *Ann Intern Med.* 2005;143(9):648–654.

27. Rigney PR. *AATB Bulletin No. 04-42-Implementation of Nucleic Acid Testing (NAT).* American Association of Tissue Banks; 2004.

28. Fishman JA, Greenwald MA, Grossi PA. Transmission of infection with human allografts: essential considerations in donor screening. *Clin Infect Dis.* 2012;55(5):720–727.

29. Wolfinbarger Jr L. *Inventor; Lifenet Research Foundation, Assignee.* Process and composition for cleaning soft tissue grafts optionally attached to bone and soft tissue and bone grafts produced thereby. US patent US6024735 A. 2000.

30. Tejwani SG, Chen J, Funahashi TT, Love R, Maletis GB. Revision risk after allograft anterior cruciate ligament reconstruction: association with graft processing techniques, patient characteristics, and graft type. *Am J Sports Med.* 2015;43(11):2696–2705.

31. Truncale KG, Cartmell JS, Syring C, Von Versen R, Ngo MD. *Inventors; Musculoskeletal Transplant Foundation, Assignee.* Soft Tissue Processing US patent US7723108 B2. 2010.

32. Moore MA, Samsell B, Wallis G, et al. Decellularization of human dermis using non-denaturing anionic detergent and endonuclease: a review. *Cell Tissue Bank.* 2015;16(2):249–259.

33. Crapo PM, Gilbert TW, Badylak SF. An overview of tissue and whole organ decellularization processes. *Biomaterials.* 2011;32(12):3233–3243.

34. Fu RH, Wang YC, Liu SP, et al. Decellularization and recellularization technologies in tissue engineering. *Cell Transpl.* 2014;23(4–5):621–630.

35. Sutton S. The sterility tests. In: Moldenhauer J, ed. *Rapid Sterility Testing.* Davis Healthcare International Publishing, LLC; 2011.

36. United States Pharmacopeia (USP). USP29: <71> Sterility Tests. http://www.pharmacopeia.cn/v29240/usp29nf24s0_c71.html.

37. Rutala WA, Weber DJ. THICPAC. *Guidel Disinfect Steriliz Healthc Facil.* 2008:2008.

38. Yuen JC, Yue CJ, Erickson SW, et al. Comparison between freeze-dried and ready-to-use AlloDerm in alloplastic breast reconstruction. *Plast Reconstr Surg Glob Open.* 2014;2(3):e119.

39. Moore MA. Inactivation of enveloped and non-enveloped viruses on seeded human tissues by gamma irradiation. *Cell Tissue Bank.* 2012;13(3):401–407.

40. Indelicato PA, Ciccotti MG, Boyd J, Higgins LD, Shaffer BS, Vangsness Jr CT. Aseptically processed and chemically sterilized BTB allografts for anterior cruciate ligament reconstruction: a prospective randomized study. *Knee Surg Sports Traumatol Arthrosc.* 2013;21(9):2107–2112.

41. Ferreira SD, Dernell WS, Powers BE, et al. Effect of gas-plasma sterilization on the osteoinductive capacity of demineralized bone matrix. *Clin Orthop Relat Res.* 2001;388:233–239.

42. Jackson DW, Windler GE, Simon TM. Intraarticular reaction associated with the use of freeze-dried, ethylene oxide-sterilized bone-patella tendon-bone allografts in the reconstruction of the anterior cruciate ligament. *Am J Sports Med.* 1990;18(1):1–10; discussion 10–11.

43. Elenes EY, Hunter SA. Soft-tissue allografts terminally sterilized with an electron beam are biomechanically equivalent to aseptic, nonsterilized tendons. *J Bone Joint Surg Am.* 2014;96(16):1321–1326.

44. White A, Burns D, Christensen TW. Effective terminal sterilization using supercritical carbon dioxide. *J Biotechnol.* 2006;123(4):504–515.

45. American Association of Tissue Banks (AATB). *American Association of Tissue Banks (AATB) Annual Survey of Accredited Tissue Banks in the United States.* McLean, VA: AATB; 2007.

46. Prodromos C, Joyce B, Shi K. A meta-analysis of stability of autografts compared to allografts after anterior cruciate ligament reconstruction. *Knee Surg Sports Traumatol Arthrosc.* 2007;15(7):851–856.

47. Sun K, Tian S, Zhang J, Xia C, Zhang C, Yu T. Anterior cruciate ligament reconstruction with BPTB autograft, irradiated versus non-irradiated allograft: a prospective randomized clinical study. *Knee Surg Sports Traumatol Arthrosc.* 2009;17(5):464–474.

48. Samsell BJ, Moore MA. Use of controlled low dose gamma irradiation to sterilize allograft tendons for ACL reconstruction: biomechanical and clinical perspective. *Cell Tissue Bank.* 2012;13(2):217–223.

49. Fanelli GC, Giannotti BF, Edson CJ. Arthroscopically assisted combined anterior and posterior cruciate ligament reconstruction. *Arthroscopy.* 1996;12(1):5–14.

50. Rihn JA, Irrgang JJ, Chhabra A, Fu FH, Harner CD. Does irradiation affect the clinical outcome of patellar tendon allograft ACL reconstruction? *Knee Surg Sports Traumatol Arthrosc.* 2006;14(9):885–896.

51. Ghodadra NS, Mall NA, Grumet R, et al. Interval arthrometric comparison of anterior cruciate ligament reconstruction using bone-patellar tendon-bone autograft versus allograft: do grafts attenuate within the first year postoperatively? *Am J Sports Med.* 2012;40(6):1347–1354.

52. Loty B, Courpied JP, Tomeno B, Postel M, Forest M, Abelanet R. Bone allografts sterilised by irradiation. Biological properties, procurement and results of 150 massive allografts. *Int Orthop.* 1990;14(3):237–242.

53. Nguyen H, Morgan DA, Forwood MR. Sterilization of allograft bone: effects of gamma irradiation on allograft biology and biomechanics. *Cell Tissue Bank.* 2007;8(2):93–105.

54. Block JE. The impact of irradiation on the microbiological safety, biomechanical properties, and clinical performance of musculoskeletal allografts. *Orthopedics.* 2006;29(11):991–996; quiz 997–998.

55. Anderson MJ, Keyak JH, Skinner HB. Compressive mechanical properties of human cancellous bone after gamma irradiation. *J Bone Joint Surg Am.* 1992;74(5):747–752.

56. Hamer AJ, Stockley I, Elson RA. Changes in allograft bone irradiated at different temperatures. *J Bone Joint Surg Br.* 1999;81(2):342–344.

57. Greaves LL, Hecker AT, Brown Jr CH. The effect of donor age and low-dose gamma irradiation on the initial biomechanical properties of human tibialis tendon allografts. *Am J Sports Med.* 2008;36(7):1358–1366.

58. Hoburg A, Keshlaf S, Schmidt T, et al. Fractionation of high-dose electron beam irradiation of BPTB grafts provides significantly improved viscoelastic and structural properties compared to standard gamma irradiation. *Knee Surg Sports Traumatol Arthrosc.* 2011;19(11):1955–1961.

59. Nichols A, Burns D, Christopher R. Studies on the sterilization of human bone and tendon musculoskeletal allograft tissue using supercritical carbon dioxide. *J Orthop.* 2009;6(2):e9.

60. Urist MR, McLean FC. Osteogenetic potency and new-bone formation by induction in transplants to the anterior chamber of the eye. *J Bone Joint Surg Am.* 1952;34-A(2):443–476.

61. Moss ML. Extraction of an osteogenic inductor factor from bone. *Science.* 1958;127(3301):755–756.

62. Bertelsen A. Experimental investigations into post-foetal osteogenesis. *Acta Orthop Scand.* 1944;15(2–4):139–181.

63. Levander G. On the formation of new bone in bone transplantation. *Acta Chir Scand.* 1934;74:425–426.

64. Huggins C. The formation of bone under the influence of epithelium of the urinary tract. *Arch Surg.* 1931;22:377–408.

65. Urist MR. Bone: formation by autoinduction. *Science.* 1965;150(3698):893–899.

66. Urist MR, Silverman BF, Büring K, Dubuc FL, Rosenberg JM. The bone induction principle. *Clin Orthop Relat Res.* 1967;53:243–283.

67. Urist MR, Strates BS. The classic: bone morphogenetic protein. *Clin Orthop Relat Res.* 2009;467(12):3051–3062.

68. McKay WF, Peckham SM, Badura JM. A comprehensive clinical review of recombinant human bone morphogenetic protein-2 (INFUSE bone graft). *Int Orthop.* 2007;31(6):729–734.

69. Teitelbaum SL. Osteoclasts: what do they do and how do they do it? *Am J Pathol.* 2007;170(2):427–435.

70. Chen G, Deng C, Li YP. TGF-beta and BMP signaling in osteoblast differentiation and bone formation. *Int J Biol Sci.* 2012;8(2):272–288.

71. Jain AP, Pundir S, Sharma A. Bone morphogenetic proteins: the anomalous molecules. *J Indian Soc Periodontol.* 2013;17(5):583–586.
72. Jimi E, Hirata S, Shin M, Yamazaki M, Fukushima H. Molecular mechanisms of BMP-induced bone formation: cross-talk between BMP and NF-κB signaling pathways in osteoblastogenesis. *Jpn Dent Sci Rev.* 2010;46(1):33–42.
73. Zhang M, Powers Jr RM, Wolfinbarger Jr L. Effect(s) of the demineralization process on the osteoinductivity of demineralized bone matrix. *J Periodontol.* 1997;68(11):1085–1092.
74. Kang J, An H, Hilibrand A, Yoon ST, Kavanagh E, Boden S. Grafton and local bone have comparable outcomes to iliac crest bone in instrumented single-level lumbar fusions. *Spine (Phila Pa 1976).* 2012;37(12):1083–1091.
75. Cammisa FP, Lowery G, Garfin SR, et al. Two-year fusion rate equivalency between Grafton DBM gel and autograft in posterolateral spine fusion: a prospective controlled trial employing a side-by-side comparison in the same patient. *Spine.* 2004;29(6):660–666.
76. Pieske O, Wittmann A, Zaspel J, et al. Autologous bone graft versus demineralized bone matrix in internal fixation of ununited long bones. *J Trauma Manag Outcomes.* 2009;3:11.
77. Skovrlj B, Guzman JZ, Al Maaieh M, Cho SK, Iatridis JC, Qureshi SA. Cellular bone matrices: viable stem cell-containing bone graft substitutes. *Spine J.* 2014;14(11):2763–2772.
78. Robertson A, Nutton RW, Keating JF. Current trends in the use of tendon allografts in orthopaedic surgery. *J Bone Joint Surg Br.* 2006;88(8):988–992.
79. Laurencin CT, Khan Y. Polymer/calcium phosphate scaffolds for bone tissue engineering. In: Ma PX, Elisseeff J, eds. *Scaffolding in Tissue Engineering.* CRC Press; 2005:253–263.
80. Murray JE. Organ transplantation (skin, kidney, heart) and the plastic surgeon. *Plast Reconstr Surg.* 1971;41:425–431.
81. Klimczak A, Siemionow M. Immunology of tissue transplantation. In: Siemionow M, Eisenmann-Klein M, eds. *Plastic and Reconstructive Surgery.* London, Springer; 2010:11–22.
82. Laing BJ, Ross DB, Meyer SR, et al. Glutaraldehyde treatment of allograft tissue decreases allosensitization after the Norwood procedure. *J Thorac Cardiovasc Surg.* 2010;139(6):1402–1408.
83. Good L, Odensten M, Pettersson L, Gillquist J. Failure of a bovine xenograft for reconstruction of the anterior cruciate ligament. *Acta Orthop.* 1989;60(1):8–12.
84. Norton L, Babensee J. Innate and Adaptive Immune responses in tissue engineering. In: Meyer U, Meyer T, Handschel J, Wesmann HP, eds. *Fundamentals of Tissue Engineering and Regenerative Medicine.* Springer-Varlag; 2009:721–745.
85. Cheng CW, Solorio LD, Alsberg E. Decellularized tissue and cell-derived extracellular matrices as scaffolds for orthopaedic tissue engineering. *Biotechnol Adv.* 2014;32(2):462–484.
86. Wu LC, Kuo YJ, Sun FW, et al. Optimized decellularization protocol including alpha-Gal epitope reduction for fabrication of an acellular porcine annulus fibrosus scaffold. *Cell Tissue Bank.* 2017;18(3):383–396.
87. Gilot GJ, Alvarez-Pinzon AM, Barcksdale L, Westerdahl D, Krill M, Peck E. Outcome of large to massive rotator cuff tears repaired with and without extracellular matrix augmentation: a prospective comparative study. *Arthroscopy.* 2015;31(8):1459–1465.
88. Gilot GJ, Attia AK, Alvarez AM. Arthroscopic repair of rotator cuff tears using extracellular matrix graft. *Arthrosc Tech.* 2014;3(4):e487–e489.
89. Burkhart SS, Denard PJ, Adams CR, Brady PC, Hartzler RU. Arthroscopic superior capsular reconstruction for massive irreparable rotator cuff repair. *Arthrosc Tech.* 2016;5(6):e1407–e1418.
90. Petri M, Warth RJ, Horan MP, Greenspoon JA, Millett PJ. Outcomes after open revision repair of massive rotator cuff tears with biologic patch augmentation. *Arthroscopy.* 2016;32(9):1752–1760.
91. Lee DK. A preliminary study on the effects of acellular tissue graft augmentation in acute Achilles tendon ruptures. *J Foot Ankle Surg.* 2008;47(1):8–12.
92. Bertasi G, Cole W, Samsell B, Qin X, Moore M. Biological incorporation of human acellular dermal matrix used in Achilles tendon repair. *Cell Tissue Bank.* 2017;18(3):403–411.
93. Choe JM, Bell T. Genetic material is present in cadaveric dermis and cadaveric fascia lata. *J Urol.* 2001;166(1):122–124.
94. Derwin KA, Baker AR, Spragg RK, Leigh DR, Iannotti JP. Commercial extracellular matrix scaffolds for rotator cuff tendon repair. Biomechanical, biochemical, and cellular properties. *J Bone Joint Surg Am.* 2006;88(12):2665–2672.
95. Agrawal H, Tholpady SS, Capito AE, Drake DB, Katz AJ. Macrophage phenotypes correspond with remodeling outcomes of various acellular dermal matrices. *Open J Regen Med.* 2012;01(03):51–59.
96. Capito AE, Tholpady SS, Agrawal H, Drake DB, Katz AJ. Evaluation of host tissue integration, revascularization, and cellular infiltration within various dermal substrates. *Ann Plast Surg.* 2012;68(5):495–500.
97. Orenstein S, Qiao Y, Kaur M, Klueh U, Kreutzer D, Novitsky Y. In vitro activation of human peripheral blood mononuclear cells induced by human biologic meshes. *J Surg Res.* 2010;158(1):10–14.
98. Lopez-Castejon G, Brough D. Understanding the mechanism of IL-1beta secretion. *Cytokine Growth Factor Rev.* 2011;22(4):189–195.
99. Mantovani A, Sica A, Sozzani S, Allavena P, Vecchi A, Locati M. The chemokine system in diverse forms of macrophage activation and polarization. *Trends Immunol.* 2004;25(12):677–686.
100. Martinez FO, Helming L, Gordon S. Alternative activation of macrophages: an immunologic functional perspective. *Annu Rev Immunol.* 2009;27:451–483.

101. Capeci CM, Turchiano M, Strauss EJ, Youm T. Osteochondral allografts: applications in treating articular cartilage defects in the knee. *Bull Hosp Joint Dis (2013)*. 2013;71(1):60–67.

102. Giannini S, Sebastiani E, Shehu A, Baldassarri M, Maraldi S, Vannini F. Bipolar fresh osteochondral allograft of the shoulder. *Joints*. 2013;1(4):150–154.

103. Black LO, Ko JK, Quilici SM, Crawford DC. Fresh osteochondral allograft to the humeral head for treatment of an engaging reverse hill-sachs lesion: technical case report and literature review. *Orthop J Sports Med*. 2016;4(11). https://doi.org/10.1177/2325967116670376.

104. Demange M, Gomoll AH. The use of osteochondral allografts in the management of cartilage defects. *Curr Rev Musculoskelet Med*. 2012;5(3):229–235.

105. Arzi B, DuRaine GD, Lee CA, et al. Cartilage immunoprivilege depends on donor source and lesion location. *Acta Biomater*. 2015;23:72–81.

106. Garrity JT, Stoker AM, Sims HJ, Cook JL. Improved osteochondral allograft preservation using serum-free media at body temperature. *Am J Sports Med*. 2012;40(11): 2542–2548.

107. Teng MS, Yuen AS, Kim HT. Enhancing osteochondral allograft viability: effects of storage media composition. *Clin Orthop Relat Res*. 2008;466(8):1804–1809.

108. Ball ST, Amiel D, Williams SK, et al. The effects of storage on fresh human osteochondral allografts. *Clin Orthop Relat Res*. 2004;(418):246–252.

109. Cook JL, Stoker AM, Stannard JP, et al. A novel system improves preservation of osteochondral allografts. *Clin Orthop Relat Res*. 2014;472(11):3404–3414.

110. Pegg DE. Principles of cryopreservation. *Methods Mol Biol*. 2015;1257:3–19.

111. Gitelis S, Cole BJ. The use of allografts in orthopaedic surgery. *Instr Course Lect*. 2002;51:507–520.

112. Song YC, Khirabadi BS, Lightfoot F, Brockbank KG, Taylor MJ. Vitreous cryopreservation maintains the function of vascular grafts. *Nat Biotechnol*. 2000;18(3): 296–299.

113. Joint Commission on Accreditation of Healthcare Organizations. *Joint Commission Transplant Safety Standards for Tissue*. TS.03.02.01; 2011.

114. American Association of Tissue Banks. *Standards for Tissue Banking*. 14th ed. 2016.

115. Bottino MC, Jose MV, Thomas V, Dean DR, Janowski GM. Freeze-dried acellular dermal matrix graft: effects of rehydration on physical, chemical, and mechanical properties. *Dent Mater*. 2009;25(9):1109–1115.

116. de Roeck NJ, Drabu KJ. Impaction bone grafting using freeze-dried allograft in revision hip arthroplasty. *J Arthroplasty*. 2001;16(2):201–206.

117. Graham RS, Samsell BJ, Proffer A, et al. Evaluation of glycerol-preserved bone allografts in cervical spine fusion: a prospective, randomized controlled trial. *J Neurosurg Spine*. 2015;22(1):1–10.

118. Pinkowski JL, Reiman PR, Chen SL. Human lymphocyte reaction to freeze-dried allograft and xenograft ligamentous tissue. *Am J Sports Med*. 1989;17(5):595–600.

119. Burchardt H, Glowczewskie F, Miller G. Freeze-dried segmental fibular allografts in azathioprine-treated dogs. *Clin Orthop Relat Res*. 1987;(218):259–267.

120. Burchardt H, Jones H, Glowczewskie F, Rudner C, Enneking WF. Freeze-dried allogeneic segmental cortical-bone grafts in dogs. *J Bone Joint Surg Am*. 1978;60(8): 1082–1090.

121. Bagherifard A, Ghandhari H, Jabalameli M, et al. Autograft versus allograft reconstruction of acute tibial plateau fractures: a comparative study of complications and outcome. *Eur J Orthop Surg Traumatol*. 2016;27(5): 665–671.

122. Lansford TJ, Burton DC, Asher MA, Lai SM. Radiographic and patient-based outcome analysis of different bone-grafting techniques in the surgical treatment of idiopathic scoliosis with a minimum 4-year follow-up: allograft versus autograft/allograft combination. *Spine J*. 2013;13(5):523–529.

123. Lasanianos N, Mouzopoulos G, Garnavos C. The use of freeze-dried cancelous allograft in the management of impacted tibial plateau fractures. *Injury*. 2008;39(10):1106–1112.

124. Stricker SJ, Sher JS. Freeze-dried cortical allograft in posterior spinal arthrodesis: use with segmental instrumentation for idiopathic adolescent scoliosis. *Orthopedics*. 1997;20(11):1039–1043.

125. Doorenweerd C, Beentjes K. *Extensive Guidelines for Preserving Specimen or Tissue for Later DNA Work*; 2012.

126. Food, Drug Administration. *Title 21 § 182.1320. Glycerin*; 2016.

127. The Soap and Detergent Association. *Glycerine: An Overivew* New York, New York. 1990.

128. Rodway I, Gander J. Comparison of fusion rates between glycerol-preserved and frozen composite allografts in cervical fusion. *Int Sch Res Not*. 2014;2014:960142.

CHAPTER 6

Biologics in Sports Medicine— Introduction

LAURA A. VOGEL, MD • MARY BETH R. MCCARTHY, BS • AUGUSTUS D. MAZZOCCA, MS, MD

INTRODUCTION

Biologic therapies have been an area of interest within sports medicine for many years as a means to maintain function in both active and aging populations. Over the last 2 decades, however, surgeon interest and industry development have significantly increased. The market for biologic therapies within orthopedic surgery was estimated to be a $3.7 billion dollar industry in 2013 and is expected to continue to increase in worth.[1]

In general, the goal of biologic therapies is enhanced healing and restoration of normal, native tissue or anatomy. Enhanced healing can be defined as improved quality of the healing tissue, decreased healing time, or improved healing rates. Examples of restoration of normal, native tissue include restoration of articular hyaline cartilage versus fibrocartilage or normal tendon to bone insertion anatomy. The variety of available biologic therapies is vast, and there is an equally large variability in the available preparations, applications, delivery systems, and outcome measurements. Biologic therapies can be used to augment other procedures or as stand-alone treatments; they can be largely divided into growth factor treatments, cell therapies, or tissue transplantations. In this chapter, we aim to provide the reader with an overview of biologic therapies in sports medicine by reviewing historical origins of biologic therapies, currently available biologics in sports medicine, and future directions for research and treatment.

HISTORICAL PERSPECTIVE

Even before the advent of cutting edge biologic therapies, surgeons have attempted to improve healing in difficult cases. Bone graft is one of the original biologic treatments. The earliest report of viable bone allograft was in 1770 by John Hunter, a Scottish surgeon and anatomist. He transplanted a bony spur from a rooster foot into its comb and found that it still grew normally owing to the rich vascular supply of the rooster's comb.[2] The first report of a successful human bone allograft transplantation was in 1879 by Sir William MacEwan, a British surgeon, in which he successfully reconstructed two-thirds of the humeral shaft of a 3 year old boy with extensive osteomyelitis.[3]

The modern concept of tissue grafting and banking began in the early 1900s. Tissue was frequently solicited from patient's friends or family, and bone was often obtained from amputees. Obtaining tissue from corpses was rarely done at that time owing to concerns regarding infection and disrupting death rites and burial rituals. The US Navy Tissue Bank was founded in 1949 and established the standard of modern tissue banks. At its inception, the bank consisted of a single small freezer in which they collected and stored surplus bone from clean cases until needed for later grafting. Issues around allograft immunogenicity and disease transmission, including human immunodeficiency virus (HIV), were prevalent in the 1960s–1980s. This led to the development of modern preservation methods and protocols for donor screening.[4] The use of human cell, tissue, and cellular and tissue-based products in the United States is regulated by the U.S. Food and Drug Administration (FDA). In order to be classified as a low-risk product (also known as 361 low-risk products vs. high-risk 351 products) that does not require specific licensing, there are four criteria that must be met. They are (1) minimal manipulation, (2) homologous use, (3) non-combination products, and (4) lack of systemic effect. These regulations affect the availability of emerging technologies to patients and clinicians in the interest of patient safety.[5]

Biologics in Orthopaedic Surgery. https://doi.org/10.1016/B978-0-323-55140-3.00006-0

CURRENT APPLICATIONS IN CLINICAL PRACTICE OF SPORTS MEDICINE
Growth Factor Therapies and Platelet-Rich Plasma

The use of single, isolated growth factors is not common in the clinical practice of sports medicine at this time, although bone morphogenetic protein 2 and 7 have shown benefits for fracture healing in clinical trials.[6,7] However, there have been a number of basic science and animal model studies investigating the effects of single, isolated growth factors in injury models that may have practical applications in sports medicine. Insulin-like growth factor I (IGF-I) has been found to be a mediator in wound healing, and Kurtz et al.[8] demonstrated that treatment with IGF-I decreased time until functional recovery and diminished the maximal functional deficit in a rat model of Achilles tendon injury. A study by Hildebrand et al.[9] investigated the role of platelet-derived growth factor-BB (PDGF-BB) and transforming growth factor β1 (TGF-β1) on healing in a rabbit model of injury to the medial collateral ligament. Their results showed improved ultimate load, energy absorbed to failure, and ultimate elongation of MCL injuries treated with PDGF-BB in a dose-dependent manner. Interestingly, addition of TGF-β1 to the model appeared to have a negative effect on MCL healing. Their group had previously demonstrated that PDGF-BB positively affected ligament fibroblast proliferation and that TGF-β1 enhanced collagen and total protein synthesis; thus the authors expected a potentiated improvement in healing with PDGF-BB and TGF-β1 treatment of MCL injuries. These counterintuitive results of MCL healing in their rabbit model exemplify the complexity of interactions between individual growth factors and difficulties in effective treatment in clinical practice; optimizing results will require not only understanding interactions between growth factors but dose- and time-dependent effects as well.

Platelet-rich plasma (PRP) was first recognized as an adhesive and hemostatic agent in the 1970s and as a source of autologous growth factors in the 1990s. In its early years, it was used to augment tissue healing within the fields of dentistry, oral maxillofacial surgery, and plastic surgery.[10] While PRP has been studied for use in almost every orthopaedic subspecialty, interest has remained strong within sports medicine owing to the potential promise of decreased recovery time and earlier return to play. Early studies of PRP were plagued by inconsistencies between preparation systems regarding cell and growth factor component concentrations. Several authors have demonstrated significant differences in commercially available systems and PRP preparation method regarding concentration of leukocytes, platelets, and growth factors.[10,11] Interestingly, there were some differences in concentration levels of PRP components in samples prepared with the same commercially available systems in the studies by Castillo et al.[10] and Mazzocca et al.[11] Classification systems of PRP by DeLong et al.[12] and Mishra et al.[13] separate preparations by platelet count, leukocyte count, and activation method in an attempt to help researchers better document and compare results. This may allow researchers to determine crucial information, such as the growth factor concentration needed to enhance healing or reduce inflammation.

PRP has been used extensively in sports medicine in the treatment of a variety of conditions such as cartilage lesions, osteoarthritis, elbow epicondylitis, ulnar collateral ligament injury, hamstring sprains, plantar fasciitis, patellar tendinopathy, Achilles tendinopathy, and rotator cuff tendinopathy. It has also been used to augment surgical procedures including ACL reconstruction, rotator cuff repair, and Achilles tendon repair.[14] PRP may also have the ability to protect against the cytotoxic effects of corticosteroids and local anesthetics on chondrocytes.[15] While there is significant variation in different preparations of PRP based on available processing systems, the generally accepted definition of PRP is "a sample of autologous blood with concentrations of platelet above baseline values."[16] The components of PRP that are clinically relevant include the concentration of platelets, white blood cells (WBC), and growth factors. Mazzucco et al.[17] reported that a platelet concentration greater than 200×10^3 platelets/µL is sufficient to produce a therapeutic effect and that concentrations 2.5 times greater than native blood have positive effects on osteoblasts and fibroblasts in vitro. Adverse effects have been reported at doses higher than 3.5 times the platelet concentration of native blood.[18] Giusti et al.[19] suggested that 1.5×10^6 platelets/µL is the optimum platelet concentration for tissue healing. Variation in platelet as well as WBC concentration can occur between repetitive blood draws from the same individual and may affect clinical outcomes after serial treatments, which are common in clinical practice.[11]

PRP can be created via a single or double spin centrifugation process that separates the liquid and solid components of blood; the processing method has significant impact on the concentration of platelets and WBCs. The effect of different preparations on cell proliferation varies based on target cell type. For example, an in vitro study showed that low platelet preparation has been shown to increase cell proliferation in osteocytes, myocytes, and tenocytes while a high platelet and high WBC preparation only increased cell proliferation in tenocytes. Furthermore, a high platelet and low WBC preparation increased proliferation in osteoblasts and tenocytes, but not in myocytes.[20] Thus, different PRP preparations may be better suited to treat some conditions over others depending on the target tissue.

The literature regarding treatment of specific conditions with various PRP preparations are detailed in depth in subsequent chapters of this book. There have been conflicting results on efficacy throughout the literature. However, trends are beginning to emerge as the literature improves. For example, current thought is that low-WBC-concentration PRP may be beneficial to avoid the inflammatory reaction associated with leukocytes and thus may be preferred in treatment of conditions such as osteoarthritis where further inflammation is undesirable.[21,22] Careful analysis of the literature and thorough reporting of techniques is paramount in optimizing outcomes of PRP treatment.

Cell Therapies

Stem cells are one generation more mature in cell lineage from germ cells. The four defining characteristics of stem cells are the following: (1) they are able to reproduce or have proliferative potential, (2) they are able to differentiate into different cell lines or have multipotentiality, (3) they are able to mobilize in situation of angiogenesis, and (4) they are able to activate and control cells within their environment or have paracrine functions.[23] The regenerative properties of bone marrow were described as early as the 1860s by a Julius Cohnheim, a German pathologist, and Emile Goujon, a French physiologist. However, it was not until the mid-1900s that Alexander Friedenstein isolated mesenchymal stem cells (MSCs) in vitro, which he called CFU-F. Subsequent researchers used his protocol and created varying terminology to describe their cell lines including marrow stromal cells, bone stem cells, and mesenchymal progenitor cells. The term mesenchymal stem cells (MSCs) was coined by Arnold Caplan in the 1990s.[24] To reduce ambiguity and variation in research and analysis of results, the International Society for Cellular Therapy introduced minimum criteria to define MSCs in a consensus statement. The criteria include four components: (1) cells must be plastic adherent in standard culture conditions, (2) cells must express CD105, CD73, and CD90 surface molecules, (3) cells must lack expression of CD45, CD34, CD14, CD11b, CD79α, CD19, and HLA-DR surface molecules, and (4) cells must be able to different to osteoblasts, adipocytes, and chondroblasts in vitro.[25]

MSCs are of the utmost interest in orthopedics, as they are the precursors to musculoskeletal cells such as chondrocytes, tenocytes, and osteoblasts. Many uses of stem cell therapy in the United States are limited by the FDA owing to classification as 351 products. They have determined that laboratory expansion of stem cells (deemed more than minimal manipulation) and subcutaneous harvesting of adipose stem cells for intraarticular injection in the knee (nonhomologous use) are both high-risk products and have strict regulations regarding their use in the United States.

Bone marrow aspirate concentration (BMAC) has gained popularity because it is one of the few FDA-approved methods for delivering stem cells.[22] BMAC is frequently formulated from iliac crest or tibial bone marrow. Techniques for harvesting MSCs from the proximal humerus have been described for use in arthroscopic rotator cuff repair.[26–28] Subacromial bursa[29] and the infrapatellar fat pad[30] have also been reported as sources of MSCs. The concentration of stem cells in BMAC formulation is low and subject to hemodilution with large volume aspiration.[22,31] The cell population in BMAC preparations is heterogenous and contains inflammatory cells, hematopoietic cells, endothelial cells, and nonviable cells. There are also growth factors present including platelet-derived growth factor, TGF-β, and bone morphogenetic proteins. BMAC has been for the treatment of osteoarthritis and focal chondral defects with relatively good results.[22,32]

Autologous chondrocyte implantation (ACI) was first described as a two stage procedure in which chondrocytes are first harvested from a patient, cultured in a laboratory, and reimplanted into a cartilage defect at a second surgery. ACI was approved by the US FDA in 1997 for treatment of focal chondral defects of the distal femur based on promising results from 159 patients in Sweden.[33] In response to issues of hypertrophy associated with the periosteal flap used in ACI, subsequent methods including second generation collagen-covered ACI (CCACI) and third generation matrix-associated ACI (MACI) were developed.[34] CCACI has been used exclusively in Europe. MACI was FDA approved for use of symptomatic full thickness cartilage defects of the knee in adults in 2016.[35] A small series with 5 year follow-up showed improvement in clinical outcome scores after treatment of cartilage defects in the knee with MACI.[36]

Tissue Therapies

Musculoskeletal human allograft tissue is used in orthopedic sports medicine for ligament reconstruction, articular cartilage reconstruction, and meniscal transplantation. There are more than 100 accredited tissue banks in the United States. The American Association of Tissue Banks (AATB) is responsible for establishing and enforcing the standards of these institutions, which supply approximately 90% of musculoskeletal allografts used in the United States.[37] While not all tissue banks are accredited through the AATB, all banks are required to register with the FDA and abide by their current good tissue practices (CGTP). These standards were implemented in May 2005 to help prevent the transmission of communicable diseases. All donor tissue undergoes screening for HIV, hepatitis B virus (HBV), hepatitis C virus (HCV), *Treponema pallidum*, and human transmissible encephalopathies.[38]

After screening and harvest, tissues that will be kept as fresh frozen grafts, such as tendon allografts, are sterilized. Sterilization methods include disinfectant washes, ultrasonics, centrifugation, γ irradiation, and carbon dioxide exposure at low temperature and pressure.[39] Sterilization procedures can vary between tissue banks and may affect the biomechanical properties of the tissue. Knowledge of a tissue banks sterilization process allows surgeons to be informed consumers and provide their patients with the safest possible allograft product. A survey from 2006 of members of the American Orthopaedic Society for Sports Medicine (AOSSM) found that 21% of respondents did not know if their allografts came from tissue banks accredited by the AATB and 46% did not know if the samples were sterilized or the specific sterilization process used.[39] After processing and packaging, some tissue, such as tendon grafts or meniscus transplants, is frozen for storage as a fresh frozen graft. Tissue that is used as a fresh graft, such as osteochondral allograft, has a window of chondrocyte viability of approximately 28 days. Testing typically takes about 14 days, which allows another 14 days for graft use.[37]

Acellular dermal matrix from human as well as bovine and porcine tissue sources has been used for augmentation of soft tissue repair such as rotator cuff repair and Achilles tendon repair.[40,41] The use of whole xenograft tissue is not standard practice in orthopaedic surgery in the United States and introduces additional concerns regarding disease transmission and immune responses.[42]

Amniotic membrane products have been used in sports medicine for cartilage restoration, ligament and tendon healing, nonoperative treatment of knee osteoarthritis, and plantar fasciitis.[43] Amniotic membrane products are a source of stem cells and avoid many of the ethical concerns over the use of fetal stem cells. As with many products discussed in this chapter, there are proprietary processing methods of different commercially available products, which may affect their efficacy in different applications. In addition to a source of stem cells, amniotic membrane products have been investigated in enhancing tendon and ligament healing. To date, the majority of studies on amniotic membrane use in musculoskeletal conditions are in basic science or animal models with only one small randomized control trial in humans demonstrating improved outcomes with amniotic membrane treatment of plantar fasciitis compared with controls.[43,44]

Particulated juvenile articular cartilage has also been used for treatment of cartilage lesions owing to the increased growth potential of juvenile chondrocytes compared with adult chondrocytes.[45] It has the benefit of being a single stage procedure unlike ACI. A case series from 2014 by Farr et al. on the treatment of articular cartilage lesions in the knee with particulated juvenile cartilage showed improved clinical outcomes and healing with a mixture of hyaline and fibrocartilage.[46]

FUTURE RESEARCH AND TREATMENT

Continued research and treatment with biologic therapies in sports medicine will likely be influenced by patient interest, market forces, and government regulation. Current areas of interest include engineered scaffolds as replacements for human allografts,[47,48] the use of peripheral blood–derived stem cells and induced pluripotent stem cells,[49] combination treatments with PRP and MSCs,[50] and PRP as an ergogenic aid[51] and patient specific bio-printed constructs.[52]

CONCLUSION

Biologic treatments will likely play an important role in sports medicine for decades to come. Patient interest and willingness to pay out of pocket for treatment is influenced by highly publicized cases of professional athletes successfully treated with biologic therapies and will remain a driving economic force in the development and use of biologic therapies. Doctors must remain stalwart custodians of their usage for appropriate indications in the interest of ethical patient care. It is important that researchers carefully define their methods, interventions, and outcome measures to best advance understanding within the field. Use of biologic therapies will continue to be influenced by regulatory bodies such as the FDA.

DISCLOSURES

Laura A. Vogel declares no conflicts of interest; Mary Beth R. McCarthy receives intellectual property royalties from Arthrex, Inc.

Augustus D. Mazzocca is a paid consultant for Arthrex, Inc. and Orthofix, Inc. and receives research support from Arthrex, Inc.

REFERENCES

1. Bray CC, Walker CM, Spence DD. Orthobiologics in pediatric sports medicine. *Orthop Clin North Am.* 2017;48(3):333–342.
2. Hernigou P. Bone transplantation and tissue engineering, part I. Mythology, miracles and fantasy: from chimera to the miracle of the black leg of Saints Cosmas and Damian and the cock of John Hunter. *Int Orthop.* 2014;38(12):2631–2638.
3. Hernigou P. Bone transplantation and tissue engineering. Part II: bone graft and osteogenesis in the seventeenth, eighteenth and nineteenth centuries (Duhamel, Haller, Ollier and MacEwen). *Int Orthop.* 2015;39(1):193–204.
4. Hernigou P. Bone transplantation and tissue engineering, part III: allografts, bone grafting and bone banking in the twentieth century. *Int Orthop.* 2015;39(3):577–587.
5. Beitzel K, Allen D, Apostolakos J, et al. US definitions, current use, and FDA stance on use of platelet-rich plasma in sports medicine. *J Knee Surg.* 2015;28(1):29–34.
6. Friedlaender GE, Perry CR, Cole JD, et al. Osteogenic protein-1 (bone morphogenetic protein-7) in the treatment of tibial nonunions. *J Bone Joint Surg Am.* 2001;83-A(suppl 1(Pt 2)):S151–S158.
7. Govender S, Csimma C, Genant HK, et al. Recombinant human bone morphogenetic protein-2 for treatment of open tibial fractures: a prospective, controlled, randomized study of four hundred and fifty patients. *J Bone Joint Surg Am.* 2002;84-A(12):2123–2134.
8. Kurtz CA, Loebig TG, Anderson DD, DeMeo PJ, Campbell PG. Insulin-like growth factor I accelerates functional recovery from Achilles tendon injury in a rat model. *Am J Sports Med.* 1999;27(3):363–369.
9. Hildebrand KA, Woo SL, Smith DW, et al. The effects of platelet-derived growth factor-BB on healing of the rabbit medial collateral ligament. An in vivo study. *Am J Sports Med.* 1998;26(4):549–554.
10. Castillo TN, Pouliot MA, Kim HJ, Dragoo JL. Comparison of growth factor and platelet concentration from commercial platelet-rich plasma separation systems. *Am J Sports Med.* 2011;39(2):266–271.
11. Mazzocca AD, McCarthy MB, Chowaniec DM, et al. Platelet-rich plasma differs according to preparation method and human variability. *J Bone Joint Surg Am.* 2012;94(4):308–316.
12. DeLong JM, Russell RP, Mazzocca AD. Platelet-rich plasma: the PAW classification system. *Arthroscopy.* 2012;28(7):998–1009.
13. Mishra A, Harmon K, Woodall J, Vieira A. Sports medicine applications of platelet rich plasma. *Curr Pharm Biotechnol.* 2012;13(7):1185–1195.
14. Hsu WK, Mishra A, Rodeo SR, et al. Platelet-rich plasma in orthopaedic applications: evidence-based recommendations for treatment. *J Am Acad Orthop Surg.* 2013;21(12):739–748.
15. Durant TJ, Dwyer CR, McCarthy MB, Cote MP, Bradley JP, Mazzocca AD. Protective nature of platelet-rich plasma against chondrocyte death when combined with corticosteroids or local anesthetics. *Am J Sports Med.* 2017;45(1):218–225.
16. Hall MP, Band PA, Meislin RJ, Jazrawi LM, Cardone DA. Platelet-rich plasma: current concepts and application in sports medicine. *J Am Acad Orthop Surg.* 2009;17(10):602–608.
17. Mazzucco L, Balbo V, Cattana E, Guaschino R, Borzini P. Not every PRP-gel is born equal. Evaluation of growth factor availability for tissues through four PRP-gel preparations: fibrinet, RegenPRP-Kit, Plateltex and one manual procedure. *Vox Sang.* 2009;97(2):110–118.
18. Graziani F, Ivanovski S, Cei S, Ducci F, Tonetti M, Gabriele M. The in vitro effect of different PRP concentrations on osteoblasts and fibroblasts. *Clin Oral Implants Res.* 2006;17(2):212–219.
19. Giusti I, Rughetti A, D'Ascenzo S, et al. Identification of an optimal concentration of platelet gel for promoting angiogenesis in human endothelial cells. *Transfusion.* 2009;49(4):771–778.
20. Mazzocca AD, McCarthy MB, Chowaniec DM, et al. The positive effects of different platelet-rich plasma methods on human muscle, bone, and tendon cells. *Am J Sports Med.* 2012;40(8):1742–1749.
21. Cerciello S, Beitzel K, Howlett N, et al. The use of platelet-rich plasma preparations in the treatment of musculoskeletal injuries in orthopaedic sports medicine. *Oper Tech Orthop.* 2013;23(2):69–74.
22. Kraeutler MJ, Chahla J, LaPrade RF, Pascual-Garrido C. Biologic options for articular cartilage wear (Platelet-Rich plasma, stem cells, bone marrow aspirate concentrate). *Clin Sports Med.* 2017;36(3):457–468.
23. Anz AW, Hackel JG, Nilssen EC, Andrews JR. Application of biologics in the treatment of the rotator cuff, meniscus, cartilage, and osteoarthritis. *J Am Acad Orthop Surg.* 2014;22(2):68–79.
24. Hernigou P. Bone transplantation and tissue engineering, part IV. Mesenchymal stem cells: history in orthopedic surgery from Cohnheim and Goujon to the Nobel Prize of Yamanaka. *Int Orthop.* 2015;39(4):807–817.
25. Dominici M, Le Blanc K, Mueller I, et al. Minimal criteria for defining multipotent mesenchymal stromal cells. The International Society for Cellular Therapy position statement. *Cytotherapy.* 2006;8(4):315–317.
26. Singh H, Voss A, Mazzocca AD, Virk MS. Biological augmentation of rotator cuff repair: platelet-rich plasma (PRP) and bone marrow aspirate (BMA). *Tech Shoulder Elbow Surg.* 2015;16(4):107–114.

27. Mazzocca AD, McCarthy MB, Chowaniec DM, Cote MP, Arciero RA, Drissi H. Rapid isolation of human stem cells (connective tissue progenitor cells) from the proximal humerus during arthroscopic rotator cuff surgery. *Am J Sports Med.* 2010;38(7):1438–1447.

28. Mazzocca AD, McCarthy MB, Chowaniec D, et al. Bone marrow-derived mesenchymal stem cells obtained during arthroscopic rotator cuff repair surgery show potential for tendon cell differentiation after treatment with insulin. *Arthroscopy.* 2011;27(11):1459–1471.

29. Utsunomiya H, Uchida S, Sekiya I, Sakai A, Moridera K, Nakamura T. Isolation and characterization of human mesenchymal stem cells derived from shoulder tissues involved in rotator cuff tears. *Am J Sports Med.* 2013;41(3):657–668.

30. Dragoo JL, Samimi B, Zhu M, et al. Tissue-engineered cartilage and bone using stem cells from human infrapatellar fat pads. *J Bone Joint Surg Br.* 2003;85(5):740–747.

31. LaPrade RF, Geeslin AG, Murray IR, et al. Biologic treatments for sports injuries II Think Tank-current concepts, future research, and barriers to advancement, Part 1: biologics overview, ligament injury. *Tendinopathy Am J Sports Med.* 2016;44(12):3270–3283.

32. Chahla J, Dean CS, Moatshe G, Pascual-Garrido C, Serra Cruz R, LaPrade RF. Concentrated bone marrow aspirate for the treatment of chondral injuries and osteoarthritis of the knee: a systematic review of outcomes. *Orthop J Sports Med.* 2016;4(1):2325967115625481.

33. Minas T. Autologous chondrocyte implantation. In: *A Primer in Cartilage Repair and Joint Preservation of the Knee.* Saint Louis: W.B. Saunders; 2011:65–119 (Chapter 7).

34. Zlotnicki JP, Geeslin AG, Murray IR, et al. Biologic treatments for sports injuries II think tank-current concepts, future research, and barriers to advancement, Part 3: articular cartilage. *Orthop J Sports Med.* 2016;4(4):2325967116642433.

35. *United States Food and Drug Administration.* December 13, 2016. Approval Letter - MACI. 2016. https://www.fda.gov/downloads/BiologicsBloodVaccines/CellularGeneTherapyProducts/ApprovedProducts/UCM533307.pdf.

36. Behrens P, Bitter T, Kurz B, Russlies M. Matrix-associated autologous chondrocyte transplantation/implantation (MACT/MACI)–5-year follow-up. *Knee.* 2006;13(3):194–202.

37. Wydra FB, York PJ, Vidal AF. Allografts. *Clin Sports Med.* 2017;36(3):509–523.

38. Wydra F, York P, Johnson C, Silvestri L. Allografts for ligament reconstruction: where are we now? *Am J Orthoped.* 2016;45(7):446–452.

39. McAllister DR, Joyce MJ, Mann BJ, Vangsness Jr CT. Allograft update: the current status of tissue regulation, procurement, processing, and sterilization. *Am J Sports Med.* 2007;35(12):2148–2158.

40. Derwin KA, Baker AR, Spragg RK, Leigh DR, Iannotti JP. Commercial extracellular matrix scaffolds for rotator cuff tendon repair. Biomechanical, biochemical, and cellular properties. *J Bone Joint Surg Am.* 2006;88(12):2665–2672.

41. Lee MS. GraftJacket augmentation of chronic Achilles tendon ruptures. *Orthopedics.* 2004;27(suppl 1):S151–S153.

42. Laurencin CT, El-Amin SF. Xenotransplantation in orthopaedic surgery. *J Am Acad Orthop Surg.* 2008;16(1):4–8.

43. Riboh JC, Saltzman BM, Yanke AB, Cole BJ. Human amniotic membrane-derived products in sports medicine: basic science, early results, and potential clinical applications. *Am J Sports Med.* 2016;44(9):2425–2434.

44. Zelen CM, Poka A, Andrews J. Prospective, randomized, blinded, comparative study of injectable micronized dehydrated amniotic/chorionic membrane allograft for plantar fasciitis–a feasibility study. *Foot Ankle Int.* 2013;34(10):1332–1339.

45. Adkisson HD, Martin JA, Amendola RL, et al. The potential of human allogeneic juvenile chondrocytes for restoration of articular cartilage. *Am J Sports Med.* 2010;38(7):1324–1333.

46. Farr J, Tabet SK, Margerrison E, Cole BJ. Clinical, radiographic, and histological outcomes after cartilage repair with particulated juvenile articular cartilage: a 2-year prospective study. *Am J Sports Med.* 2014;42(6):1417–1425.

47. Carmont MR, Carey-Smith R, Saithna A, Dhillon M, Thompson P, Spalding T. Delayed incorporation of a TruFit plug: perseverance is recommended. *Arthroscopy.* 2009;25(7):810–814.

48. Minas T. Emerging technologies. In: *A Primer in Cartilage Repair and Joint Preservation of the Knee.* Saint Louis: W.B. Saunders; 2011:219–249 (Chapter 14).

49. Li Y, Liu T, Van Halm-Lutterodt N, Chen J, Su Q, Hai Y. Reprogramming of blood cells into induced pluripotent stem cells as a new cell source for cartilage repair. *Stem Cell Res Ther.* 2016;7:31.

50. Shi WJ, Tjoumakaris FP, Lendner M, Freedman KB. Biologic injections for osteoarthritis and articular cartilage damage: can we modify disease? *Phys Sportsmed.* 2017;45(3):203–223.

51. Wasterlain AS, Braun HJ, Harris AH, Kim HJ, Dragoo JL. The systemic effects of platelet-rich plasma injection. *Am J Sports Med.* 2013;41(1):186–193.

52. Melchels FPW, Blokzijl MM, Levato R, et al. Hydrogel-based reinforcement of 3D bioprinted constructs. *Biofabrication.* 2016;8(3):035004.

CHAPTER 7

Rotator Cuff Augmentation*

JASON P. ROGERS, MD • ADAM KWAPISZ, MD, PHD • JOHN M. TOKISH, MD

INTRODUCTION

Massive rotator cuff tears are often chronic in presentation and complicated by poor tendon quality, muscular fatty atrophy, tissue retraction, and scarring. For these reasons, successful footprint repair and tendon healing may be difficult and can result in retear rate of large-to-massive rotator cuff tears as high as 70% in the elderly and an approximate 45% retear in massive rotator cuff repairs in younger cohorts[1-5] Known radiographic parameters for tear irreparability include acromiohumeral interval less than 7 mm, Goutallier grade 3–4 fatty infiltration of the infraspinatus, and a positive supraspinatus tangent sign.[6-9] Approximately 10%–40% of all rotator cuff tears are massive. In the setting of irreparability, a number of surgical treatment approaches have been suggested.[10]

There are multiple surgical treatment options for the irreparable rotator cuff tear. The patient's age, integrity of the glenohumeral joint, extent of residual shoulder function, presenting symptoms, medical comorbidities, desired activity level, and rehabilitation requirements are all important considerations. An ideal treatment should include restoration of joint function and relief of pain. Although muscle transfer remains an option in the young, laboring patient, the demanding technical aspects of this procedure, relative perioperative morbidity, and unpredictable functional outcomes, particularly in older patients, limit the indications for this procedure.[10-15]

Patch interposition (PI) and superior capsular reconstruction (SCR) have become the more commonly used reconstructive approaches[10,16,17] Patch augmentation has also been used. Examples tried have included extracellular human, porcine, and synthetic grafts, as well as autografts using fascial and long head of biceps tendon autografts. In the absence of advanced cuff tear arthropathy, there is no clear indication for one reconstructive technique over another, and there is no standard treatment approach to this challenging clinical problem.[16-19]

SUPERIOR CAPSULE RECONSTRUCTION

The treatment of the irreparable cuff tear remains a significant challenge to the shoulder surgeon. Historically, tendon transfers or shoulder hemiarthroplasty were limited goal treatment options. This option may work in older patients; however, in younger and active patients it may not give such good outcomes and may result in higher complications and reoperations rate than in older ones. Some authors suggest that Reverse Shoulder Arthroplasty (RSA) should be advocated in patients older than 65 years.[10,20-22] This is one of the reasons why many new techniques are being investigated[10,16] (Figs. 7.1 and 7.2).

Some studies have evaluated treatment options for the massive irreparable rotator cuff tear in the setting of no or minimal osteoarthritis (Fig. 7.3).[17,23-27] The concept of implanting a patch or reconstructing the superior capsule is based on restoring the fulcrum for glenohumeral joint motions.[28] The first reported approach was to fill the gap in irreparable cuff lesions with either biological or artificial grafts.[10,23,29] There have been many clinical reports of different patch techniques published; unfortunately, high rate of retears have been also reported. This corresponds with our findings that almost 40% of patch grafts tore during follow-up; on contrary, only 17% reconstructed superior capsules were torn at the last follow-up visit.[17,23,24] These results are supported by biomechanical work by Mihata et al. who reported that superior capsule reconstruction normalized superior stability of the shoulder, whereas patch grafts to the torn tendon only partially restored this stability.[30,31]

The concept of restoring glenohumeral biomechanics with patch techniques and capsule reconstruction was successfully tested on cadavers.[25,28,30] This theory is supported in the published clinical outcome studies reported herein, in which in both groups, patch filling and SCR patients had a significant and comparable increase in their ranges of motion to around 150 degrees of flexion and around 40 degrees of external rotation (ER)[17,23,24] (Fig. 7.4).

The published patient-reported outcomes did show that SCR is a promising solution.[17] Postoperative change in American Shoulder and Elbow Society score (ASES)

---

*The authors report no relationship with a commercial company that has a direct financial interest in this subject matter.

Biologics in Orthopaedic Surgery. https://doi.org/10.1016/B978-0-323-55140-3.00007-2

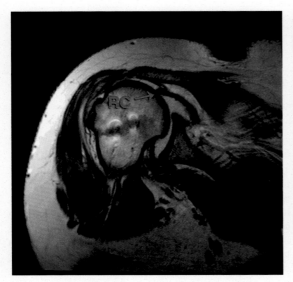

FIG. 7.1 MRI coronal view of the right shoulder with irreparable cuff tear planned to undergo superior capsule reconstruction. *RC*, rotators cuff remnant.

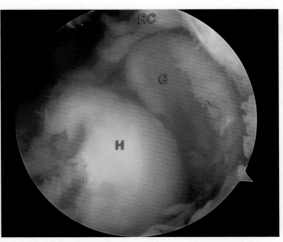

FIG. 7.3 Intraoperative arthroscopic view of the irreparable cuff tear in the right shoulder. Scope is positioned in an anterosuperolateral portal. *G*, glenoid; *H*, humeral head; *RC*, rotators cuff remnant.

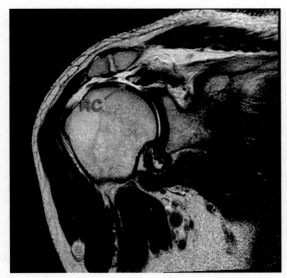

FIG. 7.2 MRI coronal view of the right shoulder with the massive cuff tear planned to undergo patch augmented repair. *RC*, rotators cuff.

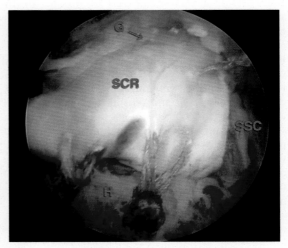

FIG. 7.4 Arthroscopic view of the completed superior capsule reconstruction performed in the right shoulder. Scope is positioned in the anterosuperolateral portal. *G*, glenoid; *H*, humeral head; *SCR*, superior capsule reconstruction graft; *SSC*, subscapularis tendon.

score for the SCR cohort was 70 points compared to 43 for patch interposition.[17,23–27,32–34] Although direct comparisons between the cohorts are limited due to heterogeneity in reported outcome scores and measures, SCR reported more favorable range of motion and functional results than PI approaches.[17,23,24] One potential explanation for this finding is the higher graft retear rate in the PI group than in SCR.[17,23,24] Admittedly, the complication rate for SCR may prove to be higher with additional outcome studies and length of follow-up.[17,25–27]

Patch Augmentation—Extracellular Matrix Patches

Previously, literature has proven that most cuff repair failure occurs at the bone to tendon interface in both large tears and medium-sized tears, which fails.[35,36] Thus successful tendon repair must produce an environment that can allow tendon to bone healing over a 12-week period, while creating uniform tension over the tendon-bone interface and preserving blood supply.[37,38] Omae and colleagues looked at the effect of acellular matrix patches on the biomechanics of the rotator cuff repair. In their cadaveric study, using single-row constructs with and without patch augmentation, the augmented groups had better pull out load to failure; however, they had less stiffness than the nonaugmented shoulders.[39] Shea et al. performed another cadaveric test of extracellular matrix (ECM) augmentation and its effect on the strength of the construct. In their study the gap formation as well as load to failure was found to be improved with ECM augmentation, and further they concluded that the addition of the ECM shared about 35% of the load felt on the native tendon.[40] The Shea study was duplicated with similar results 2 years later in a laboratory model[41] (Fig. 7.5).

In vivo studies have also been conducted to assess the effect of the ECM on an augmented rotator cuff tendon repair. In an analysis of 45 patients with massive cuff tears, Snyder and colleagues found that the use of human dermal allograft resulted in improvement of outcome measures which was significant for University of California at Los Angeles score (UCLA), Western Ontario Rotator Cuff score (WORC), and ASES[42] While these results are promising, Burkhart established years earlier that with an arthroscopic repair, massive cuff tears, with fatty changes of their muscle, could still have acceptable outcomes in the majority of cases.[43] Understanding the need for comparative analysis, multiple other studies have sought to answer the question of superiority with augmentation using ECM. In a level II study performed by Barber et al., ECM-augmented repairs were compared to standard double-row repairs of nonaugmented tears of similar size. Their results found that in addition to statistically better outcome scores, as shown in 14.5-month follow-up MRIs, the augmented repairs were healed in 85% versus the nonaugmented healed in just 40% of their cohorts.[44] In another comparative study, Gilot et al. looked at ECM augment versus no augment and used ultrasound to follow-up retear rate, along with patient-reported outcome scores. In their study, follow-up averaged 25 months, and they reported improved outcomes scores with augmentation and decreased retear rate from 26% to 10% with augmentation.[45]

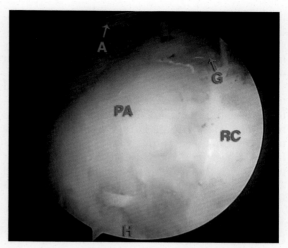

FIG. 7.5 Arthroscopic view of the completed massive tear repair with xenograft patch augmentation. Scope is positioned the anterosuperolateral portal. *A*, inferior surface of the acromion; *G*, glenoid; *H*, humeral head; *PA*, patch augmentation with a xenograft; *RC*, rotators cuff.

Patch Augmentation—Xenograft and Synthetic Augment

Xenograft and synthetic graft augmentation have also been considered for the massive rotator cuff tear (Fig. 7.1). Porcine dermal xenograft has been used to augment and as interposition graft for massive rotator cuff tears. Outcomes in level IV studies have shown promising short- to intermediate-term results on patient-reported outcomes and healing rates similar to human ECM augments with this technique.[46,47] Other attempts to augment large rotator cuff repairs have involved the use of synthetic patch graft augmentation. Most use a poly-L-lactic acid bioabsorbable patch. Results of this technique have been encouraging, out to 42 months.[48] However, the retear rate appears to parallel that of nonaugmented massive tear rates, but with good functional outcomes.[49] Ciampi et al. compared the outcomes of synthetic augmented repairs using a polypropylene patch versus augmented with collagen patch versus primary repair and no augment. At 1 year the polypropylene had the lowest retear rate by ultrasound analysis. At 3 years the synthetic augment also outperformed both the collagen augment and the primary repair, with statistical significance[50] (Fig. 7.5).

Patch Augmentation—Cellular Augments

Cellular augmentation has also been implemented in rotator cuff repair. Fascial autograft and allografts have been described as well as long head of biceps tendon autografting. Fascial allograft has shown to provide increased load to failure and longevity that may improve outcomes in massive rotator cuff repairs but warrants more investigation.[51,52]

Long head of the biceps tendon after tenotomy and tenodesis has been described as an autograft for rotator cuff repair augmentation. The biceps augment has been shown to improve outcome scores and improve tendon healing versus primary repair alone with healing percentage of 58% versus 26% as seen on follow-up MRI.[53] The biceps autograft has also been described as a manner to bridge a tendon gap to augment a repair.[54,55]

CONCLUSIONS

Only one outcome study for SCR has been published to date.[17] Supported by multiple biomechanical studies, enthusiasm for this technique has grown recently. Additional outcome studies with longer follow-up are needed to corroborate Mihata's work and examine outcome durability.[17,30,31,56] There have been multiple technical papers recently published popularizing this treatment approaches, so we should expect more clinical reports in the near future.[16,57,58] Second, among the patch grafting and RSA cohorts, there were relatively few studies that met the strict inclusion criteria for analysis.[23-27] The minimum 2-year follow-up with known osteoarthritis classification inclusion criterion is needed, however, to make clear comparisons between the treatment methods. Finally, the heterogeneity in outcome-reporting methods and arthritis classification systems between the studies makes controlled comparisons difficult. In spite of these weaknesses, this review may serve as a baseline comparison between these approaches in terms of expected outcomes after treatment for irreparable rotator cuff tears.

The treatment of the massive irreparable rotator cuff tear remains challenging. Recent advances in patch interposition, superior capsular reconstruction, and reverse shoulder arthroplasty provide promising progress in this pathology. However, in terms of patient-reported outcomes, initial postoperative SCR reports provide very promising data comparable to RSA complication rate. Further studies involving direct comparison, larger cohorts, and longer term follow-up will be necessary to determine the role of each of these treatment strategies in the treatment of massive irreparable rotator cuff tears.

REFERENCES

1. Chung SW, et al. Arthroscopic repair of massive rotator cuff tears: outcome and analysis of factors associated with healing failure or poor postoperative function. *Am J Sports Med.* 2013;41(7):1674–1683.
2. Bartl C, et al. Long-term outcome and structural integrity following open repair of massive rotator cuff tears. *Int J Shoulder Surg.* 2012;6(1):1.
3. Zumstein MA, et al. The clinical and structural long-term results of open repair of massive tears of the rotator cuff. *JBJS.* 2008;90(11):2423–2431.
4. Kim JR, et al. Clinical and radiographic outcomes after arthroscopic repair of massive rotator cuff tears using a suture bridge technique: assessment of repair integrity on magnetic resonance imaging. *Am J Sports Med.* 2012;40(4):786–793.
5. Park J-Y, et al. Clinical and ultrasonographic outcomes of arthroscopic suture bridge repair for massive rotator cuff tear. *Arthroscopy.* 2013;29(2):280–289.
6. Kissenberth MJ, et al. A positive tangent sign predicts the repairability of rotator cuff tears. *J Shoulder Elbow Surg.* 2014;23(7):1023–1027.
7. Nové-Josserand L, et al. The acromiohumeral and coracohumeral intervals are abnormal in rotator cuff tears with muscular fatty degeneration. *Clin Orthop Relat Res.* 2005;433:90–96.
8. Warner JJP, et al. Diagnosis and treatment of anterosuperior rotator cuff tears. *J Shoulder Elbow Surg.* 2001;10(1):37–46.
9. Goutallier D, et al. Fatty muscle degeneration in cuff ruptures: pre-and postoperative evaluation by CT scan. *Clin Orthop Relat Res.* 1994;304:78–83.
10. Lädermann, Alexandre, Denard PJ, Collin P. Massive rotator cuff tears: definition and treatment. *Int Orthop.* 2015;39(12):2403–2414.
11. Liem D, et al. Arthroscopic debridement of massive irreparable rotator cuff tears. *Arthroscopy.* 2008;24(7):743–748.
12. Gartsman GM. Massive, irreparable tears of the rotator cuff. Results of operative debridement and subacromial decompression. *J Bone Joint Surg Am.* 1997;79.5:715–721.
13. Rockwood CA, Williams GR, Burkhead WZ. Debridement of degenerative, irreparable lesions of the rotator cuff. *J Bone Joint Surg Am.* 1995;77(6):857–866.
14. Lee K-T, Mun G-H. A systematic review of functional donor-site morbidity after latissimus dorsi muscle transfer. *Plast Reconstr Surg.* 2014;134(2):303–314.
15. Shin JJ, et al. Pectoralis major transfer for treatment of irreparable subscapularis tear: a systematic review. *Knee Surg Sports Traumatol Arthrosc.* 2014:1–10.
16. Tokish JM, Beicker C. Superior capsule reconstruction technique using an acellular dermal allograft. *Arthrosc Tech.* 2015;4(6):e833–e839.
17. Mihata T, et al. Clinical results of arthroscopic superior capsule reconstruction for irreparable rotator cuff tears. *Arthroscopy.* 2013;29(3):459–470.
18. Kilinc AS, Ebrahimzadeh MH, Lafosse L. Subacromial internal spacer for rotator cuff tendon repair:"the balloon technique". *Arthroscopy.* 2009;25(8):921–924.

19. Senekovic V, et al. Prospective clinical study of a novel biodegradable sub-acromial spacer in treatment of massive irreparable rotator cuff tears. *Eur J Orthop Surg Traumatol.* 2013;23(3):311–316.

20. Smith CD, Guyver P, Bunker TD. Indications for reverse shoulder replacement. *J Bone Joint Surg Br.* 2012; 94(5):577–583.

21. Samuelsen BT, et al. Primary reverse shoulder arthroplasty in patients aged 65 years or younger. *J Shoulder Elbow Surg.* 2017;26(1):e13–e17.

22. Otto RJ, Clark RE, Frankle MA. Reverse shoulder arthroplasty in patients younger than 55 years: 2-to 12-year follow-up. *J Shoulder Elbow Surg.* 2017;26(5):792–797.

23. Nada AN, et al. Treatment of massive rotator-cuff tears with a polyester ligament (Dacron) augmentation. *Bone Joint J.* 2010;92(10):1397–1402.

24. Mori D, et al. Effect of fatty degeneration of the infraspinatus on the efficacy of arthroscopic patch autograft procedure for large to massive rotator cuff tears. *Am J Sports Med.* 2015;43(5):1108–1117.

25. Hartzler RU, et al. Reverse shoulder arthroplasty for massive rotator cuff tear: risk factors for poor functional improvement. *J Shoulder Elbow Surg.* 2015;24(11):1698–1706.

26. Mulieri P, et al. Reverse shoulder arthroplasty for the treatment of irreparable rotator cuff tear without glenohumeral arthritis. *J Bone Joint Surg Am.* 2010;92(15):2544–2556.

27. Wall B, et al. Reverse total shoulder arthroplasty: a review of results according to etiology. *J Bone Joint Surg Am.* 2007;89(7):1476–1485.

28. Adams CR, et al. The arthroscopic superior capsular reconstruction. *Am J Orthop.* 2016;45(5):320–324.

29. Audenaert E, et al. Reconstruction of massive rotator cuff lesions with a synthetic interposition graft: a prospective study of 41 patients. *Knee Surg Sports Traumatol Arthrosc.* 2006;14(4):360–364.

30. Mihata T, et al. Biomechanical role of capsular continuity in superior capsule reconstruction for irreparable tears of the supraspinatus tendon. *Am J Sports Med.* 2016;44(6):1423–1430.

31. Mihata T, et al. Superior capsule reconstruction to restore superior stability in irreparable rotator cuff tears a biomechanical cadaveric study. *Am J Sports Med.* 2012;40(10):2248–2255.

32. Tashjian RZ, et al. Determining the minimal clinically important difference for the American Shoulder and Elbow Surgeons score, Simple Shoulder Test, and visual analog scale (VAS) measuring pain after shoulder arthroplasty. *J Shoulder Elbow Surg.* 2017;26(1):144–148.

33. Werner BC, et al. What change in American Shoulder and Elbow Surgeons score represents a clinically important change after shoulder arthroplasty? *Clin Orthop Relat Res.* 2016;474(12):2672–2681.

34. Tashjian RZ, et al. Minimal clinically important differences in ASES and simple shoulder test scores after nonoperative treatment of rotator cuff disease. *J Bone Joint Surg.* 2010;92(2):296–303.

35. Neyton L, et al. Arthroscopic suture-bridge repair for small to medium size supraspinatus tear: healing rate and retear pattern. *Arthroscopy.* 2013;29(1):10–17.

36. Hein J, et al. Retear rates after arthroscopic single-row, double-row, and suture bridge rotator cuff repair at a minimum of 1 year of imaging follow-up: a systematic review. *Arthroscopy.* 2015;31(11):2274–2281.

37. Rodeo SA, et al. Tendon-healing in a bone tunnel. A biomechanical and histological study in the dog. *JBJS.* 1993;75(12):1795–1803.

38. Mazzocca AD, et al. Arthroscopic single-row versus double-row suture anchor rotator cuff repair. *Am Journal Sports Med.* 2005;33(12):1861–1868.

39. Omae H, et al. Biomechanical effect of rotator cuff augmentation with an acellular dermal matrix graft: a cadaver study. *Clin Biomech.* 2012;27(8):789–792.

40. Shea KP, et al. A biomechanical analysis of gap formation and failure mechanics of a xenograft-reinforced rotator cuff repair in a cadaveric model. *J Shoulder Elbow Surg.* 2012;21(8):1072–1079.

41. Ely EE, Figueroa NM, Gilot GJ. Biomechanical analysis of rotator cuff repairs with extracellular matrix graft augmentation. *Orthopedics.* 2014;37(9):608–614.

42. Wong I, Burns J, Snyder S. Arthroscopic GraftJacket repair of rotator cuff tears. *J Shoulder Elbow Surg.* 2010;19(2):104–109.

43. Burkhart SS, et al. Arthroscopic repair of massive rotator cuff tears with stage 3 and 4 fatty degeneration. *Arthroscopy.* 2007;23(4):347–354.

44. Marsella RC, et al. Identification of adenocarcinoma in effusions: a comparison of immunoperoxidase staining for monoclonal antibody B72. 3 and carcinoembryonic antigen. *Acta Cytologica.* 1990;34(4):578–580.

45. Gilot GJ, et al. Outcome of large to massive rotator cuff tears repaired with and without extracellular matrix augmentation: a prospective comparative study. *Arthroscopy.* 2015;31(8):1459–1465.

46. Giannotti S, et al. Study of the porcine dermal collagen repair patch in morpho-functional recovery of the rotator cuff after minimum follow-up of 2.5 years. *Surg Technol Int.* 2014;24:348–352.

47. Gupta AK, et al. Massive or 2-tendon rotator cuff tears in active patients with minimal glenohumeral arthritis: clinical and radiographic outcomes of reconstruction using dermal tissue matrix xenograft. *Am J Sports Med.* 2013;41(4):872–879.

48. Proctor CS. Long-term successful arthroscopic repair of large and massive rotator cuff tears with a functional and degradable reinforcement device. *J Shoulder Elbow Surg.* 2014;23(10):1508–1513.

49. Lenart BA, et al. Treatment of massive and recurrent rotator cuff tears augmented with a poly-l-lactide graft, a preliminary study. *J Shoulder Elbow Surg.* 2015;24(6): 915–921.

50. Ciampi P, et al. The benefit of synthetic versus biological patch augmentation in the repair of posterosuperior massive rotator cuff tears: a 3-year follow-up study. *Am J Sports Med.* 2014;42(5):1169–1175.

51. Baker AR, et al. Does augmentation with a reinforced fascia patch improve rotator cuff repair outcomes? *Clin Orthop Relat Res.* 2012;470(9):2513–2521.
52. McCarron JA, et al. Reinforced fascia patch limits cyclic gapping of rotator cuff repairs in a human cadaveric model. *J Shoulder Elbow Surg.* 2012;21(12):1680–1686.
53. Cho, Su N, Woong Yi J, Rhee YG. Arthroscopic biceps augmentation for avoiding undue tension in repair of massive rotator cuff tears. *Arthroscopy.* 2009;25(2):183–191.
54. Rhee YG, et al. Bridging the gap in immobile massive rotator cuff tears: augmentation using the tenotomized biceps. *Am J Sports Med.* 2008;36(8):1511–1518.
55. Obma PR. Free biceps tendon autograft to augment arthroscopic rotator cuff repair. *Arthrosc Tech.* 2013;2(4):e441–e445.
56. Schon, JM, et al. Quantitative and computed tomography anatomic analysis of glenoid fixation for superior capsule reconstruction: a cadaveric study. *Arthroscopy.* 2017;33(6):1131–1137.
57. Maximilian P, Greenspoon JA, Millett PJ. Arthroscopic superior capsule reconstruction for irreparable rotator cuff tears. *Arthrosc Tech.* 2015;4(6):e751–e755.
58. Hirahara AM, Adams CR. Arthroscopic superior capsular reconstruction for treatment of massive irreparable rotator cuff tears. *Arthrosc Tech.* 2015;4(6):e637–e641.

CHAPTER 8

Bone Loss in the Upper Extremity

MATTHEW T. PROVENCHER, MD, MC, USNR • JAKE A. FOX, BS •
ANTHONY SANCHEZ, BS • COLIN P. MURPHY, BA • LIAM A. PEEBLES, BA

INTRODUCTION

Bone loss is a serious problem that can affect any part of the body, both anatomically and functionally, and it must be considered and addressed appropriately. When examining the upper extremity specifically, an area that must be considered extensively is the glenoid and humerus that combine to create the glenohumeral joint. Hantes and Raoulis describe the shoulder as an inherently unstable ball and socket joint that is liable to a multitude of injuries, which makes it highly susceptible to dislocation.[1] In fact, the incidence rate of shoulder dislocations in the United States has been documented to be 23 injuries per 100,000 people.[2,3] The main cause of the primary shoulder dislocation events is almost always trauma related, due to the traumatic force causing the humeral head to slide out of the glenoid articular arc.[4]

The difficult aspect of glenohumeral dislocation lies in the predisposition for these injuries to become recurrent and lead to an unstable shoulder.[5-7] Recurrent instability compounds upon itself by creating further attritional bone loss. There are many factors, in addition to trauma, that lead to recurrent glenohumeral instability, such as age, hyperlaxity, glenoid bone loss, humeral head bone loss, and sex.[8-10] Oftentimes, there are multiple of these factors occurring simultaneously leading to recurrent instability, instead of one isolated factor causing a problem. When determining how to manage shoulder instability several things should be taken into consideration including, osseous defects, experience of the surgeon, and patient-related factors such as participation in athletics and work demands.[11,12]

GLENOID

The glenoid's main function is to form a rimmed barrier constraining the humeral head from dislocating. Bony lesions of the glenoid are problematic because they shorten the glenoid arc length and lessen the stability of the joint by reducing the glenoid surface contact area and its concavity (Fig. 8.1).[13] Burkhart and de

Beer were able to determine that there was a 4% failure rate for patients not containing a significant glenoid defect, while there was a 67% failure rate in patients with a significant lesion.[14] For the overall prevalence of glenoid defects in cases of recurrent anterior shoulder instability, the rate has been as high as 90%.[15] Of the 90%, 50% of the documented injuries were bony Bankart lesions and 40% were due to erosions from chronic recurrent traumatic anterior instability.

Evaluating the significance of glenoid bone loss has been controversial and indecisive as far as definitive preoperative measurements. The two most commonly used methods for measuring a glenoid defect today are the Pico method and the usage of a preinjury diameter for comparison. The Pico method determines the degree of bone loss by first creating a "normal glenoid circle" from three reference points along the intact rim of the uninjured glenoid. Then, the normal circle is placed on the pathologic glenoid, and the missing part of the normal circle can be divided by area of the inferior glenoid circle to determine the defect as a percent of the entire

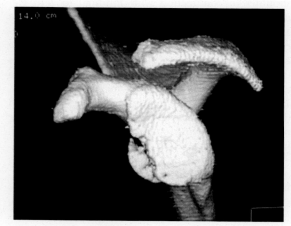

FIG. 8.1 3-Dimensional (3-D) computed tomography *en face* view of glenoid bone fragment loss. Image has undergone 3-D digital subtraction of the humeral head.

Biologics in Orthopaedic Surgery. https://doi.org/10.1016/B978-0-323-55140-3.00008-4

circle.[16] To find defect size using diameter comparison, the anterioposterior diameter of the injured glenoid is subtracted from the estimated preinjury diameter of the glenoid. Then, that number is divided by the estimated preinjury diameter. A descriptive way of describing a significant glenoid defect, as written by Lo and Burkhart, is to refer to it as an "inverted-pear" shape when viewed arthroscopically from a superior-to-inferior perspective.[17]

The general accepted numerical value for glenoid bone loss is a lesion spanning greater than 25% of the glenoid surface area. However, Gottschalk et al. conducted a systematic review recently and found that 44.7% of the recurrently unstable shoulders studied had glenoid bone loss between 5% and 20%.[18] This means that a large number of shoulders in the past may have been overlooked for potential surgical glenoid augmentation.

SURGICAL MANAGEMENT

There are several different surgical procedures to stabilize the shoulder, and the correct choice of procedure for each specific patient remains a polarizing topic in the literature. The most common debate in shoulder stabilization surgery is the comparison of the efficacy of arthroscopic and open procedures. In the 1900s and early 2000s, open procedures were thought to be the "gold" standard,[14,19] but now there is proof in the literature that there are many cases where arthroscopy offers its own advantages.[20,21]

Arthroscopic Bankart repair is an extremely successful technique for treating soft tissue injuries in the shoulder in conjunction with minimal to zero glenoid bone loss. However, when the glenoid presents a bony defect encompassing 20%–25% of the diameter of the inferior glenoid, the osseous defect must be addressed for a successful surgical outcome.[20,22,23] This is because progressive anteroinferior bone loss leads to an increased mean contact pressure and peak pressure. The neglect of the bone loss by performing solely a soft tissue Bankart repair would lead to the bone–soft tissue repair interface having to resist the extra overload, leading to a greater likelihood of repair failure.[23]

LATARJET

One of the most common and effective methods of treating shoulder instability with glenoid bone loss is the Latarjet procedure (Fig. 8.2). The Latarjet is a nonanatomic procedure involving the transfer of the horizontal limb of the coracoid process along with

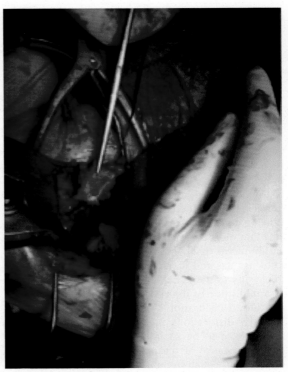

FIG. 8.2 Image of coracoid postharvesting before fixation as part of the Latarjet procedure.

the conjoint tendon to the anterior glenoid rim.[24] The traditional open procedure, which was originally proposed by Latarjet in 1954, is a successful treatment option that has been the standard for the past several decades.[25] However, in 2010, Lafosse and Boyle presented a study that aimed to conduct the Latarjet arthroscopically in order to gain the advantage of minimally invasive surgery. They operated on 100 shoulders, and outcomes revealed 91% excellent scores and 9% good scores.[26] The one limitation of this technique is it is very challenging and places several neurovascular structures at risk. Dumont et al. reported the first long-term (>5 years) results of the arthroscopic Latarjet procedure. They reported results on 64 shoulders with a mean follow-up time of 76.4 months, and they found zero true dislocations and one patient with a subluxation event.[27]

With the fairly recent advent of the arthroscopic Latarjet, there has been debate as to which technique, open or arthroscopic, is the superior method. This year Zhu and colleagues released a comparison study that included 44 patients in the open group and 46 patients in the arthroscopic group. At the final follow-up, they found all of the clinical measurements (American Shoulder and Elbow Surgeons [ASES] score, Rowe score, and range of motion [ROM]) to have no significant differences.[28] Another study by Marion et al. produced similar results in a study with 22 open and 36 arthroscopic Latarjet procedures showing that clinical outcomes between open and arthroscopic procedures were comparable after 2 years' follow-up. However, the arthroscopic procedure caused significantly less pain for the patients.[29] Both methods are viable and successful options today, so the operative decision lies in the surgeon's hands.

A new study, by Ersen et al., came out comparing the subscapularis split and subscapularis tenotomy techniques in a Latarjet procedure. They found the internal rotation durability to be significantly higher in the split group ($P=.045$) than the tenotomy group.[30] Therefore, when working with the subscapularis during a Latarjet, it should be the preferred method to use the split technique.

ILIAC CREST BONE GRAFT

The Latarjet is a successful technique, but limitations associated with its nonanatomic nature include loss of motion, arthritis, and nonunion.[31-33] An alternative to the Latarjet is the usage of an iliac crest bone graft (ICBG) to resurface the glenoid defect. Before conducting an ICBG procedure, the doctor must select to use either an allograft or autograft. An allograft is beneficial because it removes the donor-site morbidity from autogenous reconstructions and complications associated with pain and sensory disturbances.[31,34] On the other hand, an autograft has advantages in that it is osteoinductive and immunogenic. The iliac crest is the most common graft site because of easy access and procurement, low morbidity, and large quantities of both cortical and cancellous bone.[34] Warner et al.[35] described a group of 11 patients who underwent open anatomic reconstruction of the anterior glenoid with an iliac crest allograft and none of the patients reported recurrent instability. Mascarenhas et al. conducted a similar study containing 10 patients who experienced open bone graft reconstruction. Overall, the results showed no recurrent dislocations, no hardware failure, and no joint degeneracy.[36] The open method, as shown in the literature, is a highly successful technique in restoring bony glenoid anatomy.

Similar to the evolution of the Latarjet procedure, arthroscopic reconstruction with the iliac crest graft has begun to gain traction. Taverna and his colleagues recently developed an entirely arthroscopic technique without the usage of screws for anatomic glenoid

reconstruction using an iliac crest graft. This technique is important because it lessens the incisions and preserves external rotation, while preventing recurrent instability. The limitation of this procedure is that it does require expert arthroscopic technique and a long learning curve.[37]

The short-term outcomes look very promising, as the procedure has been preventing instability and causing successful union in patients. The one problem is that there has not been any literature published on the long-term outcomes, which is especially problematic because of the potential long-term issues resulting from the allograft.

DISTAL TIBIA ALLOGRAFT

In cases of glenoid bone loss where the Latarjet technique or ICBG are contraindicated or in the revision setting, distal tibial allograft (DTA) is a viable option (Fig. 8.3). DTAs are advantageous in that they provide chondral restoration of the articular surface defect in addition to osseous restoration, avoid donor-site morbidity, and are not as limited in size as coracoid grafts for reconstructing larger areas of bone loss. DTAs are also dense, weight-bearing corticocancellous bone, allowing for screw fixation with less risk of fracture as was reported in Latarjet procedures.[38] In a cadaveric study, DTA was found to have significantly higher glenohumeral contact areas than Latarjet at 60 degrees of abduction and at the abduction with external rotation (ABER) position, as well as significantly lower glenohumeral peak forces than Latarjet reconstruction in the ABER position.[39]

In clinical data, systematic review of 8 studies including 70 shoulders with recurrent anterior instability that were treated with allografts including, iliac crest, femoral head, distal tibia, glenoid, and humeral head, after a mean follow-up of 44.5 months (range 32–90), yielded results that were largely positive, with 93.4% satisfied and a mean final Rowe score of 90.6 (mean improvement of 57.5).[40] Only 9.8% of patients continued to have pain in the shoulder, 7.1% continued to experience instability (dislocation, subluxation, or apprehension), and 2.9% suffered recurrence of glenohumeral dislocation. Bony integration of the graft was achieved in 100% of shoulders without any signs of graft resorption at long-term follow-up.[40] These were excellent results for allografts in general, and the results for DTA specifically are even more encouraging. A separate outcomes study that reported on 27 patients following DTA augmentation of the anterior glenoid with an average follow-up of 45 months (range 30-60) demonstrated significant improvements in ASES score, Western Ontario Shoulder Instability (WOSI) index, and

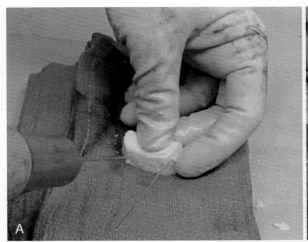 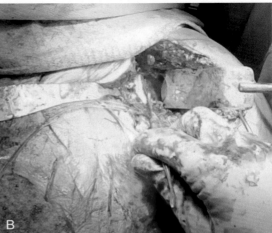

FIG. 8.3 **(A)** Distal tibial allograft having Kirschner wires inserted for provisional fixation to the glenoid defect after preparation. **(B)** Distal tibial allograft after final fixation.

Single Assessment Numerical Evaluation (SANE) score. There were no significant differences in ROM between the affected and nonaffected shoulders in any direction, and there were no signs of apprehension or cases of recurrent instability in any patients at final follow-up. Computed tomography (CT) data showed an allograft healing rate of 89% (range, 80%–100%), average allograft angle of 14.9 (range, 6.6 to 29.3), and average allograft lysis of 3% (range, 0%–25%). Notably, grafts with lesser allograft angles showed superior healing, demonstrating that optimal allograft placement results in superior bony incorporation with the native glenoid.[41] Further investigation is necessary to prove DTA efficacy in larger populations and for longer term follow-up, but initial data are promising.

HILL–SACHS LESIONS

The Hill–Sachs lesion is a compression fracture of the posterosuperolateral aspect of the humeral head that occurs when it comes into contact with the dense cortical bone of the anterior glenoid.[8] Throughout the literature, it has been noted that Hill–Sachs defects are prevalent in 67%–93% of primary anterior dislocation events and up to 100% prevalent in recurrent shoulder instability.[42–45] Recurrent dislocations are a critical issue because they continuously erode and wear down the anatomic glenohumeral constraints, leading to chronic instability.[8] In addition to wearing down the ligaments, the constant abrasion from the anterior glenoid in a dislocation causes the compression fracture on the humeral head to become larger. A larger Hill–Sachs lesion leads to postoperative recurrent instability because of the articular arc deficit, which causes engagement with the anterior glenoid rim.[46]

Grading or defining a Hill–Sachs lesion is a complex task because of the necessity to view and evaluate many different factors, such as length, depth, surface area, volume, and orientation.[47,48] Consideration of a multitude of factors stems from the hope of finding a valid predictor for when a Hill–Sachs requires surgical intervention. The typical definition of a Hill–Sachs lesion that warrants significance surgically is a bony defect covering 25% of the articular surface.[20,49] However, this percentage can decrease when considering concomitant injuries, such as a Bankart tear or bipolar bone loss.

In terms of orientation, the Hill–Sachs should be considered for surgical treatment if it lies in a position that forces it to interact with the anterior glenoid in a position of athletic function (i.e., 90 degrees of abduction and 90 degrees of external rotation).[14,23] Burkhart and de Beer first described the interaction of the humeral head with the glenoid as either "engaging" or "nonengaging."[14] If the lesion is parallel to the glenoid, it will engage and cause a higher probability of dislocation; if it is diagonal, it will make continuous articular contact and most likely not engage with the rim of the anterior glenoid. Cho et al. noted that engaging lesions are both wider and deeper than nonengaging lesions, showing a correlation between the size of the Hill–Sachs lesion and its engagement.[50]

GLENOID TRACK CONCEPT

The glenoid track was a concept first described by Yamamoto et al. in 2007.[51] They demonstrated the "track" by showing as a cadaveric arm was lifted, the glenoid shifted from the inferomedial to superolateral of the posterior articular surface of the humeral head. They measured the zone of contact to be 84% of the glenoid articular surface barring any glenoid bone loss, and Omori et al. reaffirmed Yamamoto by finding that the track covers 83% of the articular surface in vivo shoulders using 3-D magnetic resonance imaging (MRI).[52] If the lesion extends too far medially over the medial margin of the glenoid, then the risk of dislocation and engagement becomes high. The glenoid track has been known in the orthopaedic community for several years now, but its functional clinical use is just now being proven and explored in the literature.

Gyftopoulos et al.[53] were the first to relate the on-track off-track method to clinical studies by testing its ability to predict engagement during an MRI. They determined the track method to have an overall accuracy rate of 84.2% when predicting engagement during 2D-MR examination. The negative predictive value of the on-track off-track method was 91.1%, which offers reassurance its accuracy. These findings are important for clinicians because preoperative physical examination findings of increased laxity caused by torn anterior capsulolabral structures could lead to false diagnosis of engagement.[54]

Shaha et al. took the knowledge of the glenoid track to new heights in retrospective review of 57 patients who underwent arthroscopic shoulder stabilization surgery.[55] Eight patients (14%) were documented to be off-track, and 49 patients (86%) were on-track. They determined that 75% of the off-track patients experienced recurrent dislocations postoperatively, while only 8% of the on-track patients dislocated postoperatively. In a subanalysis of 30 patients with bipolar bone loss, they found seven patients with failed treatment, and six of the seven patients (86%) were off-track. The last finding presented was that the glenoid track was accurate in 89% of predictions, while using glenoid bone loss (>20%) as a predictor only offered 29% success. This study is critical to clinical practice because it validates the glenoid track, as the superior method of helping to make proper preoperative decisions in preventing recurrent instability.

The glenoid track can also be defined or measured with an expression created by De Giacomo et al.[23] The equation reads as follows: glenoid track width = 0.83D - d, where D is the diameter of the glenoid and d is the amount of glenoid bone loss (posterior radius–anterior radius). Theoretically, this method would allow the surgeon to preoperatively assess whether a Hill–Sachs lesion needs to be surgically addressed, and it has recently been validated using a biomechanical model.[56] However, the work of the likes of Gyftopoulos and Shaha is what has given clinical proof to the algorithm and theory of the glenoid track as being a necessity in clinical practice.

HUMERAL HEAD ALLOGRAFT

Bone augmentation of the humeral head has proven to be successful surgical option in repairing large Hill–Sachs lesions (>25%) without concomitant glenoid bone loss.[57,58] Its success lies in its ability to restore the humeral head articular surface, therefore increasing the surface area for contact with the glenoid and limiting possibilities of engagement. Literature has not been overly extensive on generic osteochondral allograft surgery due to the field's shift to other forms of grafting, such as iliac crest, distal tibia, and talus. One study presented by Diklic et al. in 2010 reported outcomes on 13 patients that had a humeral head lesion covering 25%–50% of the surface area, and they found nine patients to have no pain and zero restriction of activity. They also found zero of the patients to be experiencing recurrent instability at a 54-month follow-up.[59] Riff et al. also conducted osteochondral allograft reconstruction of the humeral head on nine patients and each patient was satisfied with the result and would undergo the procedure again. They concluded that allograft reconstruction is a viable and durable treatment option, especially in isolated cases of humeral head defects.[60]

In early literature, humeral head allograft procedures were done with an open procedure that was highly invasive (Fig. 8.4). In 2013, Snir and his colleagues advanced the technique by developing a purely arthroscopic approach to reconstructing a Hill–Sachs lesion with an osteochondral allograft procedure.[61] If the surgeon gets an accurate approximation of the allograft plugs, then it allows restoration of the articular surface and joint biomechanics while maintaining range of motion. In a systematic review covering 12 studies and 35 patients, Saltzman et al. showed that the allograft transplantation actually improved the range of motion (i.e., forward flexion and external rotation) and also ASES by 14 points ($P = .02$).[62] When considering other procedures, such as a remplissage or reduction, take into consideration that this technique has been shown to restore joint biomechanics in a superior fashion.[49,63]

OSTEOCHONDRAL TALUS ALLOGRAFT

Although the remplissage procedure is a viable treatment option, the resulting loss of external rotation has been

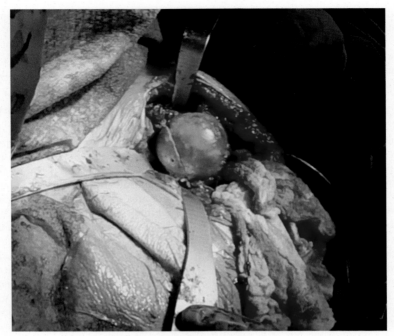

FIG. 8.4 Humeral head allograft to treat a Hill–Sachs lesion.

noted as a concern, especially in throwing athletes.[23,24] Although reconstruction through use of a humeral head allograft has been described as effective for treatment of Hill–Sachs lesions, the graft has limited accessibility and requires more precise size matching. The cartilaginous surface of the talus allograft provides for better articular contact with the glenoid bone (Fig. 8.5). The dense quality of the subchondral bone allows for more stable fixation of the graft to the humeral head. The more consistent size matching is advantageous, allowing for wider application to more patients. Talus allograft reconstruction of a reverse Hill–Sachs defect is associated with some disadvantages. There is limited availability of allografts in some regions of the world. The theoretical risk of nonunion between the humeral head and talus allograft is an additional concern; therefore, platelet-rich plasma (PRP) is used to enhance biological factors to potentially promote bony union. Future long-term studies are needed to assess the clinical efficacy of this technique.

ROLE OF PLATELET-RICH PLASMA

Platelet-rich plasma (PRP), also known as autologous conditioned plasma (ACP), is being used in an expanding range of applications. Being a blood product, PRP falls under the prevue of Food and Drug Administration's (FDA's) Center for Biologics Evaluation and Research and is regulated by the FDA's 21 CFR 1271 of the Code of Regulations. In other words, PRP is exempt from the FDA's traditional regulatory pathway owing to the 510(k) application, which allows devices that are "substantially equivalent" to a currently marketed device to come to the market. FDA 510(k) clearance allows for platelet-rich preparation production for use with bone graft materials to enhance bone graft handling properties in orthopaedic practices.[64] The elevated platelet count in PRP has been suggested in studies as necessary to stimulate targeted injured cells to proliferate.[64,65] However in an animal model study, increased platelet concentration beyond the physiologic concentration was not found to significantly improve functional graft healing.[66] Local growth factors in PRP are thought to modify the inflammatory response, which in turn may affect cell proliferation and differentiation.[67] Randomized controlled trials on the subject thus far have been virtually exclusive in investigating PRP's efficacy in the context of osteoarthritis with varying success.[68–74] In general, the gathering of data has been complicated by the lack of standardization in the preparation and dosing of PRP.[67] This is a problem that has also

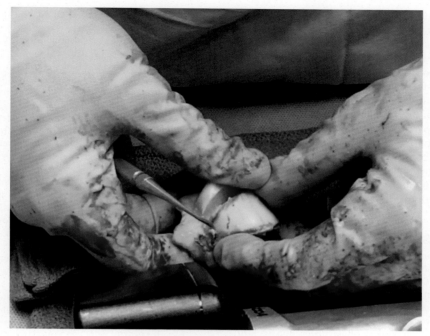

FIG. 8.5 Talus allograft being prepared.

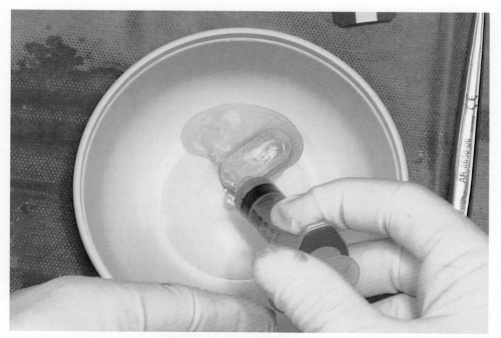

FIG. 8.6 Leukocyte-poor platelet-rich plasma (PRP), also termed autologous conditioned plasma (ACP), used to soak osteochondral allograft with the aim of augmenting healing and minimizing risk of immune rejection.

plagued bone marrow aspirate concentrate (BMAC), also termed bone marrow concentrate (BMC). Additional considerations for validating PRP treatment include finding in which applications leukocyte-rich and leukocyte-poor preparations are most effective, as they have been found to induce distinct effects,[74] as well as determining the threshold where platelet and/or factor concentration switches from being antiinflammatory to paradoxically having a proinflammatory effect as seen in studies comparing single versus double spin preparations.[68] The senior author (MTP) currently employs a leukocyte-poor PRP soak after pulsatile lavage to augment graft union and minimize the risk of graft resorption (Fig. 8.6).

REFERENCES

1. Hantes M, Raoulis V. Arthroscopic findings in anterior shoulder instability. *Open Orthop J.* 2017;11:119–132.
2. Zacchilli MA, Owens BD. Epidemiology of shoulder dislocations presenting to emergency departments in the United States. *J Bone Joint Surg Am Vol.* 2010;92(3):542–549.
3. Leroux T, Wasserstein D, Veillette C, et al. Epidemiology of primary anterior shoulder dislocation requiring closed reduction in Ontario, Canada. *Am J Sports Med.* 2014;42(2):442–450.
4. Karataglis D, Agathangelidis F. Long term outcomes of arthroscopic shoulder instability surgery. *Open Orthop J.* 2017;11:133–139.
5. Chalidis B, Sachinis N, Dimitriou C, Papadopoulos P, Samoladas E, Pournaras J. Has the management of shoulder dislocation changed over time? *Int Orthop.* 2007;31(3):385–389.
6. Chong M, Karataglis D, Learmonth D. Survey of the management of acute traumatic first-time anterior shoulder dislocation among trauma clinicians in the UK. *Ann R Coll Surg Engl.* 2006;88(5):454–458.
7. Robinson CM, Howes J, Murdoch H, Will E, Graham C. Functional outcome and risk of recurrent instability after primary traumatic anterior shoulder dislocation in young patients. *J Bone Joint Surg Am Vol.* 2006;88(11):2326–2336.
8. Provencher MT, Frank RM, Leclere LE, et al. The Hill-Sachs lesion: diagnosis, classification, and management. *J Am Acad Orthop Surg.* 2012;20(4):242–252.
9. Ramhamadany E, Modi CS. Current concepts in the management of recurrent anterior gleno-humeral joint instability with bone loss. *World J Orthop.* 2016;7(6):343–354.
10. Horst K, Von Harten R, Weber C, et al. Assessment of coincidence and defect sizes in Bankart and Hill-Sachs lesions after anterior shoulder dislocation: a radiological study. *Br J Radiol.* 2014;87(1034):20130673.
11. Gill TJ, Micheli LJ, Gebhard F, Binder C. Bankart repair for anterior instability of the shoulder. Long-term outcome. *J Bone Joint Surg Am Vol.* 1997;79(6):850–857.
12. Provencher MT, Bhatia S, Ghodadra NS, et al. Recurrent shoulder instability: current concepts for evaluation and management of glenoid bone loss. *J Bone Joint Surg Am Vol.* 2010;92(suppl 2):133–151.
13. Bhatia S, Saigal A, Frank RM, et al. Glenoid diameter is an inaccurate method for percent glenoid bone loss quantification: analysis and techniques for improved accuracy. *Arthroscopy.* 2015;31(4):608–614.e601.
14. Burkhart SS, De Beer JF. Traumatic glenohumeral bone defects and their relationship to failure of arthroscopic Bankart repairs: significance of the inverted-pear glenoid and the humeral engaging Hill-Sachs lesion. *Arthroscopy.* 2000;16(7):677–694.
15. Sugaya H, Moriishi J, Dohi M, Kon Y, Tsuchiya A. Glenoid rim morphology in recurrent anterior glenohumeral instability. *J Bone Joint Surg Am Vol.* 2003;85-A(5):878–884.
16. Baudi P, Righi P, Bolognesi D, et al. How to identify and calculate glenoid bone deficit. *La Chir degli organi Mov.* 2005;90(2):145–152.
17. Lo IK, Parten PM, Burkhart SS. The inverted pear glenoid: an indicator of significant glenoid bone loss. *Arthroscopy.* 2004;20(2):169–174.
18. Gottschalk LJ, Bois AJ, Shelby MA, Miniaci A, Jones MH. Mean glenoid defect size and location associated with anterior shoulder instability: a systematic review. *Orthop J Sports Med.* 2017;5(1):2325967116676269.
19. Kandziora F, Jager A, Bischof F, Herresthal J, Starker M, Mittlmeier T. Arthroscopic labrum refixation for posttraumatic anterior shoulder instability: suture anchor versus transglenoid fixation technique. *Arthroscopy.* 2000;16(4):359–366.
20. Garcia GH, Liu JN, Dines DM, Dines JS. Effect of bone loss in anterior shoulder instability. *World J Orthop.* 2015;6(5):421–433.
21. Archetti Netto N, Tamaoki MJ, Lenza M, et al. Treatment of Bankart lesions in traumatic anterior instability of the shoulder: a randomized controlled trial comparing arthroscopy and open techniques. *Arthroscopy.* 2012;28(7):900–908.
22. Porcellini G, Campi F, Pegreffi F, Castagna A, Paladini P. Predisposing factors for recurrent shoulder dislocation after arthroscopic treatment. *J Bone Joint Surg Am Vol.* 2009;91(11):2537–2542.
23. Di Giacomo G, De Vita A, Costantini A, de Gasperis N, Scarso P. Management of humeral head deficiencies and glenoid track. *Curr Rev Musculoskeletal Med.* 2014;7(1):6–11.
24. Boffano M, Mortera S, Piana R. Management of the first episode of traumatic shoulder dislocation. *EFORT Open Rev.* 2017;2(2):35–40.
25. Latarjet M. Treatment of recurrent dislocation of the shoulder. *Lyon Chirurgical.* 1954;49(8):994–997.
26. Lafosse L, Boyle S. Arthroscopic latarjet procedure. *J Shoulder Elbow Surg.* 2010;19(suppl 2):2–12.
27. Dumont GD, Fogerty S, Rosso C, Lafosse L. The arthroscopic latarjet procedure for anterior shoulder instability: 5-year minimum follow-up. *Am J Sports Med.* 2014;42(11):2560–2566.

28. Zhu Y, Jiang C, Song G. Arthroscopic versus open latarjet in the treatment of recurrent anterior shoulder dislocation with marked glenoid bone loss: a prospective comparative study. *Am J Sports Med*. 2017;45(7):1645–1653.
29. Marion B, Klouche S, Deranlot J, Bauer T, Nourissat G, Hardy P. A prospective comparative study of arthroscopic versus mini-open latarjet procedure with a minimum 2-year follow-up. *Arthroscopy*. 2017;33(2):269–277.
30. Ersen A, Birisik F, Ozben H, et al. Latarjet procedure using subscapularis split approach offers better rotational endurance than partial tenotomy for anterior shoulder instability. *Knee Surg Sports Traumatol Arthrosc*. 2017.
31. Young DC, Rockwood Jr CA. Complications of a failed Bristow procedure and their management. *J Bone Joint Surg Am Vol*. 1991;73(7):969–981.
32. Hovelius L, Sandstrom B, Sundgren K, Saebo M. One hundred eighteen Bristow-Latarjet repairs for recurrent anterior dislocation of the shoulder prospectively followed for fifteen years: study I–clinical results. *J Shoulder Elbow Surg*. 2004;13(5):509–516.
33. Nielson AB, Nielsen K. The modified Bristow procedure for recurrent anterior dislocation of the shoulder. Results and complications. *Acta Orthop Scand*. 1982;53(2):229–232.
34. Ahlmann E, Patzakis M, Roidis N, Shepherd L, Holtom P. Comparison of anterior and posterior iliac crest bone grafts in terms of harvest-site morbidity and functional outcomes. *J Bone Joint Surg Am Vol*. 2002;84-A(5):716–720.
35. Warner JJ, Gill TJ, O'Hollerhan JD, Pathare N, Millett PJ. Anatomical glenoid reconstruction for recurrent anterior glenohumeral instability with glenoid deficiency using an autogenous tricortical iliac crest bone graft. *Am J Sports Med*. 2006;34(2):205–212.
36. Mascarenhas R, Raleigh E, McRae S, Leiter J, Saltzman B, MacDonald PB. Iliac crest allograft glenoid reconstruction for recurrent anterior shoulder instability in athletes: surgical technique and results. *Int J Shoulder Surg*. 2014;8(4):127–132.
37. Taverna E, D'Ambrosi R, Perfetti C, Garavaglia G. Arthroscopic bone graft procedure for anterior inferior glenohumeral instability. *Arthrosc Tech*. 2014;3(6):e653–e660.
38. Provencher MT, Ghodadra N, LeClere L, Solomon DJ, Romeo AA. Anatomic osteochondral glenoid reconstruction for recurrent glenohumeral instability with glenoid deficiency using a distal tibia allograft. *Arthroscopy*. 2009;25(4):446–452.
39. Bhatia S, Van Thiel GS, Gupta D, et al. Comparison of glenohumeral contact pressures and contact areas after glenoid reconstruction with latarjet or distal tibial osteochondral allografts. *Am J Sports Med*. 2013;41(8):1900–1908.
40. Sayegh ET, Mascarenhas R, Chalmers PN, Cole BJ, Verma NN, Romeo AA. Allograft reconstruction for glenoid bone loss in glenohumeral instability: a systematic review. *Arthroscopy*. 2014;30(12):1642–1649.
41. Provencher MT, Frank RM, Golijanin P, et al. Distal tibia allograft glenoid reconstruction in recurrent anterior shoulder instability: clinical and radiographic outcomes. *Arthroscopy*. 2017;33(5):891–897.
42. Rowe CR, Zarins B, Ciullo JV. Recurrent anterior dislocation of the shoulder after surgical repair. Apparent causes of failure and treatment. *J Bone Joint Surg Am Vol*. 1984;66(2):159–168.
43. Widjaja AB, Tran A, Bailey M, Proper S. Correlation between Bankart and Hill-Sachs lesions in anterior shoulder dislocation. *ANZ J Surg*. 2006;76(6):436–438.
44. Yiannakopoulos CK, Mataragas E, Antonogiannakis E. A comparison of the spectrum of intra-articular lesions in acute and chronic anterior shoulder instability. *Arthroscopy*. 2007;23(9):985–990.
45. Welsh MF, Willing RT, Giles JW, Athwal GS, Johnson JA. A rigid body model for the assessment of glenohumeral joint mechanics: Influence of osseous defects on range of motion and dislocation. *J Biomech*. 2016;49(4):514–519.
46. Boileau P, Villalba M, Hery JY, Balg F, Ahrens P, Neyton L. Risk factors for recurrence of shoulder instability after arthroscopic Bankart repair. *J Bone Joint Surg Am Vol*. 2006;88(8):1755–1763.
47. Kurokawa D, Yamamoto N, Nagamoto H, et al. The prevalence of a large Hill-Sachs lesion that needs to be treated. *J Shoulder Elbow Surg*. 2013;22(9):1285–1289.
48. Kaar SG, Fening SD, Jones MH, Colbrunn RW, Miniaci A. Effect of humeral head defect size on glenohumeral stability: a cadaveric study of simulated Hill-Sachs defects. *Am J Sports Med*. 2010;38(3):594–599.
49. Sekiya JK, Wickwire AC, Stehle JH, Debski RE. Hill-Sachs defects and repair using osteoarticular allograft transplantation: biomechanical analysis using a joint compression model. *Am J Sports Med*. 2009;37(12):2459–2466.
50. Cho SH, Cho NS, Rhee YG. Preoperative analysis of the Hill-Sachs lesion in anterior shoulder instability: how to predict engagement of the lesion. *Am J Sports Med*. 2011;39(11):2389–2395.
51. Yamamoto N, Itoi E, Abe H, et al. Contact between the glenoid and the humeral head in abduction, external rotation, and horizontal extension: a new concept of glenoid track. *J Shoulder Elbow Surg*. 2007;16(5):649–656.
52. Omori Y, Yamamoto N, Koishi H, et al. Measurement of the glenoid track in vivo as investigated by 3-dimensional motion analysis using open MRI. *Am J Sports Med*. 2014;42(6):1290–1295.
53. Gyftopoulos S, Beltran LS, Bookman J, Rokito A. MRI evaluation of bipolar bone loss using the on-track off-track method: a feasibility study. *AJR Am J Roentgenol*. 2015;205(4):848–852.
54. Kelkar R, Wang VM, Flatow EL, et al. Glenohumeral mechanics: a study of articular geometry, contact, and kinematics. *J Shoulder Elbow Surg*. 2001;10(1):73–84.

55. Shaha JS, Cook JB, Rowles DJ, Bottoni CR, Shaha SH, Tokish JM. Clinical validation of the glenoid track concept in anterior glenohumeral instability. *J Bone Joint Surg Am Vol.* 2016;98(22):1918–1923.

56. Arciero RA, Parrino A, Bernhardson AS, et al. The effect of a combined glenoid and Hill-Sachs defect on glenohumeral stability: a biomechanical cadaveric study using 3-dimensional modeling of 142 patients. *Am J Sports Med.* 2015;43(6):1422–1429.

57. Miniaci A, Gish M. Management of anterior glenohumeral instability associated with large Hill–Sachs defects. *Tech Shoulder Elbow Surg.* 2004;5:170–175.

58. Kropf EJ, Sekiya JK. Osteoarticular allograft transplantation for large humeral head defects in glenohumeral instability. *Arthroscopy.* 2007;23(3):322.e321–e325.

59. Diklic ID, Ganic ZD, Blagojevic ZD, Nho SJ, Romeo AA. Treatment of locked chronic posterior dislocation of the shoulder by reconstruction of the defect in the humeral head with an allograft. *J Bone Joint Surg Br Vol.* 2010;92(1):71–76.

60. Riff AJ, Yanke AB, Shin JJ, Romeo AA, Cole BJ. Midterm results of osteochondral allograft transplantation to the humeral head. *J Shoulder Elbow Surg.* 2017;26(7):e207–e215.

61. Snir N, Wolfson TS, Hamula MJ, Gyftopoulos S, Meislin RJ. Arthroscopic anatomic humeral head reconstruction with osteochondral allograft transplantation for large hillsachs lesions. *Arthrosc Tech.* 2013;2(3):e289–e293.

62. Saltzman BM, Riboh JC, Cole BJ, Yanke AB. Humeral head reconstruction with osteochondral allograft transplantation. *Arthroscopy.* 2015;31(9):1827–1834.

63. Giles JW, Elkinson I, Ferreira LM, et al. Moderate to large engaging Hill-Sachs defects: an in vitro biomechanical comparison of the remplissage procedure, allograft humeral head reconstruction, and partial resurfacing arthroplasty. *J Shoulder Elbow Surg.* 2012;21(9):1142–1151.

64. Beitzel K, Allen D, Apostolakos J, et al. US definitions, current use, and FDA stance on use of platelet-rich plasma in sports medicine. *J Knee Surg.* 2015;28(1):29–34.

65. Rughetti A, Giusti I, D'Ascenzo S, et al. Platelet gel-released supernatant modulates the angiogenic capability of human endothelial cells. *Blood Transfus.* 2008;6(1):12–17.

66. Fleming BC, Proffen BL, Vavken P, Shalvoy MR, Machan JT, Murray MM. Increased platelet concentration does not improve functional graft healing in bio-enhanced ACL reconstruction. *Knee Surg Sports Traumatol Arthrosc.* 2015;23(4):1161–1170.

67. LaPrade RF, Geeslin AG, Murray IR, et al. Biologic treatments for sports injuries II think tank-current concepts, future Research, and barriers to advancement, Part 1: biologics overview, ligament injury. *Tendinopathy Am J Sports Med.* 2016;44(12):3270–3283.

68. Filardo G, Kon E, Pereira Ruiz MT, et al. Platelet-rich plasma intra-articular injections for cartilage degeneration and osteoarthritis: single- versus double-spinning approach. *Knee Surg Sports Traumatol Arthrosc.* 2012;20(10):2082–2091.

69. Kon E, Mandelbaum B, Buda R, et al. Platelet-rich plasma intra-articular injection versus hyaluronic acid viscosupplementation as treatments for cartilage pathology: from early degeneration to osteoarthritis. *Arthroscopy.* 2011;27(11):1490–1501.

70. Filardo G, Di Matteo B, Di Martino A, et al. Platelet-rich plasma intra-articular knee injections show no superiority versus viscosupplementation: a randomized controlled trial. *Am J Sports Med.* 2015;43(7):1575–1582.

71. Cole BJ, Karas V, Hussey K, Pilz K, Fortier LA. Hyaluronic acid versus platelet-rich plasma: a prospective, double-blind randomized controlled trial comparing clinical outcomes and effects on intra-articular biology for the treatment of knee osteoarthritis. *Am J Sports Med.* 2017;45(2):339–346.

72. Cerza F, Carni S, Carcangiu A, et al. Comparison between hyaluronic acid and platelet-rich plasma, intra-articular infiltration in the treatment of gonarthrosis. *Am J Sports Med.* 2012;40(12):2822–2827.

73. Patel S, Dhillon MS, Aggarwal S, Marwaha N, Jain A. Treatment with platelet-rich plasma is more effective than placebo for knee osteoarthritis: a prospective, double-blind, randomized trial. *Am J Sports Med.* 2013;41(2):356–364.

74. Smith PA. Intra-articular autologous conditioned plasma injections provide safe and efficacious treatment for knee osteoarthritis: an FDA-sanctioned, randomized, double-blind, placebo-controlled clinical trial. *Am J Sports Med.* 2016;44(4):884–891.

Preserving the Articulating Surface of the Knee

BRYAN M. SALTZMAN, MD • DAVID R. CHRISTIAN, BS • MICHAEL L. REDONDO, MA, BS • BRIAN J. COLE, MD, MBA

INTRODUCTION

Hyaline articular cartilage plays an integral role in the function of the knee joint. Isolated chondral lesions are incompletely understood, but once damaged, there is very little capacity for spontaneous healing due to intrinsically poor blood supply (Fig. 9.1). Thus, the risk of patient pain, effusions, mechanical symptoms, decreased activity and quality of life, and the possibility of progression to diffuse osteoarthritis (OA) remain a concern.[1,2] Between 30,000 and 100,000 chondral procedures are performed annually in the United States,[3] and an annual incidence growth of 5% has been reported.[4] The lesions are most commonly found in the medial compartment, followed by the patellofemoral compartment,[5] and have been theorized to occur in approximately 12% of the population.[6,7]

Numerous surgical interventions have been developed and refined over the last few decades in an attempt to preserve the articular surface of the knee. Conservative treatment options have more recently focused attention on injectable biologics in an effort to stimulate the body's natural resources and create an intraarticular milieu suitable for healing. Reparative marrow-stimulation techniques–most notably microfracture–can be used at the site of a chondral defect in an attempt to induce fibrocartilage repair tissue formation after penetration of the subchondral bone.[8,9] Restorative cartilage procedures (mosaicplasty, osteochondral allograft/autograft, particulated juvenile cartilage graft, autologous chondrocyte implantation [ACI]), by contrast, replace the native defect site with host or donor articular hyaline cartilage. These latter options have garnered more attention in the last decade as advanced efforts to provide pain relief, alter arthritic progression patterns, and hopefully delay or avoid arthroplasty.[4]

Generally, varying specifications for use exists for each of the aforementioned procedures. However, no unified consensus exists on which cartilage repair or restoration technique exhibits the most successful long-term clinical outcomes. This chapter focuses on the basic science of cartilage structure, discusses the aforementioned surgical and nonsurgical preservation techniques for the articular cartilage of the knee joint, and highlights expected future directions of study in the topic of surface cartilage defect treatment.

BASICS OF CARTILAGE STRUCTURE

Cartilage is present in various parts of the human body and it is categorized into three different types: fibrocartilage, elastic cartilage, and hyaline cartilage. Each type has a unique function, structure, and composition. Hyaline cartilage, also known as articular cartilage, covers the articular surfaces between bones to provide a load-supporting, low-friction interface. This type of cartilage has low cell density and low proliferative activity and is avascular in nature, which makes innate regeneration nearly impossible.

Hyaline cartilage is primarily composed of water, chondrocytes, and an extracellular matrix (ECM). Chondrocytes are the cellular component of this type of cartilage and are highly differentiated cells with low proliferative activity. They are found in low abundance–only 1%–5% of cartilage by volume–but have high metabolic activity because they are responsible for maintaining homeostasis within the elaborate ECM.[10] Mature chondrocytes lack cell–cell interactions and are instead surrounded by a pericellular matrix that extends radially from the cell surface. Chondrocyte function is affected by the surrounding environment including factors such as the compressive load within a joint, a phenomenon referred to as mechanotransduction.[11] The ECM is composed of water and molecules including collagen, proteoglycans, and superficial zone protein. Water is the largest component of articular cartilage, responsible for 70%–80% by weight, and interacts with the extracellular components through its polar molecular structure to provide unique biomechanical properties.[10]

Biologics in Orthopaedic Surgery. https://doi.org/10.1016/B978-0-323-55140-3.00009-6

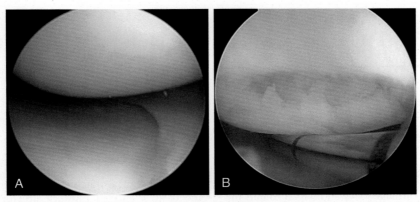

FIG. 9.1 **Articular Cartilage.** (A) Intraoperative arthroscopic images of healthy, normal knee cartilage of the femur (superior) and tibia (inferior) with normal meniscus visible (right) compared with (B) International Cartilage Restoration Society (ICRS) grade IV focal chondral defect of the femoral condyle.

There are more than 28 types of collagen identified within the human body. Type II collagen is the most prevalent type within hyaline cartilage and comprises approximately 50% of its dry weight. It is also a major component of the ECM. All types of collagen share a central core composed mostly of glycine, proline, and hydroxyproline causing the formation of a left-handed helix.[12] These individual helices further assemble into right-handed triple helix microfibrils that form larger fibrils through end-to-end fusion and lateral bundling.[12] These collagen fibrils are then arranged in different orientations in relation to the articular surface depending on their depth within the hyaline cartilage structure, and they provide stiffness to the tissue allowing it to bear weight.

The articular cartilage ECM also contains other molecules, the most prevalent of which are proteoglycans consisting of a protein core and many polysaccharides (primarily glycosaminoglycans [GAGs]) extending perpendicularly. GAGs are linear polysaccharides composed of repeating disaccharide units. The most common GAGs in hyaline cartilage are hyaluronan, dermatan sulfate, keratan sulfate, chondroitin 6-sulfate, and chondroitin 4-sulfate.[10] Hyaluronan is unique in that it is the largest GAG, does not carry a negative charge, and is able to bind strongly with aggrecan–the main proteoglycan found in articular cartilage. The strong binding between hyaluronan and aggrecan results in the formation of large proteoglycan aggregates, and a fixed negative charge within the ECM causes a significant osmotic pressure in the cartilage's interaction with synovial fluid.[10] The end result is significant accumulation of fluid and swelling, known as

the Donnan effect, that works with the collagen structure to produce the weight-bearing capability of articular cartilage.[13]

Synovial fluid directly plays an important role in maintaining the articular cartilage. Synovial fluid is composed of protein-rich plasma ultrafiltrate and hyaluronan.[10] As cartilage is avascular, the synovial fluid is responsible for providing nutrients through simple diffusion and compression–relaxation cycles during weight-bearing. It also contains a protein called "superficial zone protein"—or lubricin—which is also present on the surface of hyaline cartilage and contributes to the lubrication and ease of joint movement.[10] Additionally, synovial fluid contributes to the load-bearing capacity by increasing its viscosity in response to pressure.

Articular cartilage is divided based on depth and composition into four structural zones: the superficial zone, the middle or transitional zone, the deep or radial zone, and the calcified zone.[10] The outermost layer of cartilage is covered by the *lamina splendens*, which is a layer of proteins thought to be produced by the accumulation of proteins from synovial fluid that acts as a protective, low-friction layer for the cartilage.[14] Immediately deep to that is the superficial layer of cartilage, which is densely packed with collagen fibers oriented parallel to the articulating surface and with a low concentration of proteoglycans.[10] Chondrocytes in the superficial layer are flat in shape and also oriented parallel to the articulating surface. They produce proteins to lubricate the articular surface such as lubricin, which are not present in deeper zones.[10] The middle zone is responsible for 40%–60% of cartilage thickness and has the highest concentration of proteoglycans. It has low cellular density, and its most prevalent ECM component is type II collagen arranged in arches.[15] The chondrocytes here are round and produce a large amount of type II collagen and proteoglycans, specifically aggrecan. The deep zone has a lower cell density than the superficial or middle zones and contains type II collagen fibers oriented perpendicular to both the subchondral bone and articular surface. The chondrocytes in the deep zone appear elongated and are oriented parallel to the collagen fibers.[10] Finally, the calcified zone contains hydroxyapatite and acts as a transitional zone between the cartilage and subchondral bone.[10]

Injury to the articular surface can occur secondary to trauma of the joint causing disruption of the cartilage and formation of a focal chondral defect. The deeper cartilage layers, or possibly the subchondral bone, become exposed leading to pain, stiffness, and loss of function. If left untreated, focal chondral defects can progress to OA over time due to further degeneration of the surrounding cartilage. OA is caused by a combination of degenerative and abnormal remodeling processes within the cartilage in response to repetitive stress. Cartilage has low proliferative capacity making these processes nearly irreversible. Changes in the ECM begin in the superficial zone with the appearance of erosions, fissures, and fibrillation. The disruption of the collagen network results in a loss of proteoglycans that eventually inhibits its biomechanical function. The innate type II cartilage shows decreased fiber diameter while the type I cartilage concentration increases, representing the formation of fibrocartilage. Fragmentation continues until the subchondral bone becomes exposed, which allows direct force to be applied to the bone causing remodeling and thickening. Chondrocytes also undergo a series of changes during the development of OA including proliferation and pericellular matrix remodeling.[10] Eventually, the chondrocytes die and release necrosis factors that induce apoptosis of surrounding chondrocytes. This leads to further degradation of the cartilage structure and eventual exposure of the subchondral bone.

ORTHOBIOLOGIC INJECTIONS
Hyaluronic Acid

Hyaluronic acid (HA) is naturally present throughout the human body but specifically is found within articular cartilage and synovial fluid. As OA progresses, the synovial fluid shifts toward lower-molecular-weight HA, leading to a decrease in its viscoelastic properties. Lower-molecular-weight HA is also strongly associated with higher levels of pain. Intraarticular HA injections have been used for many years as a treatment for OA directed at replenishing the concentration of HA and increasing the average molecular weight.

Intraarticular HA injections are most commonly believed to reduce symptoms of OA through mechanisms of chondroprotection.[16] Within the joint, HA binds to cluster of differentiation 44 (CD44) and inhibits the expression of interleukin (IL)-1β, consequently inhibiting the synthesis of matrix metalloproteinases that have catabolic enzymatic activity toward collagen fibers causing the destruction of articular cartilage. The HA-CD44 binding pathway also augments chondroprotection through decreased apoptosis of chondrocytes, allowing preserved synthesis of the cartilage ECM and slowed degeneration. The current literature suggests that higher-molecular-weight HA is more effective at inducing these mechanisms of chondroprotection than lower-molecular-weight HA.[16] Additionally, intraarticular HA injections have been shown to increase the synthesis and impair the degradation of aggrecan, thus slowing the progression of OA. Many studies have also suggested an antiinflammatory effect through decreased synthesis of IL-8, IL-6, prostaglandin-E_2 (PGE_2), and tumor necrosis factor-α (TNFα), in addition to the decrease in IL-1β. Some studies suggest a mechanical mechanism of action by increasing the viscosity of synovial fluid, which provides increased lubrication of the articular surface, and shock absorption.[16] Few studies have reported that HA decreases the extent of subchondral bone changes in addition to functioning as an analgesic.

Intraarticular HA injections have shown variable outcomes in the current medical literature. Several studies and metaanalyses report statistically significant improvement in pain and function scores in patients with OA receiving HA injections while others suggest no difference between treatment and placebo. Also highly debated is whether the observed statistical difference is clinically relevant, as often times it has not exceeded the minimum clinically important difference (MCID).[17] The efficacy of high-molecular-weight HA versus low-molecular-weight HA for treatment of OA has been discussed with some reports suggesting improved pain reduction with high-molecular-weight HA while others report no difference at all. While these studies have investigated the short-term benefit, recent literature suggests no difference in time to knee surgery or arthroplasty in patients receiving low-, medium-, or high-molecular-weight HA.[18] Owing to the variable results in the medical literature, the current American Academy of Orthopaedic Surgeons (AAOS) guidelines

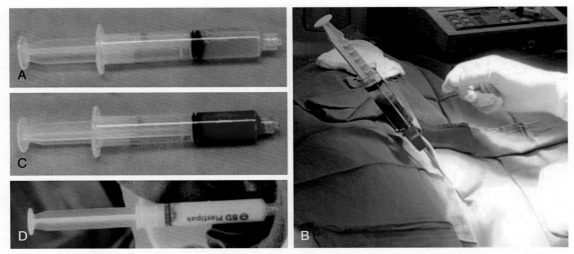

FIG. 9.2 **Orthobiologic Injections.** (A) 10 cc syringe containing approximately 5 cc of platelet-rich plasma (PRP) isolated from a venous blood sample. (B) Bone marrow aspiration from the right iliac crest. (C) 10 cc syringe containing approximately 5 cc of bone marrow aspirate concentrate (BMAC) prepared after centrifugation of bone marrow aspirate (BMA). (D) 10 cc syringe containing approximately 8 cc of adipose tissue and adipose-derived stem cell prepared from adipose tissue collected during liposuction.

state that a recommendation cannot be made for the use of intraarticular HA injections for OA.

Platelet-Rich Plasma

Platelet-rich plasma (PRP) is plasma containing supraphysiologic levels of platelets and platelet-derived growth factors used as a therapeutic modality for treatment of symptomatic cartilage defects and OA. PRP is produced from a patient's venous blood that has been centrifuged to isolate the platelets, plasma, and growth factors (Fig. 9.2). Platelets produce α granules, which contain many growth factors including transforming growth factor-β (TGF-β), fibroblast growth factor (FGF), and platelet-derived growth factor (PDGF).[19] These growth factors have been found to be involved in tissue repair, and the goal is that PRP injections in theory could contribute to cartilage regeneration.

Recent in vitro and in vivo studies have shown that PRP functions by inducing cartilage regeneration and decreasing inflammation. Chondrocytes treated in vitro with PRP have shown increased proliferation and increased synthesis of type II collagen and GAGs.[20] Additionally, in vitro studies have shown that PRP inhibits nuclear factor-κB (NF-κB), which is a transcription factor for the expression of proinflammatory and catabolic cytokines IL-1β and

TNFα.[20] In vivo, synovial fluid samples aspirated at 12 and 24 months after PRP injections trended toward decreased levels of IL-1β and TNFα, although the difference compared with treatment with HA was not statistically significant.[21]

The existing literature varies in terms of PRP preparation technique, platelet concentration, white blood cell concentration, amount injected into the joint, and presence of an activating agent such as calcium chloride. The therapeutic range for platelet concentration is thought to be between two and six times higher than physiologic levels.[20] A recent systematic review of six level I studies found significant improvement in clinical outcomes and Western Ontario and McMaster Universities Osteoarthritis Index (WOMAC) scores on OA patients treated with PRP when compared with HA at 3–12 months after injection.[22] Very few studies have investigated outcomes past 1 year, but the available data suggest a decline in outcomes between 1 and 2 years after injection.[20] The nuances of ideal PRP preparation to help maximize efficacy have begun to be elucidated in recent years, however. A systematic review of nine level I and level II studies that differentiated between leukocyte-rich and leukocyte-poor PRP found significant improvement in OA patients treated with leukocyte-poor PRP compared with HA or placebo but not with leukocyte-rich PRP. These data support the need for standardization of PRP preparations in order to maximize efficacy in all patients.[23]

Bone Marrow–Derived Stem Cells

Mesenchymal stem cells (MSCs) have been of great interest for use in cartilage restoration and repair owing to their inherent regenerative potential. Bone marrow aspiration (BMA) has become one of the preferred techniques of acquiring MSCs, but stem cells only account for 0.001%–0.01% of nucleated cells in bone marrow.[24] It is typically concentrated, usually through centrifugation, to produce bone marrow aspirate concentrate (BMAC) with higher concentrations of MSCs. Once concentrated, BMAC is then injected into the joint of interest either as an isolated treatment or augmentation to surgical treatment.

In addition to MSCs, bone marrow also contains high levels of growth factors and cytokines including vascular endothelial growth factor (VEGF), PDGF, TGF-β, and bone morphogenic protein 2 and 7 (BMP-2, BMP-7), which are known to have anabolic and antiinflammatory effects.[25] Although PRP contains these same growth factors, BMAC has significantly higher concentrations.[26] This mixture of growth factors has been identified to play a variety of roles in the cartilage regeneration capabilities of BMAC. VEGF and PDGF both promote angiogenesis, which increases the blood supply to the subchondral bone and normally avascular cartilage to promote regeneration.[26] TGF-β and BMP both play a role in the chondrogenic differentiation of MSCs, which then synthesize type II collagen and GAGs.[26] Collectively, the MSCs and accompanying molecules promote cartilage regeneration at the articular surface.

The results of intraarticular BMAC joint injections are promising both as an isolated treatment and as augmentation to procedures such as osteochondral collagen scaffolds. When compared with matrix induced chondrocyte implantation (MACI) for patellofemoral chondral lesions, significant improvement was seen in both groups, but MACI outcomes declined between years 1 and 2 whereas BMAC outcomes continued to improve.[27] Additionally, chondral lesions treated with BMAC showed complete coverage in 80% of patients.[25] When used in conjunction with collagen scaffolds to treat chondral defects, the repaired lesions showed better tissue similarity to surrounding hyaline cartilage by both magnetic resonance imaging (MRI) and histology compared with controls.[25,28] As a whole, the existing literature suggests that the treatment of chondral lesions with MSCs in BMAC provides good outcomes as either an isolated or combined treatment.

Adipose-Derived Mesenchymal Stem Cells

Adipose tissue also contains MSCs termed adipose-derived mesenchymal stem cells (ASCs), which were first described in 2001.[29] These cells have been found to have endodermal, mesodermal, and ectodermal proliferative potential, making them a great candidate to aid in cartilage restoration. ASCs are obtained via liposuction, and the adipose sample is then purified to isolate the stem cells. The stem cell concentration has typically been found to be significantly higher than that of BMAC.[29]

Similar to both PRP and BMAC, ASCs have been shown in vitro and in animal studies to have antiinflammatory and chondroprotective characteristics.[30,31] The exact mechanism has not been elucidated, but they appear to be activated by inflammation and in part modulate inflammation and cartilage remodeling through prostaglandin E2 (PGE$_2$).[30,31] The initial results of treating chondral defects with ASCs have been promising in relation to both clinical symptoms and lesion appearance. The first randomized control trial performed by Jo et al. found that intraarticular ASC injections in OA patients provide significant clinical improvement and cartilage regeneration observed by both MRI and second-look arthroscopy.[32] There also appears to be a dose-dependent effect for ASCs that will be critical, as its preparation becomes standardized.[33] Further investigation is needed to determine the long-term outcomes, but intraarticular ASCs provide a promising therapeutic avenue for symptomatic chondral lesions and OA.

MARROW STIMULATION/MICROFRACTURE

Microfracture (MFx) is a common surgical procedure used in the treatment of focal chondral defects of the knee (Fig. 9.3). The technique relies on marrow stimulation from the subchondral bone allowing the recruitment of MSCs for the formation of fibrocartilage repair.[34] However, the outcomes of MFx surgery have been variable. Short-term clinical outcomes (<24 months) for MFx surgeries have been shown to have a high efficacy for small chondral lesions regardless of whether traumatic or degenerative etiology.[35,36] A seminal systematic review including 3122 patients by Mithoefer et al. demonstrated that the average knee function scores remained above the preoperative level and that the short-term clinical improvement rate of MFx surgeries was 75%–100%.[37]

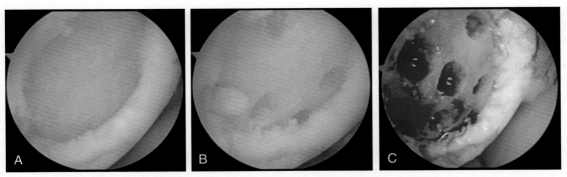

FIG. 9.3 **Microfracture Surgery.** Intraoperative arthroscopic photographs of a right knee medial femoral condyle focal chondral defect (A) treated with mircofracture surgery (B), (C).

However, these same authors also demonstrated that the long-term outcomes of MFx showed reduced durability over time. After 24 months postoperatively, 47%–80% of MFx patients reported functional decline from their original improvements.[37] Moreover, 67%–86% of subjects reported a decline in long-term improvement rate after 24 months.[37] In another review by Steinwachs et al., this decline in long-term clinical outcomes occurred even sooner (18 months postoperatively) in older patients and in patients with larger defects (>2.5 cm²).[38]

Long-term outcomes in high activity level patients, such as athletes, have also been questionable. A prospective study by Gobbi et al. followed athletes in order to measure their improvement after MFx.[39] The participants demonstrated an improved Tegner activity scale at 2 years postoperatively, yet 80% of the athletes in the study progressively declined in sport activity at final follow-up.[39] In two studies following National Basketball Association (NBA) patients who underwent MFx, a significant correlation was observed between MFx and decreased minutes per game, decreased player efficiency rating, or points per game.[40,41] More importantly, 21% of the NBA players treated with MFx did not return to professional competition in the NBA.[40] The predominant causal factors for poor long-term clinical outcome include inadequate clot stability and the concept that fibrocartilage is not the ideal replacement for defects in the articular cartilage, as it by comparison is soft and has a decreased ability to tolerate with shear stresses. Ultimately, this decreases the longevity and the outcomes seen with the MFx technique.[42]

Recently, new innovations in augmentation strategies for MFx have been developed. A current advancement in MFx augmentation includes fixation of a collagen synthetic matrix over the drilled subchondral bone to act as an exogenous scaffold. The MSCs brought to the surface by MFx drilling interact with the collagen scaffold enhancing clot stability and MSC adhesion, organization, and differentiation into chondrocytes.[42] The collagen-based scaffold's intent is to promote and maintain the chondrocytic phenotype and type II collagen synthesis to ultimately fill the defect with regenerated natural hyaline-like cartilage.[43] These MFx augmentation techniques seek to use potential autologous sources of cartilage regeneration in a fast, one-step, inexpensive procedure.[44]

Most of the collagen scaffold augmentations of MFx provide equal or better short-term clinical outcomes when compared with MFx alone.[44–46] Autologous matrix induced chondrogenesis (AMIC; ChondroGide), the arguably most well-studied collagen scaffold worldwide, uses a collagen type-III/I matrix bilayer matrix to serve as its natural scaffold.[42] AMIC short-term outcomes at follow-up of 1 and 2 years have been demonstrated to be as effective as MFx.[47] In a prospective randomized-controlled study by Anders et al., patients with a mean defect size of 3.4 cm² were randomized and treated either with MFx alone or an AMIC technique.[48] Clinical outcomes (modified Cincinnati and International Cartilage Restoration Society [ICRS] score) were evaluated in 30 patients at 1 year and 27 patients at 2 years postoperatively. Clinical outcomes were significantly improved at 1 and 2 years postoperatively for all techniques used with no statistical difference between the techniques.[48] However, AMIC has also exhibited promise in eliminating the two major weaknesses of MFx: long-term clinical outcomes and the ability to successfully treat larger size defects. The evidence for long-term clinical outcomes for AMIC is sparse, yet promising. A prospective randomized-controlled trial of 47 patients (mean defect size 3.6 ± 1.6 cm²) treated either with MFx or AMIC demonstrated improved outcomes in all cohorts at 2 years postoperatively; however, a significant and progressive score degradation was observed in the MFx group.[49] At that 2-year mark, only 11%–22% of all patients in the study described their knee function as abnormal, while at 5-year follow-up the percentage of MFx patients rose to 66%, whereas the percentage remained stable at 6%–7% for AMIC patients.[49] Additionally, Schiavone et al. displayed a potential future for the use of AMIC in larger articular cartilage defects.[50] The study examined a median defect size of 4.3 cm² (range, 2.9–8 cm²) at median follow-up of 7 years. The results demonstrated a significant improvement from a mean international knee documentation committee (IKDCR) score of 31.7 (±8.9) points preoperatively to 80.6 (±5.3) and a significant improvement in Lysholm test when comparing preoperative score to final follow-up.

MFx and exogenous scaffolds can be further augmented by the use of PRP. Little is currently known about the addition of PRP to collagen graft augmented MFx procedures, but some evidence has shown that PRP can aid in recruitment of bone marrow MSCs from the underlying subchondral bone.[51] BioCartilage (Arthrex Inc., Naples, FL) is a novel technique that combines a dehydrated allograft cartilage ECM scaffold and the addition of PRP.[44] The ECM is made up of type II collagen, proteoglycans, and cartilaginous growth factors, which are components of native articular cartilage.[44] Few peer-reviewed studies on BioCartilage outcomes are available, but in a study by Fortier et al.[43] the authors reported that BioCartilage-treated knee lesions had significantly higher ICRS repair scores when compared with MFx alone at 2, 6, and 13 months postoperatively via repeat arthroscopy in equine models. Furthermore, when histology was examined, BioCartilage-repaired defects had significantly better formation of type II collagen than the control defects.[43] The increase in type II collagen allows hyaline-like cartilage to regenerate within the defect, which is optimal for repair.[43]

CHONDROCYTE IMPLANTATION INDICATIONS AND OUTCOMES

While the aforementioned procedures result in fibrocartilage formation, which has biomechanical characteristics inferior to that of native cartilage, the following cartilage restoration procedures actually replace hyaline cartilage by cell-based implantation or osteochondral grafting, with or without the subchondral bone, using host or donor articular cartilage.[52] These procedures include single-stage (mosaicplasty, osteochondral allograft/autograft, particulated juvenile cartilage graft) and two-stage (ACI) interventions. Not unexpectedly, regardless of technique, those patients who are younger, more active, with shorter preoperative symptom duration, fewer prior cartilage procedures, without concurrent ligamentous or meniscal deficiency, and with smaller isolated defects on the medial femoral condyle have the greatest expectations for superior outcomes.[8] In the evaluation of these often complex patients, the orthopaedic surgeon must perform a thorough history and physical examination. It is necessary to identify the location and duration of symptoms, presence of knee swelling or instability, and a patient's goals of care. Concomitant pathology of the meniscus, ligament(s), or mechanical axis must be addressed in a concurrent or staged fashion in order to provide a biomechanically sound environment for chondrocyte implantation surgery.

Osteochondral Autograft

Osteochondral autograft, also known as osteoarticular transfer system (OATS), includes whole-tissue transfer of cancellous autograft bone, normal subchondral bone tidemark, and mature hyaline articular cartilage, which immediately provides a new, functional chondral surface. This allows for a more rapid rehabilitation than the fibrocartilage maturation process of MFx or the cell-based maturation of ACI.[53] The technology is beneficial in the treatment of full-thickness lesions. Either one single, large plug or multiple smaller plugs (known as mosaicplasty) of osteochondral tissue are transferred from non–weight-bearing areas (i.e., the periphery of the femoral condyles or superolateral/superomedial femoral trochlea) to the site of chondral loss.[54] While osteochondral autografting can be technically difficult, its durability and successful outcomes particularly in high-demand patient populations makes it a popular option in the surgeon's armamentarium.[2] In general, clinical outcomes up to 17 years postoperatively have demonstrated good to excellent results in more than 90% of patients with defects between 1 and 5 cm² in size.[55] However, morbidity including pain and discomfort at the donor/harvest site of the autograft is a concern.[55]

Depending on defect location, size, ability to obtain perpendicular access, and surgeon experience, the lesions can be managed via all-arthroscopic or open techniques.[2] The donor tissue is gathered by positioning the harvesting tool perpendicular to the cartilage surface, impacting to a depth of 10-mm, and removing the intact plug.[56] The recipient site is prepared to accept the donor plug using a corresponding recipient core harvester, curettes, and/or motorized shavers to obtain stable vertical margins. The graft is gently inserted and impacted in a press-fit manner, so it is flush with the native surrounding cartilage. Harvest plugs should be

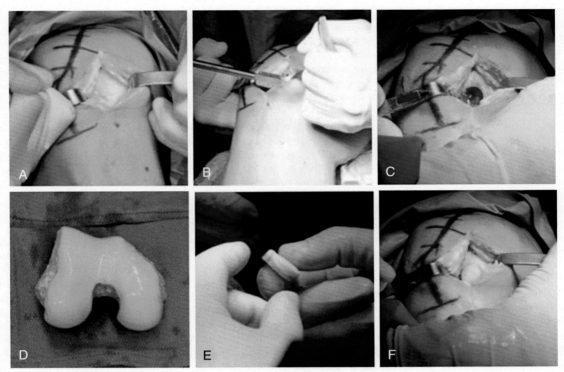

FIG. 9.4 **Osteochondral Allograft.** Intraoperative photographs of a (A) right knee medial medial femoral condyle focal chondral defect being (B) reamed to excise (C) the chondral defect. The (D) allograft tissue is then prepared to create (E) an osteochondral plug that is then (F) implanted to reconstruct the articular surface.

limited to 3–4 cm² in size to avoid donor site morbidity and to allow the donor surface to reconstitute.[56] After osteochondral autograft transplantation, the strongest MRI finding that correlates with clinical outcomes are defect fill and repair tissue structure, highlighting the importance of this reconstitution process.[57] While osteochondral lesions between 1 and 8 cm² have been treatment by this technique, those lesions with <2 cm² are associated with superior outcomes.[54]

Hangody and Fules[58] reported their findings from 597 femoral condyles and 76 tibial plateaus treated by osteochondral autograft mosaicplasty. At up to 10 years postoperatively, 92% of patients undergoing femoral condyle treatment had good or excellent results, with 87% good/excellent findings for those with tibial plateau treatment. Solheim et al.[59] found higher failure rates in patients who were women, over 40 years of age, and with defect size >3 cm² in their evaluation of 73 patients between 5 and 14 years postoperatively. Systematic review of nine studies with 607 patients by Lynch et al.[60] demonstrated significant improvements,

with return to sport as early as 6 months after surgery, and superior results for lesions <2 cm². Pareek et al.[54] systematically reviewed 10 studies with a total of 610 patients (mean defect size, 2.6 cm²) with an average age of 27.0 years at the time of surgery. At a long-term mean 10.2 years' follow-up, 72% of patients demonstrated successful outcomes, and the reoperation rate was 19%. IKDC and Lysholm scores improved significantly, but there was no improvement in Tegner score over the long-term despite a return-to-sport rate of 85%. The authors noted that increased age, greater numbers of previous surgical procedures, and increasing defect size correlated with risk of failure.

Osteochondral Allograft

Osteochondral allograft transplantation allows treatment of chondral lesions that are too large (>2 cm²) to be effectively treated with OATS and can be performed in a single-stage unlike ACI (Fig. 9.4). Plain radiographs are used for sizing purposes to find a matching donor.[61] This allows for transfer of size-matched cartilage and subchondral

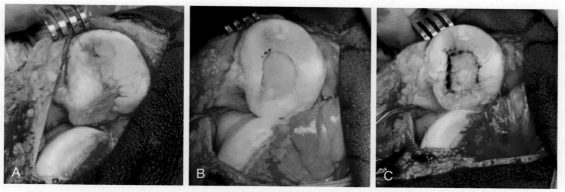

FIG. 9.5 Autologous Chondrocyte Implantation. Intraoperative photographs of a (A) chondral defect of the left patella in which (B) the cartilage defect is debrided and (C) treated with autologous chondrocyte implantation.

bone into osteochondral lesions of the knee. It provides a good salvage option for failed prior cartilage restoration procedures as well.[61] However, concerns with allograft use persist, including the risk for disease transmission, graft availability, technical difficulty, cost, and the long-term viability of cadaver chondrocytes and graft resorption.[56,62] The highest level of chondrocyte viability is seen with fresh osteochondral allografts, with storage times ideally <24 days,[61,63] and while frozen allografts demonstrate lower disease transmission rates, they additionally have inferior biological and biomechanical properties than their fresh allograft counterparts.[64]

Advantages of this technique include the one-step procedure, large defect sizes that can be addressed, salvage ability of the procedure, and restoration of both subchondral bone and surface hyaline cartilage.[65] The highest rates of success are seen with younger patients, normal or corrected malalignment, unipolar lesions, and defects with <1 year of symptomatic duration.[66] Patients younger than 25 years of age with preoperative symptoms <1 year of duration have a higher rate of return to sport following allograft transplantation than their counterparts.[67] Further disadvantages include mismatch of graft contour to the native joint, risk of disease transmission, and graft availability.[65] Negative prognostic factors for osteochondral allograft outcomes include patient age >50 years, 2 + prior surgeries, preoperative symptom duration >1 year, bipolar lesions, limb malalignment, and Workers' Compensation status.[68–70] One of the major limitations of osteochondral allograft may be with patellofemoral lesions, as this technology has not had great success within this compartment of the knee.[71]

Chahal et al.[72] systematically reviewed 19 studies with 644 knees at a mean follow-up of 58 months, which underwent osteochondral allograft transplantation of the knee. Most grafts identified were procured fresh (61%), and the most common indication for transplantation was posttraumatic injury (38%). Nearly half (46%) of patients had concurrent procedures, and the mean defect size was 6.3 cm² across all included studies. The overall failure rate was 18%, but outcomes were overall favorable with high satisfaction rates at this intermediate follow-up. The authors reported superior outcomes in younger patients with unipolar lesions and shorter symptomatic duration. De Caro et al.[73] found similar success for osteochondral allograft in their systematic review, with overall excellent results achieved, improvement in clinical scores, a survivorship rate of 89% at 5 years postoperatively, and a high rate of return to sport. While bony integration was typically achieved, the authors found that cartilage integration was scant or failed to occur, particularly with frozen grafts.

Assenmacher et al.[65] found similar findings with systematic review of long-term outcome studies, where five studies totaling 291 patients demonstrated significant improvement in all clinical outcome scores. At 12.3 years postoperatively, the mean failure rate was 25%, and 72% of these failures were for conversion to arthroplasty. The reoperation rate was 36%. Patellofemoral lesions were associated with decreased clinical improvement and greater reoperation rates.

Autologous Chondrocyte Implantation

ACI works by the induction of hyaline-like cartilage formation, and while it previously had been considered a second-line treatment option, recent evidence suggests that its use as a primary intervention in certain patients is warranted (Fig. 9.5).[74] ACI may be the most appropriate option for young, active patients with a relatively short duration of preoperative symptoms, a large full-thickness surface chondral defect (>4 cm²), and no prior cartilage procedures.[8,75] Ideal candidates also have minimal or no involvement of the subchondral bone.

ACI treatment of focal cartilage defects in the patellofemoral as well as tibiofemoral compartments has evolved tremendously since first being utilized in 1994.[8,76] Increasing generations have incorporated a periosteal cover, a collagen membrane cover, and several three-dimensional scaffolds with varying means of fixation to contain the chondrocytes.[8] The procedure requires two stages: first, autologous chondrocytes are harvested via chondral biopsy samples and are cultured and amplified in vitro. The chondral biopsy is commonly performed at the superolateral edge of the lateral femoral condyle, the superomedial edge of the medial femoral condyle, or the intercondylar notch in order to obtain about 200–300 mg of tissue.[75] Up to 48 million cells can be obtained via standard cell culture means.[75] Secondarily, 3–8 weeks later, these cultured cells are implanted at the focal defect site. The cultured chondrocytes are most commonly implanted via arthrotomy, but all-arthroscopic techniques have been described.[77]

The first-generation procedure included implantation of the cultured chondrocytes under a periosteal patch with resorbable sutures and fibrin glue. The second-generation technique suspends the cultured cells with a membrane of type I/III collagen. Third-generation techniques utilize an ECM chondroinductive/-conductive scaffold to which the cultured cells attach, and this is implanted at the time of surgery.[74] The periosteal graft used to contain the autogenous cells has been a source of required reoperation in order to debride hypertrophic tissue in as may as 50% of cases in some reports.[78] The patellofemoral joint is at particularly high risk for such a complication. Adverse effects of the procedure have included joint stiffness and periosteal hypertrophy requiring revision procedures.[79] The use of a type I/III absorbable collagen membrane in second-generation ACI versus native periosteum in first-generation means has demonstrated a reduction in reoperation rate of 80% for symptomatic graft hypertrophy.[80] Third-generation ACI techniques simplify the procedure and have lower complication rates and superior graft quality than the preceding generations.[81] Second- and third-generation ACI demonstrate accelerated weight-bearing protocols over the first-generation technique.[82] As an additional tool, characterized chondrocyte implantation utilizes a genetic profile marker score to optimize the phenotype of the cultured cartilage tissue.[83]

While ACI has demonstrated significant improvements in large-sized (>4 cm²) full-thickness chondral defects of young adults at short- and mid-term follow-up, less evidence exists for the long-term course in these patients. However, MRI and histologic data suggest that ACI techniques restore nearly native cartilage appearance. The strongest MRI findings after ACI that correlate with clinical outcomes are graft hypertrophy and repair tissue signal.[57]

Long-term outcomes have shown durability of ACI at up to 11 years postoperatively.[84] Systematic review of high-level evidence evaluating ACI[8] suggests that there is a trend for ACI to demonstrate improved outcomes in comparison with MFx, but no conclusion could be made with regards to differences with osteochondral autograft transplantation. Biopsies after ACI continue to show maturation for up to 24 months postoperatively, but the timing of maturation of cartilage repair and its clinical correlation is still somewhat ambiguous.[85] In the patellofemoral joint, ACI with patellofemoral osteotomy has shown significantly greater improvements in multiple clinical domains when compared with ACI in isolation, without any significant differences in the rate of total complications.[86]

A systematic review by DiBartola et al.[87] evaluated ACI in the adolescent knee, and identified five studies with 115 patients at a mean 16.2 years of age with chondral defect size of mean 5.3 cm². At a mean 52.3 months postoperatively, all studies reported improvement in clinical outcome measures, with graft hypertrophy being the most common complication (7.0%) and shorter duration of preoperative symptoms being the only identifiable variable that influenced outcomes. Peterson et al.[88] published on long-term follow-up of 224 patients with first-generation ACI at 10–20 years postoperatively. They reported that 92% were satisfied with their outcome and would have the procedure performed again.

Particulated Minced Cartilage

Implantation of minced cartilage allows for a single-stage application technique of natural chondral tissue. This technology is appropriate for the treatment of chondral defects without significant bone loss.[89] The minced pieces of hyaline cartilage are often supplemented within a scaffold delivery system.[62] Lesion should be contained and between 1 and 6 cm², patient BMI below 35 kg/m², chondral defect grade 3 or higher, and subchondral bone relatively nonedematous.[90] The most commonly reported adverse effects after this type of treatment are joint stiffness and effusion, with reoperation most commonly occurring for graft delamination and hypertrophy.[90]

Cartilage autograft implantation system (CAIS) procedure includes harvesting of cartilage from a non–weight-bearing area of the knee through a CAIS harvester, followed by dispersion of the minced cartilage pieces onto a copolymer foam scaffold, stabilization with a fibrin sealant, and stapling into the defect site with resorbable polydioxanone staples.[62] While the technology has shown promise histologically and through imaging in large animal studies, human studies confirming its efficacy are limited at this time. By contrast, DeNovo NT Graft ("Natural Tissue Graft," Zimmer Inc., Warsaw, IN/ISTO Technologies Inc., St. Louis, MO) includes particulated allograft cartilage tissue from juvenile (<13-year-old) donors. The minced cartilage is implanted at the time of surgery and stabilized with fibrin glue adhesive,[62] and does not stimulate any immunogenic response.[91] It has an ~40-day shelf life.[89]

While clinical data are somewhat limited, there are some data published with promising clinical outcomes and histologic findings with hope for increased restorative and proliferative potential.[90] Tompkins et al.[92] reported on use of DeNovo in the patella for defects of a mean $2.4 \pm 1.2\,cm^2$ size at an average of 28 months postoperatively. While 2 of 15 grafts required debridement because of hypertrophy, mean fill on MRI was 89%. Farr et al. demonstrated a favorable type II/I collagen ratio on immunohistochemistry biopsies in 25 patients who underwent DeNovo NT treatment; at 2 years postoperatively, there were no reoperations required in this cohort.[93] However, the long-term efficacy of this technology in terms of cartilage histology and symptomatic relief remains to be seen. Ultimately, further high-level human studies are necessary to better scrutinize the technology and corroborate the promising basic science and animal study findings.

COMPARISONS OF SURGICAL INTERVENTIONS

ACI has shown a slower clinical response when compared with osteochondral autograft, which is not unexpected given the immediate presence of hyaline cartilage with the latter as compared with the remodeling process that occurs with the former.[8] Mundi et al.[94] performed a metaanalysis of 12 randomized trials with a cumulative 765 patients and a mean lesion size of $3.9 \pm 1.3\,cm^2$. The authors reported no significant difference in functional outcomes or pain at

intermediate-term follow-up for marrow stimulation, ACI, and osteochondral autograft transfer techniques, despite all generally showing efficacy in treatment.

Harris et al.[8] conducted a systematic review of level I and II studies comparing ACI with either MFx or osteochondral autograft. In three of seven studies comparing ACI with MFx, clinical outcomes were superior with ACI after 1–3 years postoperatively, one study demonstrated superior results 2 years after MFx, and the final three studies demonstrated no differences in these interventions after 1–5 years. With both procedures, younger patients with shorter duration of preoperative symptoms and fewer prior surgeries demonstrated the best outcomes. The authors noted that clinical outcomes after MFx deteriorated after 1.5–2 years postoperatively. In the identified studies comparing ACI with osteochondral autograft, equivalent short-term clinical outcomes were identified although in the two relevant studies there was more rapid improvement with the latter. Equivalent outcomes were noted between open and all-arthroscopic techniques of ACI, but complication rates after open, periosteal cover, first-generation ACI was higher in four studies. The authors ultimately reported that a chondral defect size of $>4\,cm^2$ was predictive of superior outcomes with ACI over either MFx or osteochondral autograft.[8]

Osteochondral autograft has shown through systematic review to have superior clinical results, less reoperation, a higher rate of return to sport, and maintenance of sports function when compared with MFx. However, outcome improvements were not different from ACI, yet the latter had a lower failure rate at 10-year follow-up.[60]

In a systematic review of 44 studies, Krych et al.[53] evaluated 2549 patients with an average age of 35 years to assess the optimal surgical cartilage restoration treatment of chondral defects in athletic populations. The authors found that return to sport at some level was 76% overall but that the greatest return rate was after osteochondral autograft (93%; at a mean 5.2 months postoperatively), followed by osteochondral allograft (88%; at a mean 9.6 months), ACI (82%; at a mean 11.8 months), and MFx (58%; at a mean 9.1 months). However, there may be a selection bias in these findings in terms of patient age and lesion sizes of those treated with autograft.

Schrock et al.[79] compared the functional outcomes and cost-effectiveness of MFx, osteochondral autograft transplantation, and first- and second-generation ACI. They found all to be effective surgical procedures with increases in functional outcomes scores at short-term follow-up, with second-generation ACI having statistically greater improvements than the others. Interestingly, MFx was found to be the most cost-effective treatment, and first-generation ACI, the least cost-effective.

FUTURE DIRECTIONS

The current focus on healthcare costs and cost-efficacy in treatment options is likely to play a role in future study and implementation of treatment options. Restrictions imposed by the Food and Drug Administration (FDA) have made further progress difficult in some respects as well in this field of orthopedics. It is clear that collaborative efforts with multicenter research and standardization of treatment regimens will be important to furthering this area of study. Additionally, collaboration among engineers, scientists, and orthopedic surgeons will continue to help spur further technologic advancements.[95]

Combination therapies of the aforementioned cartilage surgery and orthobiologics must be evaluated more closely to better replicate the native cartilage and joint homeostasis.[95] Additional methods of ACI including matrix ACI with growth factors are still evolving in an effort to improve the bioscaffold for implanted chondrocytes and produce type II collagen closer to native cartilage.[75] Continued efforts are expected with production of three-dimensional, ECM bioscaffolds as acellular sheets, layered scaffolds, hydrogels, and decellularized osteochondral allografts given their cytocompatibility and positive influence on stem cell behavior including growth, differentiation, migration and viability in the setting of cartilage restoration.[96] Future investigations may also include gene therapy, using biologic factors to suppress proinflammatory cytokines.[97]

The use of cell sources (i.e., bone marrow MSCs, umbilical cord cells, embryonic stem cells, and ASCs) in isolation and with the aforementioned cartilage regeneration procedures will continue to receive research attention and efforts.[89] The use of amniotic membrane products for cartilage restoration is gaining momentum in the last decade. As a source of pluripotent cells, this technology provides a highly organized collagen, antifibrotic and antiinflammatory product, which may be beneficial when utilized as an alternate tissue engineering scaffold for MSCs or delivery of chondrocytes or by chondrogenic differentiation or proliferation.[98] Although, no human studies are available to date, as the preliminary studies have been performed in animal models and through in vitro research. As the regulatory process around these amniotic membrane products continues to evolve, so will the clinical applications in cartilage restoration efforts.

CONCLUSIONS

Isolated, symptomatic chondral or osteochondral defects of the knee are a challenging pathology for orthopaedic surgeons to combat. The multitude of current surgical and nonsurgical options used to address these cartilage injuries underscores the notion that surgeons do not yet have a conclusion on which is superior to its counterparts. Continued research efforts are necessary to better understand the appropriate settings, mechanisms of application, and patient populations for the aforementioned orthobiologics and surgical techniques.[99] Independent of the treatment option being utilized, successful outcomes are contingent on proper patient selection and appropriate indications.[89] Every patient's treatment regimen should be individualized based on age, lesion size, patient activity and preference, and treatment costs.[97]

Joint injections with orthobiologic agents work to decrease symptoms caused by inflammation and joint viscosity. However, disease-modifying effects are not readily evident.[89] No orthobiologic or cartilage procedure can entirely reproduce the native structure and function of true hyaline cartilage.[89] From a surgical standpoint, smaller lesions ($<2\,cm^2$) are best treated with MFx or osteochondral autograft, with the latter showing more durable outcomes in higher demand patients. Lesions of intermediate size ($2-4\,cm^2$) can be treated well in general by ACI or osteochondral autografting, but lesions considered large ($>4\,cm^2$) have evidence to support use of ACI or osteochondral allograft.[2]

REFERENCES

1. Alford JW, Cole BJ. Cartilage restoration, part 1: basic science, historical perspective, patient evaluation, and treatment options. *Am J Sports Med*. 2005;33:295–306.
2. Richter DL, Tanksley JA, Miller MD. Osteochondral autograft transplantation: a review of the surgical technique and outcomes. *Sports Med Arthrosc Rev*. 2016;24:74–78.
3. Montgomery SR, Foster BD, Ngo SS, et al. Trends in the surgical treatment of articular cartilage defects of the knee in the United States. *Knee Surg Sports Traumatol Arthrosc*. 2014;22(9):2070–2075.
4. McCormick F, Harris JD, Abrams GD, et al. Trends in the surgical treatment of articular cartilage lesions in the United States: an analysis of a large private-payer database over a period of 8 years. *Arthroscopy*. 2014;30(2):222–226.

5. Ciccotti MC, Kraeutler MJ, Austin LS, et al. The prevalence of articular cartilage changes in the knee joint in patients undergoing arthroscopy for meniscal pathology. *Arthroscopy.* 2012;28:1437–1444.

6. Aroen A, Loken S, Heir S, et al. Articular cartilage lesions in 993 consecutive knee arthroscopies. *Am J Sports Med.* 2004;32:211–215.

7. Basad E, Ishaque B, Bachmann G, Sturz H, Steinmeyer J. Matrix-induced autologous chondrocytes implantation versus microfracture in the treatment of cartilage defects of the knee: a 2-year randomized study. *Knee Surg Sports Traumatol Arthrosc.* 2010;18:519–527.

8. Harris JD, Siston RA, Pan X, Flanigan DC. Autologous chondrocyte implantation: a systematic review. *J Bone Joint Surg Am.* 2010;92:2220–2233.

9. Steadman JR, Rodkey WG, Briggs KK. Microfracture to treat full-thickness chondral defects: surgical technique, rehabilitation, and outcomes. *J Knee Surg.* 2002;15:170–176.

10. Camarero-Espinosa S, Rothen-Rutishauser B, Foster EJ, Weder C. Articular cartilage: from formation to tissue engineering. *Biomat Sci.* 2016;4:734–767.

11. Szafranski JD, Grodzinsky AJ, Burger E, Gaschen V, Hung HH, Hunziker EB. Mechanotransduction: effects of compression on deformation of intracellular organelles and relevance to cellular biosynthesis. *Osteoarthr Cartil.* 2004;12:937–946.

12. Eyre DR. Collagens and cartilage matrix homeostasis. *Clin Orthop Relat Res.* 2004;(suppl 427):S118–S122.

13. Cohen NP, Foster RJ, Mow VC. Composition and dynamics of articular cartilage: structure, function and maintaining healthy state. *J Orthop Sports Phys Ther.* 1998;28:203–215.

14. Thambyah A, Broom N. On how degeneration influences load-bearing in the cartilage–bone system: a microstructural and micromechanical study. *Osteoarthr Cartil.* 2007;15:1410–1423.

15. Hunziker EB, Michel M, Studer D. Ultrastructure of adult human articular cartilage matrix after cryotechnical processing. *Microsc Res Tech.* 1997;37(4):271–284.

16. Altman RD, Manjoo A, Fierlinger A, Niazi F, Nicholls M. The mechanism of action for hyaluronic acid treatment in the osteoarthritic knee: a systematic review. *BMC Musculoskelet Disord.* 2015;16:321–331.

17. O'Hanlon CE, Newberry SJ, Booth M, et al. Hyaluronic acid injection therapy for osteoarthritis of the knee: concordant efficacy and conflicting serious adverse events in two systematic reviews. *Syst Rev.* 2016;5:186–197.

18. Shewale AR, Barnes CL, Fischbach LA, Ounpraseuth ST, Painter JT, Martin BC. Comparison of low-, moderate-, and high-molecular-weight hyaluronic acid injections in delaying time to knee surgery. *J Arthroplasty.* 2017;32(10):2952–2957.

19. Abrams GD, Frank RM, Fortier LA, Cole BJ. Platelet-rich plasma for articular cartilage repair. *Sports Med Arthrosc Rev.* 2013;21:213–219.

20. Laver L, Marom N, Dnyanesh L, Mei-Dan O, Espregueira-Mendes J, Gobbi A. PRP for degenerative cartilage disease: a systematic review of clinical studies. *Cartilage.* 2017;8(4):341–364.

21. Cole BJ, Karas V, Hussey K, Merkow DB, Pilz KP, Fortier LA. Hyaluronic acid versus platelet-rich plasma: a prospective, double-blind randomized controlled trial comparing clinical outcomes and effects on intraarticular biology for the treatment of knee osteoarthritis. *Am J Sports Med.* 2017;45:339–346.

22. Meheux CJ, McCulloch PC, Lintner DM, Varner KE, Harris JD. Efficacy of intra-articular platelet-rich plasma injections in knee osteoarthritis: a systematic review. *Arthroscopy.* 2016;32:495–505.

23. Riboh JC, Saltzman BM, Yanke AB, Fortier L, Cole BJ. Effect of leukocyte concentration M on the efficacy of platelet-rich plasma in the treatment of knee osteoarthritis. *Am J Sports Med.* 2016;44:792–800.

24. Kasten P, Beyen I, Egermann M, et al. Instant stem cell therapy: characterization and concentration of human mesenchymal stem cells in vitro. *Eur Cells Mater.* 2008;16:47–55.

25. Chahla J, Dean CS, Moatshe G, Pascual-Garrido C, Cruz RS, LaPrade RF. Concentrated bone marrow aspirate for the treatment of chondral injuries and osteoarthritis of the knee: a systematic review of outcomes. *Ortho J Sports Med.* 2016;4:1–8.

26. Holton J, Imam M, Ward J, Snow M. The basic science of bone marrow aspirate concentrate in chondral injuries. *Orthop Rev.* 2016;8:80–84.

27. Gobbi A, Chaurasia S, Karnatzikos G, Nakamura N. Matrix-induced autologous chondrocyte implantation versus multipotent stem cells for the treatment of large patellofemoral chondral lesions: a nonrandomized prospective trial. *Cartilage.* 2015;6:82–97.

28. Krych AJ, Nawabi DH, Farshad-Amacker NA, et al. Bone marrow concentrate improves early cartilage phase maturationof a scaffold plug in the knee: a comparative magnetic resonance imaging analysis to platelet-rich plasma and control. *Am J Sports Med.* 2016;44:91–98.

29. Kasir R, Vernekar VN, Laurencin CT. Regenerative engineering of cartilage using adipose-derived stem cells. *Regen Eng Transl Med.* 2015;1:42–49.

30. ter Huurne M, Schelbergen R, Blattes R, et al. Anti-inflammatory and chondroprotective effects of intraarticular injection of adipose-derived stem cells in experimental osteoarthritis. *Arthritis Rheum.* 2012;64:3604–3613.

31. Manferdini C, Maumus M, Elena G, et al. Adipose-derived mesenchymal stem cells exert antiinflammatory effects on chondrocytes and synoviocytes from osteoarthritis patients through prostaglandin E2. *Arthritis Rheum.* 2013;65:1271–1281.

32. Jo CH, Lee YG, Shin WH, et al. Intra-articular injection of mesenchymal stem cells for the treatment of osteoarthritis of the knee: a proof-of-concept clinical trial. *Stem Cells.* 2014;32:1254–1266.

33. Pak J, Lee JH, Kartolo WA, Lee SH. Cartilage regeneration in human with adipose tissue-derived stem cells: current status in clinical implications. *BioMed Res Int.* 2016;5:192–200.

34. Case JM, Scopp JM. Treatment of articular cartilage defects of the knee with microfracture and enhanced microfracture techniques. *Sports Med Arthrosc.* 2016;24(2):63–68. https://doi.org/10.1097/JSA.0000000000000113. PMID: 27135288.

35. Erggelet C, Vavken PJ. Microfracture for the treatment of cartilage defects in the knee joint—a golden standard?. *Clin Orthop Trauma.* 2016;7(3):145–152. https://doi.org/10.1016/j.jcot.2016.06.015. PMID: 27489408.

36. Falah M, Nierenberg G, Soudry M, Hayden M, Volpin G. Treatment of articular cartilage lesions of the knee. *Int Orthop.* 2010;34(5):621–630. https://doi.org/10.1007/s00264-010-0959-y. PMID: 20162416.

37. Mithoefer K, McAdams T, Williams RJ, Kreuz PC, Mandelbaum BR. Clinical efficacy of the microfracture technique for articular cartilage repair in the knee: an evidence-based systematic analysis. *Br Am J Sports Med.* 2009;37(10):2053–2063. https://doi.org/10.1177/0363546508328414. PMID: 19251676.

38. Steinwachs MR, Guggi T, Kreuz PC. Marrow stimulation techniques. *Injury.* April 2008;39(suppl 1):S26–S31. https://doi.org/10.1016/j.injury.2008.01.042. PMID:18313469.

39. Gobbi A, Nunag P, Malinowski K. Treatment of full thickness chondral lesions of the knee with microfracture in a group of athletes. *Knee Surg Sports Traumatol Arthrosc.* 2005;13(3):213–221. PMID:15146311.

40. Cerynik DL, Lewullis GE, Joves BC, Palmer MP, Tom JA. Outcomes of microfracture in professional basketball players. *Knee Surg Sports Traumatol Arthrosc.* 2009;17(9):1135–1139. https://doi.org/10.1007/s00167-009-0765-5. PMID:19296083.

41. Namdari S, Baldwin K, Anakwenze O, Park MJ, Huffman GR, Sennett BJ. Results and performance after microfracture in national basketball association athletes. *Am J Sports Med.* 2009;37(5):943–948. https://doi.org/10.1177/0363546508330150. PMID:19251677.

42. Lee YH, Suzer F, Thermann H. Autologous matrix-induced chondrogenesis in the knee: a review. *Cartilage.* 2014;5(3):145–153. https://doi.org/10.1177/1947603514529445. PMID: 26069694.

43. Fortier LA, Chapman HS, Pownder SL, et al. BioCartilage improves cartilage repair compared with microfracture alone in an equine model of full-thickness cartilage loss. *Am J Sports Med.* 2016;44(9):2366–2374. https://doi.org/10.1177/0363546516648644. PMID:27298478.

44. Abrams GD, Mall NA, Fortier LA, Roller BL, Cole BJ. BioCartilage: background and operative technique. *Operative Tech Sports Med.* 2013;21(2):116–124.

45. Gille J, Behrens P, Volpi P, et al. Outcome of autologous matrix induced chondrogenesis (AMIC) in cartilage knee surgery: data of the AMIC registry. *Arch Orthop Trauma Surg.* 2013;133(1):87–93. https://doi.org/10.1007/s00402-012-1621-5. PMID:23070222.

46. Kusano T, Jakob RP, Gautier E, Magnussen RA, Hoogewoud H, Jacobi M. Treatment of isolated chondral and osteochondral defects in the knee by autologous matrix-induced chondrogenesis (AMIC). *Knee Surg Sports Traumatol Arthrosc.* 2012;20(10):2109–2115. PMID: 22198419.

47. Siclari A, Mascaro G, Gentili C, Cancedda R, Boux E. A cell-free scaffold-based cartilage repair provides improved function hyaline-like repair at one year. *Clin Orthop Relat Res.* 2012;470(3):910–919. https://doi.org/10.1007/s11999-011-2107-4. PMID: 21965060.

48. Anders S, Volz M, Frick H, Gellissen J. A randomized, controlled trial comparing autologous matrix-induced chondrogenesis (AMIC®) to microfracture: analysis of 1- and 2-year follow-up data of 2 centers. *Open Orthop J.* 2013;7:133–143. https://doi.org/10.2174/1874325001307010133. PMID: 23730377.

49. Volz M, Schaumburger J, Frick H, Grifka J, Anders S. A randomized controlled trial demonstrating sustained benefit of Autologous Matrix-Induced Chondrogenesis over microfracture at five years. *Int Orthop.* 2017;41(4):797–804. https://doi.org/10.1007/s00264-016-3391-0. PMID: 28108777.

50. Schiavone Panni A, Del Regno C, Mazzitelli G, D'Apolito R, Corona K, Vasso M. Good clinical results with autologous matrix-induced chondrogenesis (Amic) technique in large knee chondral defects. *Knee Surg Sports Traumatol Arthrosc.* 2017. https://doi.org/10.1007/s00167-017-4503-0. PMID: 28324152.

51. Patel S, Dhillon MS, Aggarwal S, Marwaha N, Jain A. Treatment with platelet-rich plasma is more effective than placebo for knee osteoarthritis: a prospective, double-blind, randomized trial. *Am J Sports Med.* 2013;41(2):356–364. https://doi.org/10.1177/0363546512471299. PMID: 23299850.

52. Bobic V, Noble J. Articular cartilage—to repair or not to repair. *J Bone Joint Surg Br.* 2000;82:165–166.

53. Krych AJ, Pareek A, King AH, Johnson NR, Stuart MJ, Williams III RJ. Return to sport after the surgical management of articular cartilage lesions in the knee: a meta-analysis. *Knee Surg Sports Traumatol Arthrosc.* 2017;25(10):3186–3196.

54. Pareek A, Reardon PJ, Maak TG, Levy BA, Stuart MJ, Krych AJ. Long-term outcomes after osteochondral autograft transfer: a systematic review at mean follow-up of 10.2 years. *Arthroscopy.* 2016;32(6):1174–1184.

55. Hangody L, Dobos J, Balo E, Panics G, Hangody LR, Berkes I. Clinical experiences with autologous osteochondral mosaicplasty in an athletic population: a 17-year prospective multicenter study. *Am J Sports Med.* 2010;38:1125–1133.

56. Brophy RH, Wojahn RD, Lamplot JD. Cartilage restoration techniques for the patellofemoral joint. *J Am Acad Orthop Surg.* 2017;25(5):321–329.

57. Blackman AJ, Smith MV, Flanigan DC, Matava MJ, Wright RW, Brophy RH. Correlation between magnetic resonance imaging and clinical outcomes after cartilage repair surgery in the knee: a systematic review and meta-analysis. *Am J Sports Med.* 2013;41(6):1426–1434.

58. Hangody L, Fules P. Autologous osteochondral mosaicplasty for the treatment of full-thickness defects of the weight-bearing joints: ten years of experimental and clinic experience. *J Bone Joint Surg Am*. 2003;85-A(suppl 2):25–32.

59. Solheim E, Hegna J, Oyen J, et al. Results at 10 to 14 years after osteochondral autografting (mosaicplasty) in articular cartilage defects in the knee. *Knee*. 2013;20:287–290.

60. Lynch TS, Patel RM, Benedick A, Amin NH, Jones MH, Miniaci A. Systematic review of autogenous osteochondral transplant outcomes. *Arthroscopy*. 2015;31(4):746–754.

61. Zouzias IC, Bugbee WD. Osteochondral allograft transplantation in the knee. *Sports Med Arthrosc Rev*. 2016;24:79–84.

62. McCormick F, Yanke A, Provencher MT, Cole BJ. Minced articular cartilage—basic science, surgical technique, and clinical application. *Sports Med Arthrosc Rev*. 2008;16:217–220.

63. Williams SK, Amiel D, Ball ST, et al. Prolonged storage effects on the articular cartilage of fresh human osteochondral allografts. *J Bone Joint Surg Am*. 2003;85:2111–2120.

64. Allen RT, Robertson CM, Pennock AT, et al. Analysis of stored osteochondral allografts at the time of surgical implantation. *Am J Sports Med*. 2005;33:1479–1484.

65. Assenmacher AT, Pareek A, Reardon PJ, Macalena JA, Stuart MJ, Krych AJ. Long-term outcomes after osteochondral allograft: a systematic review at long-term follow-up of 12.3 years. *Arthroscopy*. 2016;32(10):2160–2168.

66. Chui K, Jeys L, Snow M. Knee salvage procedures: the indications, techniques and outcomes of large osteochondral allografts. *World J Orthop*. 2015;6(3):340–350.

67. Gudas R, Gudaite A, Pocius A, et al. Ten-year follow-up of a prospective, randomized clinical study of mosaic osteochondral autologous transplantation versus microfracture for the treatment of osteochondral defects in the knee joint of athletes. *Am J Sports Med*. 2012;40(11):2499–2508.

68. Gross AE, Shasha N, Aubin P. Long-term follow-up of the use of fresh osteochondral allografts for posttraumatic knee defects. *Clin Orthop Relat Res*. 2005;435:79–87.

69. Krych AJ, Robertson CM, Williams III RJ. Return to athletic activity after osteochondral allograft transplantation in the knee. *Am J Sports Med*. 2012;40:1053–1059.

70. Levy YD, Gortz S, Pulido PA, McCauley JC, Bugbee WD. Do fresh osteochondral allografts successfully treat femoral condyle lesions? *Clin Orthop Relat Res*. 2013;471:231–237.

71. Torga Spak R, Teitge RA. Fresh osteochondral allografts for patellofemoral arthritis: long-term followup. *Clin Orthop Relat Res*. 2006;444:193–200.

72. Chahal J, Gross AE, Gross C, et al. *Arthroscopy*. 2013;29(3):575–588.

73. De Caro F, Bisicchia S, Amendola A, Ding L. Large fresh osteochondral allografts of the knee: a systematic clinical and basic science review of the literature. *Arthroscopy*. 2015;31(4):757–765.

74. Welch T, Mandelbaum B, Minas T. Autologous chondrocyte implantation: past, present, and future. *Sports Med Arthrosc Rev*. 2016;24:85–91.

75. Gillogly SD, Wheeler KS. Autologous chondrocyte implantation with collagen membrane. *Sports Med Arthrosc Rev*. 2015;23:118–124.

76. Brittberg M, Lindahl A, Nilsson A, Ohlsson C, Isaksson O, Peterson L. Treatment of deep cartilage defects in the knee with autologous chondrocyte implantation. *N Engl J Med*. 1994;331:889–895.

77. Marcacci M, Kon E, Zaffagnini S, et al. Arthroscopic second-generation autologous chondrocyte implantation. *Knee Surg Sports Traumatol Arthrosc*. 2007;15:610–619.

78. Gillogly SD, Arnold R. Autologous chondrocyte implantation and anteromedialization for isolated patellar articular cartilage lesions: 5- to 11-year follow-up. *Am J Sports Med*. 2014;42:912–920.

79. Schrock JB, Kraeutler MJ, Houck DA, McQueen MB, McCarty EC. A cost-effectiveness analysis of surgical treatment modalities for chondral lesions of the knee. *Orthop J Sports Med*. 2017;5(5):2325967117704634.

80. Gomoll AH, Probst C, Farr J, et al. Use of a type I/III bilayer collagen membrane decreases reoperation rates for symptomatic hypertrophy after ACI. *Am J Sports Med*. 2009;37S:20–23.

81. Zhang C, Cai Y, Lin X. Autologous chondrocyte implantation: is it likely to become a savior of large-sized and full-thickness cartilage defect in young adult knee? *Knee Surg Sports Traumatol Arthrosc*. 2016;24:1643–1650.

82. Goyal D, Goyal A, Keyhani S, Lee EH, Hui JHP. Evidence-based status of second- and third-generation autologous chondrocyte implantation over first generation: a systematic review of level I and II studies. *Arthroscopy*. 2013;29(11):1872–1878.

83. Saris DB, Vanlauwe J, Victor J, et al. Characetrized chondrocyte implantation results in better structural repair when treating symptomatic cartilage defects of the knee in a randomized controlled trial versus microfracture. *Am J Sports Med*. 2008;36:235–246.

84. Peterson L, Brittberg M, Kiviranta I, Akerlund EL, Lindahl A. Autologous chondrocyte transplantation. Biomechanics and long-term durability. *Am J Sports Med*. 2002;30:2–12.

85. Gikas P, Morris T, Carrington R, Skinner J, Bentley G, Briggs T. A correlation between the timing of biopsy after autologous chondrocyte implantation and the histological appearance. *J Bone Joint Surg Br*. 2009;91:1172–1177.

86. Trinh TQ, Harris JD, Siston RA, Flanigan DC. Improved outcomes with combined autologous chondrocyte implantation and patellofemoral osteotomy versus isolated autologous chondrocyte implantation. *Arthroscopy*. 2013;29(3):566–574.

87. DiBartola AC, Wright BM, Magnussen RA, Flanigan DC. Clinical outcomes after autologous chondrocyte implantation in adolescents' knees: a systematic review. *Arthroscopy*. 2016;32(9):1905–1916.

88. Peterson L, Vasiliadis HS, Brittberg M, et al. Autologous chondrocyte implantation: a long-term follow-up. *Am J Sports Med*. 2010;38:1117–1124.

89. Yanke AB, Chubinskaya S. The state of cartilage regeneration: current and future technologies. *Curr Rev Musculoskelet Med*. 2015;8:1–8.

90. Riboh JC, Cole BJ, Farr J. Particulated articular cartilage for symptomatic chondral defects of the knee. *Curr Rev Musculoskelet Med*. 2015;8:429–435.

91. Adkisson HD, Martin JA, Amendola RL, et al. The potential of human allogeneic juvenile chondrocytes for restoration of articular cartilage. *Am J Sports Med*. 2010;38:1324–1333.

92. Tompkins M, Hamann JC, Diduch DR, et al. Preliminary results of a novel single-stage cartilage restoration technique: particulated juvenile articular cartilage allograft for chondral defects of the patella. *Arthroscopy*. 2013;29:1661–1670.

93. Farr J, Tabet SK, Margerrison E, Cole BJ. Clinical, radiographic, and histological outcomes after cartilage repair with particulated juvenile articular cartilage: a 2-year prospective study. *Am J Sports Med*. 2014;42(6):1417–1425.

94. Mundi R, Bedi A, Chow L, et al. Cartilage restoration of the knee: a systematic review and meta-analysis of level I studies. *Am J Sports Med*. 2015;44(7):1888–1895.

95. Zlotnicki JP, Geeslin AG, Murray IR, et al. Biologic treatments for sports injuries II think tank—current concepts, future research, and barriers to advancement, part 3: articular cartilage. *Orthop J Sports Med*. 2016;4(4):1–11.

96. Monibi FA, Cook JL. Tissue-derived extracellular matrix bioscaffolds: emerging applications in cartilage and meniscus repair. *Tissue Eng*. 2017;23(4):386–398.

97. Richter DL, Schenck RC, Wascher DC, Treme G. Knee articular cartilage repair and restoration techniques: a review of the literature. *Sports Health*. 2015;8(2):153–160.

98. Riboh JC, Saltzman BM, Yanke AB, Cole BJ. Human amniotic membrane-derived products in sports medicine: basic science, early results, and potential clinical applications. *Am J Sports Med*. 2016;44(9):2425–2434.

99. Anz AW, Hackel JG, Nilssen EC, Andrews JR. Application of biologics in the treatment of the rotator cuff, meniscus, cartilage, and osteoarthritis. *J Am Acad Orthop Surg*. 2014;22:68–79.

CHAPTER 10

Orthobiologics in Osteoarthritis

THIERRY PAUYO, MD, FRCSC • JAMES P. BRADLEY, MD

INTRODUCTION

The development of osteoarthritis (OA) precipitates an irreversible cascade of degenerative changes affecting the hyaline articular cartilage. It is projected to affect more than 20% of adults in North America and Europe by 2020.[1,2] The burden of disease of OA on the affected patient population ranges from pain to severe functional limitation. With the increased prevalence of OA in the aging population, more than one-third of adults older than 60 years have radiographic evidence of knee OA.[3] Currently, nonsurgical treatments such as topical or oral nonsteroidal antiinflammatory drugs (NSAIDs), intraarticular steroid injection, or hyaluronic acid (HA) have produced mixed results in pain reduction and functional improvement.[1] These pharmacologic treatments target the catabolic cytokines and inflammatory mediators that are integral to OA's pathophysiologic process of degrading cartilage, synovium, and bone.[4] Although these treatment modalities have proven to be effective in short-term symptom relief, they have not been shown to stop, prevent, or reverse disease progression. A thorough evaluation of the current literature surrounding the role of biologics in OA will be discussed in the following section, which is included to help the treating physician understand how to appropriately utilize this new treatment option.

THE CLINICAL CHALLENGE

The articular hyaline cartilage is composed of chondrocytes and the extracellar matrix (ECM), which mainly includes type II collagen, proteoglycan, and water. The irreversible loss of type II collagen observed during OA progression is attributed to the absence of vasculature and innervation to its microstructure.[5] There is a need to transcend the current symptom relief treatment modalities and provide opportunities to stop and possibly reverse the OA process. Novel biologic treatment modalities have emerged to provide alternative process in decreasing inflammation and cytokines and possibly reverse the collagen and cell population lost. These new biologic treatment options include platelet-rich plasma (PRP) and stem cells and express potential regenerative properties and antiinflammatory modulating effects.

ORTHOBIOLOGICS
Platelet-Rich Plasma

Over the past few years, the advances in our understanding of the pathophysiology of OA have peaked, stimulating a growing interest in biological aids to disease modulation. The biologic factors recently studied to alter articular cartilage degeneration mainly focused on stem cells and PRP. PRP has been used to enhance soft tissue repairs such as Achilles tendon and rotator cuff repair and also to aid in the treatment of osteoarthritis and cartilage pathology.[6,7] PRP provides a unique treatment modality given that it has been shown to have a successful modulatory effect on inflammation and healing through molecules such as interleukin 1B and of TGF-B.[8,9] Over the last decade, the preparation of PRP has been greatly simplified and is often done in clinical setting.

The procedure consists on drawing whole blood from the patient with a venipuncture. The whole blood is then put through a centrifugation process that effectively concentrates the platelets. The supernatant contains a high concentration of platelets (150,000–350,000), which release a numerous amount of growth factors upon activation. This process concentrates growth factors and cytokines modulator above physiologic levels, which can then be sterilely injected in the joint. The sizable amount of signaling proteins, growth factors, and chemokines are theorized to potentiate and enhance tissue repair process.[10] More specifically, PRP modulates inflammation and vascular pathology and is a precursor to cell migration, proliferation, and differentiation.[1,11]

In the adult joint, the chondrocyte in cartilage do not have the capacity to divide or proliferate leading to an incapacity to regenerate after injury or demise.[12] Cartilage regeneration is therefore contingent on cell migration of precursor cells to the articular surface with the capacity to differentiate into the appropriate ECM

Biologics in Orthopaedic Surgery. https://doi.org/10.1016/B978-0-323-55140-3.00010-2

structure.[1] These precursor cells have been found in surrounding soft tissue, such as the synovium, fat pad, and the subchondral bone.[13-15]

Outcomes

The application of PRP in the clinical setting to treat OA has been extensively studied and shown to be efficacious at symptoms relief. In a study of 115 osteoarthritic knees treated with three intraarticular injections of PRP, Kon et al. showed an improvement in the posttreatment clinical scores at 6 and 12 months.[16] They found the maximal symptom relief at 6 months with a subsequent significant, but reduced, improvement at 12 months post PRP injections. In a randomized double-blind trial of Duif et al. 58 knees were randomized to either intraarticular PRP during arthroscopy versus control.[17] They found initial improvements in pain and assessment of life quality (SF-36) at 6 months but equal results at 12 months. In a midterm follow-up, Gobbi et al. performed a prospective randomized control trial of 119 knees, which either receive one cycle of three intraarticular injections of PRP or two cycles, 1 year apart, of three PRP injections.[18] They found a significant reduction in pain and improvement in function at 12 months post PRP injection, and they also found continued improvement at 18 months by annual repetition of the PRP intraarticular treatment.

Furthermore, in a systematic review of overlapping meta-analysis, Campbell et al. demonstrated that intraarticular injection of PRP in the treatment of OA provides symptoms relief up to 12 months.[19] In addition, they concluded that PRP injections should be considered in patients with early knee OA.[20] While intraarticular injections of PRP have been shown to provide short-term symptomatic relief and improvement of function, there is little evidence demonstrating that PRP reverses osteoarthritis degeneration of bone and cartilage. To investigate if PRP had molecular intraarticular effect beyond inflammation modulation, Sundman et al. performed a laboratory analysis of soft tissue harvested from OA knees, which were subjected to PRP or HA.[21] They found PRP to be effective at both stimulating endogenous HA production and decreasing cartilage catabolism.

Other evidence supports the role of PRP as modulator of the intraarticular inflammatory response. Furthermore, recent evidence has promoted the use of leukocyte-poor PRP to decrease the damaging effect of cytokines and proteases releases by the white cells.[22,23]

Stem Cells

Stem cell–based treatment approaches aimed to create, replace, repair, or improve diseased tissue have recently emerged.[22] The stems cells are generally characterized by undifferentiated cells expressing an ability to self-renew and also to differentiate into specific cell types; this allows maintenance of tissue homeostasis through repair.[23] The multipotent stems such as mesenchymal stems cells (MSCs) have the capacity to differentiate into particular cell lineage and are widely used in research secondary to regulations.[24,25] MSCs have been utilized and implanted both in an autologous and in an allograft setting. MSCs can be harvested from bone marrow aspirate, synovium, periosteum, adipose tissue, and postnatal umbilical cords.[26-30] Furthermore, the MSCs are precursor cells that can differentiate into chondrogenic, osteogenic, and adipogenic cells and are theorized to improve intrinsic regenerative and reparative functions of tissue such as cartilage.[31,32]

The MSCs are thought to potentiate reparative healing and regeneration of tissue through a plethora of characteristics such as cellular proliferation, antiinflammatory modulation, antiapoptosis, and antimicrobial.[23] The regenerative and antiinflammatory properties of MSCs have stimulated the investigation of novel approaches in altering the normal disease progression in OA.

The utilization of stem cells as a treatment approach in cartilage injury is increasing both in basic science and in clinical studies.[33] The basic science setting has demonstrated that stem cells can be effectively delivered to the knee cartilage either through implantation with a scaffold or from direct intraarticular injection. Fortier et al. have shown in an equine model that stem cells from bone marrow concentrate injected intraarticularly were superior in knee cartilage regeneration than microfracture alone.[34]

In the clinical setting, Wong et al. investigated autologous bone marrow-derived MSCs in unicompartmental OA of the knees undergoing high tibial osteotomies and microfracture. In the randomized controlled trial, they investigated 58 knees in which 28 knees received MSCs 3 weeks postoperatively. They found an improvement in both clinical scores at 2 years and healing imaging scores at 1 year in knee treated with MSCs.[35] In another study evaluating the role of MSCs in OA, Koh et al. performed intraarticular injection of MSCs into 30 elderly patients.[36] They saw a significant improvement in all clinical outcomes measures at 12 months and 2 years post treatment. Another randomized control trial investigated the use of intraarticular injection of allograft stem cells in patients with OA unresponsive to conservative treatment.[37] They found that, at 12 months, the MSCs-retreated knees had better pain score and functional outcomes score than the control knees. Lastly, Saw et al. investigated in a randomized control trial the regenerative properties of cartilage subjected to autologous blood-derived stem cells.[38] At 2 years' follow-up, the intraarticular stem cell injection in combination with HA produced an improvement in imaging scoring cartilage regeneration.

The safety of injecting stem cell in the intraarticular environment has been well studied. Hendrich et al. performed intraarticular injection of autologous bone marrow stem cells in 101 consecutive patients and found no complications or malignant transformation.[39] Malignant transformation of stem cells has been observed in prolonged culture of MSCs; short-term culture has proven to be neoplastic free.[40,41] Centeno et al. found no neoplastic occurrence after intraarticular injection of limited cultured MSCs in knee at 15 months.

Bone Morphogenic Protein
Another biologic that has been widely studied is bone morphogenic protein-7 (BMP-7). It came under scientific scrutiny because of a theorized anabolic effect on cartilage synthesis and ECM components while inhibiting catabolic molecules such as interleukin-1 (IL-1).[42,43] Badlani et al. demonstrated less cartilage degradation in rabbit anterior cruciate ligament (ACL)–injured knee compared with controls. In a double-blind multicenter controlled trial, Hunter et al. evaluated four cohorts of patients with knee OA found a trend toward a dose-dependent improvement in pain.

CONCLUSION
The use of biologic in the treatment of OA of the knee represents an unprecedented approach to this rising worldwide public health problem. Although the research in the field is still in its infancy, it appears that leukocyte-poor PRP and MSCs provide pain relief and improved function on a short-term basis. It appears that some research endeavors are producing early signs of cartilage repair; however, much more work is needed to obtain a definitive answer. The treating physician should be aware of the current literature in order to best advise their patients in the utilization of biologics in the treatment of OA.

REFERENCES
1. Andia I, Abate M. Knee osteoarthritis: hyaluronic acid, platelet-rich plasma or both in association? *Expert Opin Biol Ther.* 2014;14(5):635–649.
2. Divine JG, Zazulak BT, Hewett TE. Viscosupplementation for knee osteoarthritis: a systematic review. *Clin Orthop Relat Res.* 2007;455:113–122.
3. Dillon CF, Rasch EK, Gu Q, Hirsch R. Prevalence of knee osteoarthritis in the United States: arthritis data from the third National Health and Nutrition Examination Survey 1991-94. *J Rheumatol.* 2006;33(11):2271–2279.
4. de Rezende MU, de Campos GC, Pailo AF. Current concepts in osteoarthritis. *Acta Ortop Bras.* 2013;21(2):120–122.
5. Aigner T, Kim HA. Apoptosis and cellular vitality: issues in osteoarthritic cartilage degeneration. *Arthritis Rheum.* 2002;46(8):1986–1996.
6. Warth RJ, Dornan GJ, James EW, Horan MP, Millett PJ. Clinical and structural outcomes after arthroscopic repair of full-thickness rotator cuff tears with and without platelet-rich product supplementation: a meta-analysis and meta-regression. *Arthroscopy.* 2015;31(2):306–320.
7. Cai YZ, Zhang C, Lin XJ. Efficacy of platelet-rich plasma in arthroscopic repair of full-thickness rotator cuff tears: a meta-analysis. *J Shoulder Elbow Surg.* 2015;24(12):1852–1859.
8. Namazi H. Rotator cuff repair healing influenced by platelet-rich plasma construct augmentation: a novel molecular mechanism. *Arthroscopy.* 2011;27(11):1456; author reply 1456–1457.
9. Randelli P, Randelli F, Ragone V, et al. Regenerative medicine in rotator cuff injuries. *Biomed Res Int.* 2014;2014:129515.
10. Andia I, Abate M. Platelet-rich plasma: underlying biology and clinical correlates. *Regen Med.* 2013;8(5):645–658.
11. Andia I, Maffulli N. Platelet-rich plasma for managing pain and inflammation in osteoarthritis. *Nat Rev Rheumatol.* 2013;9(12):721–730.
12. Loeser RF. Aging and osteoarthritis: the role of chondrocyte senescence and aging changes in the cartilage matrix. *Osteoarthritis Cartilage.* 2009;17(8):971–979.
13. Karystinou A, Dell'Accio F, Kurth TB, et al. Distinct mesenchymal progenitor cell subsets in the adult human synovium. *Rheumatology (Oxford, England).* 2009;48(9):1057–1064.
14. Manferdini C, Maumus M, Gabusi E, et al. Adipose-derived mesenchymal stem cells exert antiinflammatory effects on chondrocytes and synoviocytes from osteoarthritis patients through prostaglandin E2. *Arthritis Rheum.* 2013;65(5):1271–1281.
15. de Vries-van Melle ML, Narcisi R, Kops N, et al. Chondrogenesis of mesenchymal stem cells in an osteochondral environment is mediated by the subchondral bone. *Tissue Eng Part A.* 2014;20(1–2):23–33.
16. Kon E, Buda R, Filardo G, et al. Platelet-rich plasma: intraarticular knee injections produced favorable results on degenerative cartilage lesions. *Knee Surg Sports Traumatol Arthrosc.* 2010;18(4):472–479.
17. Duif C, Vogel T, Topcuoglu F, Spyrou G, von Schulze Pellengahr C, Lahner M. Does intraoperative application of leukocyte-poor platelet-rich plasma during arthroscopy for knee degeneration affect postoperative pain, function and quality of life? A 12-month randomized controlled double-blind trial. *Arch Orthop Trauma Surg.* 2015;135(7):971–977.

18. Gobbi A, Lad D, Karnatzikos G. The effects of repeated intra-articular PRP injections on clinical outcomes of early osteoarthritis of the knee. *Knee Surg Sports Traumatol Arthrosc.* 2015;23(8):2170–2177.

19. Campbell KA, Saltzman BM, Mascarenhas R, et al. Does intra-articular platelet-rich plasma injection provide clinically superior outcomes compared with other therapies in the treatment of knee osteoarthritis? A systematic review of overlapping meta-analyses. *Arthroscopy.* 2015;31(11):2213–2221.

20. Campbell KA, Erickson BJ, Saltzman BM, et al. Is local viscosupplementation injection clinically superior to other therapies in the treatment of osteoarthritis of the knee: a systematic review of overlapping meta-analyses. *Arthroscopy.* 2015;31(10):2036–2045.e2014.

21. Sundman EA, Cole BJ, Karas V, et al. The anti-inflammatory and matrix restorative mechanisms of platelet-rich plasma in osteoarthritis. *Am J Sports Med.* 2014;42(1):35–41.

22. Hogan MV, Walker GN, Cui LR, Fu FH, Huard J. The role of stem cells and tissue engineering in orthopaedic sports medicine: current evidence and future directions. *Arthroscopy.* 2015;31(5):1017–1021.

23. DeLong JM, Bradley J. *The Current State of Stem Cell Therapies in Sports Medicine, Operative Techniques in Orthopedic.* Elsevier; 2016.

24. Fortier LA. Stem cells: classifications, controversies, and clinical applications. *Vet Surg.* 2005;34(5):415–423.

25. Wei X, Yang X, Han ZP, Qu FF, Shao L, Shi YF. Mesenchymal stem cells: a new trend for cell therapy. *Acta Pharmacol Sin.* 2013;34(6):747–754.

26. Filardo G, Madry H, Jelic M, Roffi A, Cucchiarini M, Kon E. Mesenchymal stem cells for the treatment of cartilage lesions: from preclinical findings to clinical application in orthopaedics. *Knee Surg Sports Traumatol Arthrosc.* 2013;21(8):1717–1729.

27. Veronesi F, Giavaresi G, Tschon M, Borsari V, Nicoli Aldini N, Fini M. Clinical use of bone marrow, bone marrow concentrate, and expanded bone marrow mesenchymal stem cells in cartilage disease. *Stem Cells Dev.* 2013;22(2):181–192.

28. Wolfstadt JI, Cole BJ, Ogilvie-Harris DJ, Viswanathan S, Chahal J. Current concepts: the role of mesenchymal stem cells in the management of knee osteoarthritis. *Sports Health.* 2015;7(1):38–44.

29. Pastides P, Chimutengwende-Gordon M, Maffulli N, Khan W. Stem cell therapy for human cartilage defects: a systematic review. *Osteoarthritis Cartilage.* 2013;21(5):646–654.

30. Yoshiya S, Dhawan A. Cartilage repair techniques in the knee: stem cell therapies. *Curr Rev Musculoskelet Med.* 2015;8(4):457–466.

31. Caplan AI. Adult mesenchymal stem cells: when, where, and how. *Stem Cells Int.* 2015;2015:628767.

32. De Ugarte DA, Morizono K, Elbarbary A, et al. Comparison of multi-lineage cells from human adipose tissue and bone marrow. *Cells Tissues Organs.* 2003;174(3):101–109.

33. Anderson JA, Little D, Toth AP, et al. Stem cell therapies for knee cartilage repair: the current status of preclinical and clinical studies. *Am J Sports Med.* 2014;42(9):2253–2261.

34. Fortier LA, Potter HG, Rickey EJ, et al. Concentrated bone marrow aspirate improves full-thickness cartilage repair compared with microfracture in the equine model. *J Bone Joint Surg Am.* 2010;92(10):1927–1937.

35. Wong KL, Lee KB, Tai BC, Law P, Lee EH, Hui JH. Injectable cultured bone marrow-derived mesenchymal stem cells in varus knees with cartilage defects undergoing high tibial osteotomy: a prospective, randomized controlled clinical trial with 2 years' follow-up. *Arthroscopy.* 2013;29(12):2020–2028.

36. Koh YG, Choi YJ, Kwon SK, Kim YS, Yeo JE. Clinical results and second-look arthroscopic findings after treatment with adipose-derived stem cells for knee osteoarthritis. *Knee Surg Sports Traumatol Arthrosc.* 2015;23(5):1308–1316.

37. Vega A, Martin-Ferrero MA, Del Canto F, et al. Treatment of knee osteoarthritis with allogeneic bone marrow mesenchymal stem cells: a randomized controlled trial. *Transplantation.* 2015;99(8):1681–1690.

38. Saw KY, Anz A, Siew-Yoke Jee C, et al. Articular cartilage regeneration with autologous peripheral blood stem cells versus hyaluronic acid: a randomized controlled trial. *Arthroscopy.* 2013;29(4):684–694.

39. Hendrich C, Franz E, Waertel G, Krebs R, Jager M. Safety of autologous bone marrow aspiration concentrate transplantation: initial experiences in 101 patients. *Orthop Rev.* 2009;1(2):e32.

40. Tolar J, Nauta AJ, Osborn MJ, et al. Sarcoma derived from cultured mesenchymal stem cells. *Stem Cells (Dayton, Ohio).* 2007;25(2):371–379.

41. Centeno CJ, Schultz JR, Cheever M, et al. Safety and complications reporting update on the re-implantation of culture-expanded mesenchymal stem cells using autologous platelet lysate technique. *Curr Stem Cell Res Ther.* 2011;6(4):368–378.

42. Badlani N, Oshima Y, Healey R, Coutts R, Amiel D. Use of bone morphogenic protein-7 as a treatment for osteoarthritis. *Clin Orthop Relat Res.* 2009;467(12):3221–3229.

43. Fibel KH, Hillstrom HJ, Halpern BC. State-of-the-art management of knee osteoarthritis. *World J Clin Cases.* 2015;3(2):89–101.

CHAPTER 11

Biologics in Orthopedic Surgery: Ligament Reconstruction in the Knee

KATHERINE COYNER, MD • JAMIE FRIEDMAN, MD • COLIN PAVANO, BA

KNEE ANATOMY AND BIOMECHANICS

The knee joint is the largest and most complex joint in the human body. The ligaments of the knee, which provide structural stability to the joint, are particularly vulnerable to injury. The knee consists of two bony articulations, one between the femur and the tibia creating the tibiofemoral joint, and one between the patella and femur creating the patellofemoral joint. The primary function of the knee ligaments is to control normal kinematics, to stabilize the knee, and to prevent abnormal displacement and rotation that may damage articular surfaces. Ligaments of the knee function as the most important static stabilizers and are composed of collagen, elastic, and reticular fibers. Parallel collagen-fiber bundles enable ligaments to bare axially directed tensile loads.

The ligament-to-bone interface is divided into four zones: (1) the ligament substance, (2) fibrocartilage matrix, (3) mineralized fibrocartilage, and (4) bone.[1] This composition is designed to reduce the chance of failure by distributing stress at the bone ligament interface in a gradual fashion.

Fig. 11.1 represents the load-elongation curve for tensile failure of the anterior cruciate ligament (ACL) illustrated by Cabaud.[2] The figure illustrates the ability of the ligament to resist tensile loading. As more load is applied to the knee, ligament fibers straighten, and the ligament elongates. The slope of the curve represents the stiffness of the ligament, whereas the area under the curve represents energy absorbed by the ligament. The initial portion of the graph labeled "clinical test" represents the amount of stiffness that can be elicited during a clinical examination of the knee. The second portion of the graph labeled "physiologic load" is a near linear relationship between load and joint displacement and is characterized by the elastic deformation of the ligament. The yield point represents the point of load beyond which injury to the ligament occurs, followed by a steep drop in load which represents failure of the ligament.

Cruciate Ligaments

The cruciate ligaments consist of a highly organized collagen matrix that accounts for approximately three-fourth of their dry weight. The majority of the collagen is of type I (90%), and the remainder is type III (10%).[3] The cruciate ligaments are named for their attachments on the tibia and are essential for knee joint function.[4-7] They act to stabilize the knee joint and prevent antero-posterior displacement of the tibia on the femur. The presence of numerous sensory endings also implies a proprioceptive function. They receive the majority of their blood supply from the middle geniculate artery.

The ACL originates from the medial surface of the posterior lateral femoral condyle and courses anteriorly, distally, and medially to the tibial attachment, which is a wide depressed area anteriolateral to the medial tibial spine in the intercondylar fossa. The average length of the ligament is 38 mm, and the average width is 11 mm.[8] The ACL is the primary static stabilizer against anterior tibial translation. Biomechanical testing has shown that the ACL provides an average anterior translation restraint of 87.2% of the applied load at 30 degrees flexion and 85.1% at 90 degrees flexion.[9] The ACL consists of two bundles, the anterome-dial bundle which is tight during knee flexion, and the posterolateral bundle which is tight during knee extension.[10] The ACL also plays a lesser role in resisting internal rotation. The maximum tensile strength of the ACL is approximately 1725+/− 270N.[11]

The posterior cruciate ligament (PCL) originates from the lateral surface of the posterior medial femoral condyle in the intercondylar notch, courses distally, and attaches to the tibia in a depression, posterior to the intraarticular surface of the tibia and extends distally 1 cm. The PCL has an average length of 38 mm and an average width of 13 mm.[8,12] The PCL is considered the primary stabilizer of the knee because it is located close to the central axis of the rotation of the joint and is almost twice as strong as the ACL.[7,12-15] The PCL has been shown to provide approximately 95% of the total restraint to posterior translation of the tibia on the

Biologics in Orthopaedic Surgery. https://doi.org/10.1016/B978-0-323-55140-3.00011-4
Copyright © 2019 Elsevier Inc. All rights reserved.

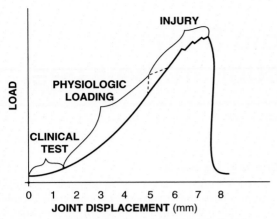

FIG. 11.1 Load-elongation curve for the tensile failure of the ACL. *ACL*, anterior cruciate ligament. (Data from: Cabaud HE. Biomechanics of the anterior cruciate ligament. *Clin Orthop Relat Res*. 1983; 172:26–31.)

femur.[9] It consists of an anterolateral and posteromedial bundle. The anterolateral bundle forms the majority of the PCL and is taut during knee flexion, whereas the posteromedial bundle is smaller and is taut during knee extension.[16] Injuries to the PCL are less common than injuries to the ACL and usually result from hyperextension or an anterior blow to a flexed knee. Of significant degenerative changes that involve the medial compartment, 90% of cases have been associated with chronic PCL injuries.[13]

Collateral Ligaments

The medial collateral ligament (MCL or tibial collateral ligament) connects the medial epicondyle of the femur to the medial tibia and serves to stabilize the knee specifically during valgus knee stress. The MCL consists of superficial and deep portions. The superficial MCL, as described by Brantigan and Voshell,[17] consists of parallel and oblique portions. The anterior parallel fibers arise from the sulcus of the medial epicondyle of the femur and consist of heavy, vertically orientated fibers coursing distally to insert on the medial surface of the tibia. This insertion is on average 4.6 cm inferior to the tibial articular surface and is just posterior to the insertion of the pes anserine. The posterior oblique ligament and deep fibers of the MCL run from the medial epicondyle and blend to form the posteromedial knee joint capsule. The superficial MCL functions as the primary restraint against valgus stress, a restraint to external rotation of the tibia, and a weak restraint to anterior tibial translation in ACL-deficient knees.[18,19]

The parallel fibers of the superficial MCL are under tension from full extension to 90 degrees of flexion but become maximally taut at 45–90 degrees of flexion. The deep MCL extends from the femur to the midportion of the peripheral margin of the meniscus and tibia. Anteriorly, the deep MCL is clearly separated from the superficial MCL by a bursa, but posteriorly the layers blend together. The deep MCL also functions as a weak secondary stabilizer against valgus stress.

The lateral collateral ligament (LCL or fibular collateral ligament) serves as restraint during varus stress of the knee. The LCL originates on the lateral epicondyle of the femur just anterior and distal to the origin of the gastrocnemius. It runs beneath the lateral retinaculum to insert on the head of the fibula, where it blends with the insertion of the biceps femoris. In biomechanical studies the LCL provides 55% varus restraint at 5 degrees of knee flexion and 69% restraint at 25 degrees of knee flexion. There is decreased varus resistance from the posterolateral capsule as the knee is flexed, leading to an increase in total varus restraint by the LCL.[20]

Other Ligaments

Another important ligament of the knee is the medial patellofemoral ligament (MPFL), which serves to stabilize the patella. The MPFL connects the medial border of the patella to the femur and prevents lateral translation of the patella. Anteriorly, the transverse ligament (or anterior intermeniscal ligament) of the knee connects the anterior edges of the medial and lateral menisci. The transverse ligament prevents anterior translation of both menisci during knee extension. Collectively, the posterolateral corner (PLC) also plays a role in knee stability. The static stabilizers of the PLC include the LCL, the popliteus tendon, and the popliteofibular ligament.[21] The PLC functions primarily to resist varus force, as well as posterolateral rotation of the tibia, especially when the cruciate ligaments are deficient. Cruciate tears often accompany PLC injuries, as both are strong stabilizers of the knee.

GRAFT OPTIONS FOR ACL RECONSTRUCTION IN 2018

As ACL reconstruction surgeries have become more frequent, the graft options have also expanded to include traditional autografts and allografts as well as synthetic grafts and xenografts. Autografts involve the use of the patient's own tissue, including options such as hamstring, patellar, and quadriceps tendons. Allografts are donated tissue from cadavers, which also include hamstring, patellar, and quadriceps tendons in addition to achilles and tibialis anterior/posterior tendons. Synthetic grafts, which may be composed of various materials such as Gore-Tex, polypropylene, and so forth, are a less popular option but are an area of future research in ACL reconstruction. Finally, xenografts are similar structures found in a different species which may be used rather than a human cadaveric donor. In choosing the appropriate graft for a patient, many characteristics are taken into consideration including the patient's age, level of activity, and comorbidities.

Hamstring Autograft

Hamstring autografts are frequently used by harvesting the patient's ipsilateral semitendinosus and/or gracilis tendons from their sight of insertion on the tibia.[22] Hamstring tendon grafts are often harvested through the same incision through which the surgeon drills the tibial tunnel for the ACL reconstruction, which decreases donor-site morbidity and improves cosmesis. In a study by Gupta et al.,[23] patients treated with a hamstring autograft experienced less postoperative pain for up to 6 hours than those treated with bone patellar tendon bone (BPTB) autografts. However, 6–48 h after operation, patients treated with either hamstring or BPTB autografts showed similar pain on a visual analog scale. Hamstring tendons tend to have less long-term postoperative pain associated with them than other autografts such as BPTB autografts, which have been correlated with kneeling pain.[24–31] A meta-analysis revealed 17.4% kneeling pain in the patellar tendon group compared with 11.5% kneeling pain in the hamstring group.[4] Numerous studies have compared the strength of various graft types. Hamner et al.[32] demonstrated quadruple hamstring tendon grafts to have greater strength and stiffness than patellar tendon grafts during biomechanical analyses (quadruple hamstring tensile load = 4090 N; stiffness, 776 N/m).

Downsides to the hamstring autograft include graft-harvesting morbidity related to sore hamstrings and subsequent weakened knee flexion. The deficit in knee flexion is thought to be more significant at greater flexion angles.[33] Aune et al.[26] found this knee flexion deficit to be statistically significant at the 6-, 12-, and 24-month follow-up when compared to patellar tendon grafts ($P < .01$; mean flexion at 240 degrees/s relative to unaffected side in hamstring group = 80%–90% compared with near 100% in patellar tendon group). Patients who undergo hamstring autograft must often adhere to a longer, more cautious recovery. The reason for this is because the graft lacks the bony component similar to that of the BPTB graft, requiring more time for integration into the native femur and tibia.[34] Rodeo

et al.[35] reported that soft tissue–bone grafts such as the hamstring graft incorporate into the subject's bone within 8–12 weeks, which is about 2–6 weeks longer than grafts containing bone.[11,36] In addition, Brophy et al.[37] analyzed the Multicenter Orthopaedic Outcome Network (MOON) data from 2002 to 2005 and demonstrated an increased risk of infection postoperatively in hamstring autografts when compared with that in BPTB autografts (odds ratio [OR] = 4.6 [95% confidence interval (CI) = 1.2 to 17.9; $P = .026$).

Bone Patella Tendon Bone Autograft

BPTB autografts consist of harvesting the patient's ipsilateral middle third of the patellar tendon with adjacent bone from the patella and tibia. The inclusion of bone plugs in the autograft provides bone-to-bone healing and is thought to have faster incorporation than other soft tissue graft types.[24,26] For this reason, some argue that the use of BPTB autografts for ACL reconstruction is better suited for young, highly active patients desiring a quick recover to high-intensity sports.[24]

Significant kneeling pain and decreased knee extension due to quadriceps weakness postoperatively are two downsides to the BPTB autograft. Corry et al.[38] showed that at 1-year postoperatively, 55% of patients who received a BPTB autograft experienced kneeling pain compared with 6% of patients who received a hamstring autograft. At 2 years, the number for BPTB autograft patients experiencing kneeling pain dropped to 31% and remained at 6% in hamstring autograft patients. A 21-study meta-analysis revealed 17.4% kneeling pain in the patellar tendon group compared with 11.5% kneeling pain in the hamstring group.[25] Some argue that kneeling pain can be decreased by implementing a more rigorous rehabilitation program. Researchers found less patellofemoral pain with an accelerated rehab, attributing the improvement to early range of motion and quadriceps strengthening.[39] Corry et al.[38] also demonstrated a significant amount of thigh atrophy compared to the contralateral leg with BPTB grafts, indicating a decreased extensor mechanism at 1 year after surgery. This difference, however, was no longer significant at 2-year follow-up. BPTB graft harvesting also introduces the risk of fracture in the proximal tibia and patella. Other complications include damage to the patellar articular cartilage, increased risk of patella tendon rupture, and risk of damage to the saphenous nerve below the patella.[24,34,40] Though the BPTB autograft may offer a quicker return to high-intensity activity, pain with kneeling, quadriceps weakness, and harvest morbidity must be considered when using a BPTB autograft.

The choice between the two most popular autografts for ACL reconstruction, BPTB versus hamstrings, remains a debate today. Poehling-Monaghan et al.[41] performed a systematic review of 12 publications investigating ACL graft choice and found no statistically significant differences between the BPTB and hamstring autografts in regard to manual laxity or graft failure rates. Manual laxity was measured via Lachman and pivot-shift tests, and instrumental laxity was measured using a KT-1000 arthrometer. They did find that BPTB grafts were associated with increased kneeling pain as well as an increased frequency of osteoarthritis after 5 years. In terms of clinical outcomes measured by International Knee Documentation Committee (IKDC), Lysolm, and Tegner scores, no significant difference was noted between hamstring and BPTB autografts. In another meta-analysis, Samuelsen et al.[42] found a small increased risk in graft rupture requiring revision in hamstring grafts compared to BPTB grafts (2.84% compared to 2.80% in the BPTB grafts), with a number needed to treat of 235.

Quadriceps Autograft

Although less common, quadriceps autograft has shown to be another viable option for ACL reconstruction, and in recent times, it has been gaining popularity. Slone et al.[43] performed a systematic literature review of 14 studies and found the quadriceps tendon autograft to be a safe, reproducible, and versatile graft in regard to ACL reconstruction. The quadriceps tendon is harvested from the patient's ipsilateral knee using an anterior approach proximal to the patella. In a study by Lee et al.[44] with patients treated with hamstring autografts versus quadriceps autografts, they were found to have similar knee joint stability and functional outcomes postoperatively. The quadriceps tendon autograft had a better outcome in terms of knee flexion than the hamstring graft. Chen et al.[45] found only mild harvest-site tenderness in a group of 12 patients who received a quadriceps autograft at 18-month follow-up, and Fulkerson et al.[46] reported no quadriceps morbidity in their 28-patient study.

The quadriceps graft can be difficult to harvest as the bone is denser, curved, and in close proximity to the suprapatellar pouch.[24] The lack of long-term quadriceps tendon studies has made it a less popular choice than other autograft options, though it is gaining popularity in both research and usage.[43,47–50] It remains clear that more research including direct comparison studies between BPTB, hamstring, and quadriceps autograft tendons for ACL reconstruction is needed to provide a better understanding of outcomes.

Allograft

An alternative to using a patient's own tissue is allograft from cadaveric tissue. Typical allografts include patellar, hamstring, quadriceps, achilles, or tibialis anterior/posterior tendons from a cadaveric donor.[51] The benefits of allograft for ACL reconstruction include decreased morbidity and postoperative pain because the tissue is not harvested from the patient. The lack of donor-site morbidity may also increase the esthetic outcome for the patient, as there are no additional incisions made for graft harvesting.[34] Allografts are associated with shorter surgery time, smaller incisions, less postoperative pain, and hence a quicker return to activities of daily living.[52] Shino et al.[53] reported good to excellent results in 94% of patients receiving an Achilles or peroneal tendon allograft at a 3-year follow-up interval. Indelicato et al.[54] reported 93% of patients with a Lachman score of grade I or less and 78% having a negative pivot shift receiving a BPTB allograft at 27 months of follow-up. At a 3- to 5-year follow-up, Harner et al.[55] found similar outcomes comparing allograft and BPTB autograft ACL reconstructions. Allografts tend to be used more often in ACL revisions and have provided a useful alternative to autograft options. However, longer follow-up studies have shown some downsides to using allograft for ACL reconstruction. For example, the MOON data analyses by Kaeding et al.[56] indicated a 5.2 times greater risk of retear in allograft reconstructions than that in BPTB autografts (OR = 5.20; 95% CI: 2.60–10.44; $P < .01$). In addition, other MOON data analyses indicated the use of allograft in young patients as the only predictor for retear in a 2497-patient cohort.[57]

The quality of allograft tissue is variable due to different company and processing standards. Allografts are harvested from cadaveric donors and treated using a variety of techniques including cryopreservation and gamma irradiation for sterilization.[24] The sterilization process may affect the structural stability of the tissue. For example, >3 millirad (mrad) can result in weakening of the graft tissue, which limits sterilization techniques to using <3 mrad.[58] Another concern in allograft tissue is the risk of infection. There have been three reported cases of disease transmission from ACL BPTB allografts, including HIV and Hepatitis C Virus (HCV).[58,59] Allograft tissue is also slower to heal than autograft tissue and can be associated with an immune response because it is foreign to the patient's body.[60] Kaeding et al.[61] demonstrated that allografts were associated with a four times higher failure rate than autografts for ACL reconstruction in the pediatric population (age range of 10–19), putting their efficacy into question for younger patients. Though these disadvantages exist, allograft remains a viable option for select ACL reconstructions in modern orthopedic practice, especially in patients older than 40 years, with multiple ligament reconstructions, and revision procedures. Kuechle et al.[62] reported 96% of 28 patients over the age of 40 years who received an ACL allograft (either freeze-dried fascia lata or Achilles tendon) to have a 0–1 Lachman test, KT-1000 arthrometer readings within 5.5 mm of the contralateral knee, and 55% achieved the same or better preoperative activity level measured by IKDC classification.

There have been extensive studies evaluating the best graft choice for ACL reconstruction. In a meta-analysis of 21 studies including 1348 patients, Freedman et al.[25] reported an overall failure rate of 1.9% in BPTB autografts compared with 4.9% in the hamstring autograft group. BPTB autografts remain the most widely used graft type to date.[63] Patellar tendon autografts are recommended especially for younger, competitive athletes looking for a quicker return to sports. The bone-to-bone healing in BPTB may offer an advantage over other graft types in the young, active patient. Soft tissue grafts including the hamstring are also successful and have continued to grow in popularity as they offer high tensile strength, less donor-site morbidity, and consistent patient satisfaction.[24,26–29,64] Allografts are used less frequently yet have proven to be successful in select patients. One study examined patients receiving soft tissue ACL allografts and reported that 79 of 84 patients returned to a desired activity level postoperatively.[65] Allografts are successful in older, less active patients due to their lack of harvest morbidity and easier rehabilitation, with a longer healing time being more accepted by this demographic.[24,66]

Large multicenter data sets such as the MOON cohort have provided valuable insight into the performance and outcomes of various ACL graft choices in the recent years. The MOON cohort analyses[37] suggest a decreased risk of infection with BPTB autografts (0.3%) compared with hamstring autografts (1.3%) and all types of allografts (1.0%). It also concluded that there is a significantly increased risk of retear with allografts when compared with BPTB autografts.[56] A MOON study of 2683 patients found that 3.2% of BPTB autografts, 4.6% of hamstring autografts, and 6.9% of allografts tore over the course of a 2-year follow-up. Though a higher percentage of hamstring grafts suffered retear than BPTB autografts, this did not reach statistical significance ($P = .12$).[56] Ultimately large database studies, such as those using the MOON cohort, provide objective data that surgeons can use when deciding what is the best ACL graft choice for the patient.

Synthetics and Xenograft

To date, synthetic graft and xenograft reconstructions have not had much success; however, they are still an area for further research in ACL graft technology. Legnani et al.[67] provided a review of literature of artificial grafts in 2010, in which they recognized carbon grafts as the first synthetic graft form. The carbon grafts were eventually abandoned due to serious sequelae including early rupture, inflammatory synovitis, and deposition in the liver. Polytetrafluorethylene (PTFE) grafts followed and were implemented in clinical trials. After initial positive results, Paulos et al.[68] demonstrated a 76% complication rate in PTFE grafts. Eventually in 1993 the PTFE graft was removed from the market after reports of complications, including inguinal lymph node involvement.[69] The Dacron polyester graft, introduced in 1989, also reached clinical trials but was removed from the market due to various studies demonstrating rupture, increased knee osteoarthritis, and synovitis.[67,70] Other synthetics such as the Kennedy ligament augmentation device have shown complication rates up to 63%, including increased infection risk.[71,72]

A synthetic graft that has shown some promise is the Ligament Advanced Reinforcement System (LARS) ligament.[67] The LARS ligament is composed of polyethylene terephthalate and contains sutures intended to allow growth inside the joint space.[67] Lavoie et al.[73] followed up 47 patients who underwent ACL reconstruction with the LARS ligament and found favorable postoperative results. Patients reported satisfaction with activities of daily living, recreational ability, and postoperative pain levels; however, patients on average did not reach preinjury activity levels. Jia et al.[74] performed a 7-year follow-up in patients with a LARS ligament ACL graft and found an overall complication rate of 2.2%. They found decreased knee laxity measured by KT-1000 arthrometer, improved Lysholm scores, and an 87% return to sport. Given these outcomes, they deemed the LARS ligament ACL reconstruction graft to have a good prognosis. In another study comparing outcomes of artificial ligaments such as the LARS ligament, Jia et al.[75] found the clinical outcomes and complication rates for synthetic grafts to be similar to those of BPTB and hamstring autograft ACL reconstructions.

Xenografts, or grafts from another species used for human implantation, are currently being investigated. A study by Zaffagnini et al.[76] attempted to find a method to reduce the immunological reaction associated with xenograft placement in a different species. They have demonstrated that treatment with alpha-galactosidase can decrease the immune reaction associated with non–self-antigen alpha-Gal found in the porcine ligament.

After a 2-year follow-up of three patients receiving the "Z-Lig device" which uses this concept, they observed a subjective improvement in Tegner scores, and one-legged hop tests postoperatively indicated functional return to a high level versus the unoperated knee at 12 and 24 months. Most importantly, blood tests of all three patients showed the absence of major anti-Gal and anti–non-Gal antibodies, demonstrating successful attenuation of the biological immune reaction to the foreign ligament. Further research into producing and testing a viable synthetic or xenograft ligament for ACL reconstruction is necessary before they may be considered a reliable graft option.

BIOLOGY OF HEALING AFTER ACL RECONSTRUCTION

A successful ACL reconstruction not only relies on adequate graft choice, technique, and execution by the surgeon but also the biologic healing of the graft. Depending on the type of graft used, there are known processes of healing in which the patient's body incorporates the new graft. Grafts that contain bone, such as the BPTB and quadriceps tendons, rely on bone-to-bone healing, specifically the incorporation of new bone into the tunnels created in the native femur and tibia. Other grafts, such as the hamstrings tendon, a soft tissue graft, rely on tendon-to-bone healing, a different biological healing process. Both methods have proven to be effective in ACL reconstruction, and it is important for the surgeon to recognize the various processes of healing so that they may facilitate the patient's recovery.

Tendon-to-Bone Healing

Tendon-bone healing is paramount to the success of a reconstruction when an autograft or allograft is entirely of soft tissue. For example, the popular hamstring graft undergoes tendon-to-bone healing, which requires the healing of a newly introduced tendinous structure to the femoral and tibial bone tunnels. Cole et al.[77,78] characterize the tendon-to-bone healing as either a compression or suspension fixation. Compression fixation secures the tendon at its bony insertion point, and suspension fixation uses fixation distant from the insertion site, such as the cortical periosteal or endosteal surface, cancellous, or cortical bone. Many researchers have shown that the native ACL insertion into bone can be broken down into four zones: (1) ligament, (2) unmineralized fibrocartilage, (3) mineralized fibrocartilage, and (4) bone.[79–81] Genin et al.[82] describe this transition, characterized by the increasing stiffness in

collagen-fiber alignment and increased mineralization. In ACL reconstruction, the tendon graft is directly fixed into a bone tunnel creating a direct graft tendon-to-bone interface or bone-to-bone interface for BPTB and quadriceps grafts.

There are three phases of ACL graft soft tissue integration: (1) early, (2) proliferative, and (3) ligamentization.[83,84] Cuti et al.[84] describe an initial "early" phase, characterized by graft necrosis, hypocellularity, and blood vessel formation in an animal model. This phase typically lasts from weeks 1–4 postoperatively. The graft necrosis stimulates a cytokinetic and cellular response, drawing in neutrophils and macrophages via the release of tumor necrosis factor-a, interleukin 1-b, and interleukin 6.[65,85–89] These cells work to eliminate waste and continue to release cytokines to facilitate the inflammatory response.[79,90] The formation of granulation tissue fills the gap between the bone and the graft and is rich in vascular endothelial growth factor (VEGF) and fibroblast growth factor, promoting revascularization and recruitment of fibroblasts, respectively.[91]

The "proliferative" phase of healing is characterized by increased cellularity during weeks 4–12 and includes the presence of mesenchymal stem cells that help to facilitate graft remodeling.[65,89] Scheffler et al.[89] described an invasion of myofibroblasts that takes place toward the end of the proliferative phase. The fibroblasts replace granulation tissue and exert tension on the cellular and extracellular matrix, restoring the "ligament-like" tension during the healing process.[92] As the healing process continues, macrophages release transforming growth factor-beta (TGF-β), facilitating the creation of a fibrovascular scar that connects the graft to the native bone. These perpendicular type III collagen fibers are called "Sharpey-like fibers."[79,91,93] These bundles function to resist shear stress placed on the graft during the early phase of rehabilitation.[79] At week four of a rabbit study, Liu et al.[93] noted a dense connective tissue matrix joining the bone to the soft tissue hallucis longus tendon graft, and at 6 weeks, there was a fibroblastic cellularity with longitudinal collagen organization. At 8 weeks postoperatively in rabbit models, Kanazawa et al.[91] found that type III collagen is deposited around the fibroblast-like cells that move toward the center of the healing semitendinosus tendon. Throughout the proliferative phase, bone tunnel remodeling also takes place, characterized by osteoblast activity producing new bone to fill the void of the tunnels.

Many studies have examined the mechanical stability of ACL grafts postoperatively. At weeks 6–8 postoperatively, several studies show that the graft is at its weakest mechanical point. Some suggest that this decreased mechanical stability can be attributed to the disorganized collagen network that is laid down during the healing process. This collagen network starts to become organized late in the healing process, when the graft begins to resemble a native ACL.[94,95] At this point in rehabilitation, the graft must be loaded carefully to avoid compromise, but appropriate loading is required to ensure the continuation of graft integrity.[94,96–98]

The final phase of ACL graft healing involves "ligamentization" of the tendon. At approximately 12 weeks, the graft finally starts to resemble a native ACL in strength.[84] It is important to note, however, that the new ACL graft never truly replicates a native ACL because it has a different histologic and morphologic appearance. Hypercellularity and vascularization during the proliferative phase decreases to levels similar to those of the native ACL by 6–12 months in animal models.[35,94,99–101] In a biochemical study by Marumo et al.,[102] longitudinally oriented collagen fibers and spindle-shaped cells were observed at 4–6 months postoperatively. They believe that the ligamentization process can continue for up to 1 year. As Cole et al.[77] noted, the entire healing process plateaus at approximately 6 months postoperatively. A small margin void of bridging collagen or mineralization between tendon and bone can even remain.[103] Suspensory fixation methods can even exhibit granulation tissue and irregular bone without collagen ingrowth between the graft and native bone for up to 6–14 months.[77,104]

Bone-to-Bone Healing

Compared with soft tissue grafts, ACL grafts containing bone heal by a different mechanism, similar to fracture healing. Grafts that undergo this type of healing include BPTB and quadriceps because they are harvested with a bone plug. Direct contact between the bone tunnels in the tibia/femur with the ACL graft bone plug provides a site for bone-to-bone healing. Once the bone plug and native bone are in contact, the formation of new bone begins. Inflammatory cells, mesenchymal stem cells (MSCs), and chemotactic agents are abundant in the bone-to-bone interface.[105] Granulation tissue forms and macrophages remove cellular debris as the osteoclasts continue to resorb bone.[105] Osteoblasts eventually lay down osteoid, which is then mineralized to form new bone. This process can take anywhere from 6 to 12 months after ACL reconstruction.[105–107]

Tomita et al.[108] performed a randomized trial observing the intraosseous graft healing between a doubled flexor digitorum superficialis and a BPTB graft in canine ACL reconstructions. At 3 weeks postoperatively

from BPTB autografts, they observed the anterior portion of the bone plug and tunnel interface filled with granulation tissue, whereas the posterior bone plug was in direct contact with the bone tunnel wall.[108] On high-power magnification, they noticed few collagen fibers surrounding the intraosseous tendon portion, osteocyte necrosis throughout the bone plug (excluding the superficial layer), and limited change in the tendon-to-bone junction of the graft itself.[108] At 6 weeks, the granulation tissue in the anterior gap remained, the posterior gap demonstrated new bone formation, and Sharpey's fibers began to bridge the space between the bony wall and the intraosseous tendon portion of the graft. Also, the bone plug of the BPTB graft showed new bone formation and anchoring to the bone tunnel wall. A decrease in cartilaginous cells in the bone-to-tendon interface was also noted.[108] At 12 weeks, more bony integration was seen in the posterior gap, perpendicular collagen fibers were increased in number, and granulation tissue in the anterior gap remained at levels similar to soft tissue ACL grafts.[108] At 3 and 6 months postoperatively, the BPTB graft demonstrated a higher ultimate failure load than the flexor tendon graft, demonstrating its potentially quicker healing potential and early strength.

BIOLOGIC AUGMENTATION IN ACL RECONSTRUCTION

The use of biologic augmentation in ACL reconstruction is a developing and controversial topic in orthopedic surgery. The most commonly studied biologic agent is platelet-rich plasma (PRP), an autologous blood product with increased concentration of platelets compared with whole blood. Platelets have been isolated as a valuable biologic agent due to the inherent growth factors known to stimulate tissue healing. Another novel biologic agent undergoing orthopedic research is stem cells, primarily MSCs acquired from bone marrow adipose. There are numerous in vitro and animal studies on this topic, but clinical evidence is still lacking, as the concept is relatively new.

Most clinical studies regarding PRP in ACL reconstruction have focused on clinical outcomes, bone tunnel enlargement, the graft-bone interface, and ACL graft maturation.[109,110] Functional scores have primarily been assessed by physical examination, KT-1000/2000 testing, the Lysholm scale, Western Ontario and McMaster Universities Osteoarthritis Index (WOMAC) stiffness scale, and so forth. Advanced imaging by computed tomography (CT) and magnetic resonance imaging (MRI) has been used to evaluate bone tunnels, the graft-bone interface, and ACL graft maturation.

Clinical outcomes have been measured using various methods including functional scores, objective examination findings, and in some studies, return to sports. Del Torto et al.[111] noted no significant difference in objective IKDC scores between patients with a platelet-rich fibrin matrix added to the hamstring autograft versus the control. However, they did find a significant difference in subjective IKDC scores. Because the patients were not blinded, this could be due to patient-reporting bias. Valenti et al.[112] also noted no difference in objective IKDC scores when comparing platelet-rich growth factor (PRGF) using a single-spin method without leukocytes, a PRP spin with leukocytes, and a control. Their study also found no difference in objective functional tests including knee range of motion, muscle torque, and KT-1000. There was, however, a notable difference in decreased postoperative effusion for the PRFG group, which has been demonstrated in other studies as well.[113] Interestingly, Darabos et al.[114] used an intraarticular injection of autologous conditioned serum consisting of cytokines and growth factors on the day of ACL surgery (day 0), day 1, day 6, and day 10, and they also found a decrease in postoperative effusion with an associated decreased WOMAC stiffness subscore after 1 year compared to placebo patients. The authors attributed this to the known anti-inflammatory effects of cytokines and growth factors that are found in PRP. This study also found that interleukin-1B synovial concentration, a marker of inflammation, was lower on postoperative day 10 for the ASC-injected patients than that for placebo-injected patients, further supporting an anti-inflammatory effect of using a platelet adjunct. One study using platelet-leukocyte gel applied to the hamstring autograft noted better anterioposterior stability using KT-2000 arthrometer at the 6-month evaluation.[115] Conversely, other studies have negated this finding, claiming that there is no difference in stability as measured by the Lachman test or KT-1000.[116–118] At this time, only data for a short-term follow-up of 2 years or less exist. Therefore, more studies are needed to understand whether the use of PRP provides a long-term difference in clinical outcomes for ACL reconstruction.

Can We Improve Graft-to-Bone Healing?

An important aspect in the success of ACL reconstruction is the incorporation of the graft into the native knee during healing. The graft is placed through femoral and tibial bone tunnels during surgery. Poor graft-bone healing can cause early postoperative failure of the reconstruction.

Bone tunnel widening

Bone tunnel widening is a phenomenon seen after ACL reconstruction. Although this may not be significant in clinical outcomes, widened bone tunnels add complexity to revision surgery, sometimes requiring staged operations. Some believe it occurs more in hamstring than patellar autografts and with extracortical fixation due to mechanical etiologies.[119,120] Others believe that it is due to biologic factors activated by drilling through bone to create tunnels for graft insertion.[121] Therefore biologic agents have been considered as a means to decrease bone tunnel enlargement postoperatively. Mirzatoloogei et al.[122] found no difference in bone tunnel widening at 3 months postoperatively after hamstring autograft with PRP application to both femoral and tibial tunnels. Vadala et al.[116] agreed with this finding using similar operative and biologic techniques, finding no difference in tunnel enlargement. However, a few studies did find a significant difference with decreased tunnel enlargement after application of PRP measured by CT at approximately 1 year postoperatively.[109,123] It is thought that improved graft-bone integration may decrease bone tunnel enlargement. Therefore the size of postoperative bone tunnels may be a prognostic sign of better graft incorporation. There have been no studies that correlate bone tunnel widening directly to worse outcomes, but it is a significant factor when considering ACL revision for graft failure.

Orrego et al.[124] did a randomized control study comparing the use of platelet concentrate placed onto the hamstring autograft versus using a bone plug harvested from the tibial tunnel and placed by interference fit in the femoral tunnel, and the combination of both on the effect of bone tunnel widening as well as graft-bone interface. They demonstrated a significant difference in decreased bone tunnel widening using the bone plug, but no difference with platelet concentrate or the combination of both was found. It is unclear whether this is due to a decrease in the number of cytokines causing osteolysis of the bone or a reduction in mechanical motion which may attribute to tunnel widening. MRI was also used to detect signal intensity around the graft, which characterizes tendon integration. They found no difference between any groups at 6 months. This was consistent with other studies that found no difference in postoperative MRIs of ACL reconstructions using platelet augmentation versus no augmentation.[117,125,126]

Vascularity

Another principal factor in graft-bone integration is revascularization during the healing phase. Vogrin et al.[127] did a study focusing on the revascularity of the graft-bone interface as well as intraarticular graft substance using platelet gel with the hamstring autograft. He noted that there was a significant increase in vascularization at the osteoligamentous junction at 4–6 weeks of the ACL grafts with platelet augmentation compared with the control but with a relatively decreased vascularity at 10–12 weeks postoperatively. He attributed this change to the replacement of vascular tissue with hypovascular collagenous scar tissue in the zone between the graft and the bone tunnels, which suggests normal graft healing. The control group had a slightly higher vascularity at the second follow-up point than that at the first, for which they concluded a slower healing process in the control group than in the augmented group. There was no difference in healing of the intraarticular segment of the graft. Another study by Rupreht et al.[128] supported a similar finding with increased vascularity of the tibial tunnel. They found that locally applied PRP gel to the hamstring tendon autograft reduced tendon-bone interface edema in the first postoperative month on MRI. They also found an increase in vascular density and microvessel permeability in the tibial tunnel in the first couple of months postoperatively. These findings of decreased edema and increased vascularity of the tibial tunnel support the use of PRP on ACL reconstruction to aid in graft incorporation.

Stem cells

Stem cells derived from the bone marrow are another biologic agent with healing potential that is a newer concept and much less studied than PRP. MSCs are multipotent cells, which have the ability to differentiate into several different musculoskeletal structures such as cartilage, bone, muscle, tendon, and ligament. For this reason, they are under investigation for their healing potential in ACL reconstruction. As of right now, there are many in vitro and animal studies published with various promising results; however, very little clinical data exist on this topic.

There have been several animal studies focusing on stem cell augmentation for ACL reconstruction.[129] Lim et al.[130] used bone marrow stem cells (BMSCs) to coat hamstring autografts during rabbit ACL reconstruction and found a greater number of chondrocytes at the tendon-bone junction with a subsequent mature zone of cartilage than the control with only mature scar tissue. Other animal studies have shown similar benefits, with the administration of BMSCs demonstrating increased collagen expression and decreased catabolic proteins after ACL reconstruction, which also signifies improved tendon-bone healing.[117,118] In addition to

these histologic discoveries, there are also animal studies showing a positive effect on mechanical strength by testing load to failure of BMSC-enhanced grafts compared with the control grafts.[130,131] These animal studies may represent superior healing potential of ACL grafts with BMSC augmentation, but clinical trials are needed to further validate these results.

Silva et al.[132] attempted to use adult noncultivated bone marrow stem cells to improve the healing time of the tendon-bone interface in the femoral tunnel during hamstring allograft ACL reconstruction. They performed an anterior iliac bone crest aspiration of the patient during surgery in a commercially available kit to isolate the stem cells. Half of the concentrate was injected into the graft, and the other half was injected into the femoral tunnel. MRIs were obtained at 3 months and measured for signal intensity at the graft-bone interface. They found no difference in graft incorporation compared with the control. Although BMSCs have been shown to accelerate the healing of the graft-bone junction in animal models, clinical studies to date have been unable to reproduce these results.

Can We Improve the Biology of the Graft?

Improving the biology of an ACL graft is a topic of interest, particularly in graft remodeling and maturation. Using biologic augmentation to expedite graft maturation would allow for quicker healing and potentially improve clinical outcomes while decreasing the risk of early failure. Orrego et al.[124] not only studied bone tunnel widening as previously mentioned but also investigated graft maturation by assessing signal intensity within the graft, with a low-intensity signal indicating graft maturation. At 6 months of follow-up, there was a significant difference in graft maturation in the platelet concentrate group compared with the control group. Another study injected PRP after surgical portals were closed and compared the MRIs with those of patients who did not receive the injection. They found increased maturation on MRI signal intensity at 4 and 6 months, but no statistical significance at 12 months.[133] Radice et al.[134] applied PRP gel to BPTB autografts and measured maturation by MRI heterogeneity. This study reported a shortened time by 48% (179 days) to reach graft maturation compared with the control (369 days). One could infer that this means potential graft healing in almost half of the time with PRP as an adjunct. Although MRI is a practical method to obtain objective data on graft maturation, there may be some interobserver error. Furthermore, there are several studies that claim there is no difference in graft maturation when evaluated by MRI.[118,120,135] Rather than relying on MRI studies to evaluate graft maturation, Sanchez et al.[136] published a study of second-look arthroscopy at 6–24 months after surgery with direct evaluation and histologic analysis of previous ACL grafts with and without PRGFs. They compared graft thickness and apparent tension, which were reviewed by blinded observers, and found that the ACL grafts treated with biologic augmentation rated higher, but this did not reach statistical significance. The histology was evaluated using the Ligament Tissue Maturity Index of Murray et al.[137] and found the grafts with PRGF to have more mature tissue. Interestingly, they noticed a new connective tissue formed around the graft, which occurred more frequently in grafts augmented by PRGF. This highly vascular envelope became denser over time until it was nearly indistinguishable from the original graft. All these patients required a second-look surgery for other intraarticular pathology, which is not part of standard ACL reconstruction postoperative care. Therefore this study had a limited number of patients, and they may not be generalizable to ACL patients without postoperative pathology. A second-look arthroscopic surgery does provide the most direct and objective analysis; therefore this information is important. However, graft maturation has not been directly related to clinical outcomes in any of these studies and therefore may be clinically insignificant.

Undoubtedly, there is still significant controversy on the topic of biologic agent augmentation with ACL reconstruction. The results of clinical outcomes, graft-to-bone healing, and ACL graft biology are inconclusive at this time. However, using these biologic agents has not shown to cause harm; therefore more research is warranted to better define the beneficial qualities of biologic augmentation in ACL reconstruction.

Can We Improve Healing of Partial Tears?

Partial ACL tears represent only about 10%–28% of ACL tear patients,[138] yet there are ongoing discussions in the orthopedic community regarding the treatment of incomplete tears. When compared with other ligaments of the knee, the ACL has poor ability for primary healing, usually requiring intervention to facilitate a full recovery.[139] As described by Dallo et al.,[139] the synovial fluid of the knee joint has inhibitory properties preventing fibrin-platelet clot formation and fibroblast recruitment, which results in poor primary healing potential.[139-142] In an attempt to overcome the poor healing potential of partial ACL tears, the efficacy and viability of biologic augmentation is a topic of growing interest. Though not yet popular in 2018, biologics may offer a potential option for treatment of incomplete ACL tears in the future. Options for augmentation include PRP injection, biologic scaffolds, and stem cell therapy.

Platelet-rich plasma

The use of PRP is common in other orthopedic procedures, and although some research exists regarding the use of PRP in combination with reconstruction procedures, there is limited literature regarding its sole efficacy in partial ACL repairs. PRP is known to contain various growth factors that help to facilitate the healing and blood clot formation process, including TGF-β1, platelet-derived growth factor (PDGF), VEGF, and basic fibroblast growth factor. The PDGF and TGF-β1 specifically facilitate recruitment of fibroblasts and collagen growth,[139] which enhances the healing of damaged connective tissue. Seijas et al.[143] described a study involving 19 patients with previous partial ACL tears. Patients were assessed via diagnostic arthroscopy, and a senior surgeon with experience in ligamentoplasty assessed the integrity of the remnant ACL bundle. All 19 patients demonstrated a complete rupture of the anteromedial bundle with an intact posterolateral bundle and therefore were included in the study. Four milliliters of PRGF was injected in the proximal and middle portion of the intact bundle, as well as in the articular space. They found that 16 patients who received the injection returned to their previous level of playing sports on national and international soccer teams at an average of 12.33 weeks for Tegner 10 and 16.2 weeks for Tegner 9 patients. At the 1-year MRI follow-up, complete ligamentization was seen in all cases, and at the 2-year follow-up, all patients had no sign of instability. In a canine model by Bozynski et al.,[144] subjects with partial ACL tears treated with PRP had better postoperative outcomes in terms of pain, effusions, function, and range of motion than groups treated with Non-steroidal anti-inflammatory drugs (NSAIDs) only. These differences, however, were not statistically significant. In a similar study by Cook et al.,[145] canines with partially transected ACLs as well as meniscal lesions were treated with leukoreduced PRP injections and observed alongside a control group treated with saline injections. Within 1 week, decreased pain and increased range of motion was noted in the PRP group, and within 5 weeks, there was an improvement in subject lameness, kinetics, and function. However, at the 6-month period, the differences in outcomes when compared with the control group were not statistically significant. Owing to limited research and lack of statistical significance, there is not enough evidence to recommend the treatment of incomplete ACL tears with PRP injections alone.

Murray et al.[146] performed a porcine-based experiment in which the animal ACLs were completely transected and treated with PRP injections. They observed no benefit of the PRP injections, hypothesizing that the formed clot dissolves in the joint space precluding activity at the site of healing. This is likely due to the intraarticular presence of urokinase plasminogen activator which increases plasmin, leading to fibrin degredation.[141,142,147] Ultimately, this finding has steered the field toward exploring the option of PRP combined with biologic scaffolds to hold the PRP material near the intended site of healing.

PRP plus collagen scaffold

The use of PRP injections in combination with a biologic scaffold to hold the injection to the site of healing has shown some promising outcomes in its infancy. Dunn et al.[148] initially described a collagen-fiber scaffold used for ACL reconstruction procedures that allows better fibroblast attachment and proliferation as well as increased collagen synthesis. This scaffold provides a location for fibroblasts to proliferate and lay down collagen fibers near the site of injury, thereby improving healing directly near the site of the injured ACL. Combining targeted healing with the enhanced regenerative potential of PRP injections has shown potential to improve the healing of incomplete tears. Vavken et al.[142] described the combination of a collagen scaffold with PRP. They demonstrated that fibroblasts respond to platelet concentrate, leading to increased proliferation and collagen production. In a canine model, Murray et al.[149] found that partial central ACL defects treated with a collagen scaffold and platelets resulted in improved biomechanical properties after healing compared to the no treatment group. Interestingly, they observed similarities between the healing of a partial ACL tears treated with collagen platelets with scaffolding and a patellar tendon graft on a histologic level.[142] Studies such as these have demonstrated that partial ACL tear healing is more efficient when PRP and a biologic scaffold are used in tandem rather than separately.[139] In 2016, Murray et al.[150] described the bridge-enhanced ACL repair procedure (BEAR procedure). The technique involves suture repair of the ligament combined with a bioactive scaffold that fills in the gap between the torn ligament fragments. The BEAR scaffold consists of extracellular matrix proteins including collagen from bovine tissue which has been treated to remove DNA content to less than 50 ng per milligram of scaffold. It is a highly hydrophilic material, allowing absorption of up to 5 times its weight in fluid. They predicted that the implantation of the graft

into the intraarticular space would not result in significant inflammation or infection and that it would lead to similar early postoperative outcomes compared with ACL reconstruction using an autologous hamstring graft. The BEAR scaffold is not cross-linked similar to other biologic scaffolds. Murray et al.[151] believed this would allow cells to more easily permeate and implant into the scaffold. In turn, the increased permeability leads to improved resorption of the material, therefore decreasing inflammatory immune reactions. The BEAR scaffold is also highly processed to remove any remaining bovine DNA that can serve as a potential immune trigger, which was demonstrated in preclinical testing.[150,151] In their nonrandomized study, 10 patients received the BEAR treatment, and 10 received standard ACL reconstruction with hamstring autograft. Results showed similar outcomes among the two groups using measurements such as effusion, pain, Lachman tests, and MRI analysis of ligament continuity. At 3 months, the BEAR group showed better hamstring strength than the hamstring autograft reconstruction group (mean ± standard deviation: $77.9 \pm 14.6\%$ vs. $55.9 \pm 7.8\%$ of the contralateral side; $P < .001$). Success of the BEAR technique in initial testing may demonstrate its readiness for further testing in a larger cohort of patients. A potential downside to the experiment by Murray et al. is that only patients with greater than 50% of the ACL tibial remnant were included in the study. This makes it difficult to extrapolate successful results to more severe tissue resorption or patients with less than 50% of the ACL tibial remnant intact.

Murray et al.[152] went one step further to consider the addition of thrombin to the PRP-collagen scaffold for further testing. In vivo, thrombin improves the healing process by increasing fibroblast growth and collagen synthesis. They found that a low concentration of thrombin added to the PRP-collagen scaffold can aid in recruitment of inflammatory cells but was not beneficial at high concentrations. Further research is required to identify the benefit of adding low concentrations of thrombin to a PRP-collagen scaffold to aid in the repair of partial ACL tears.

Though studies demonstrating the improved healing of partial ACL tears using PRP and collagen scaffolds are promising in canine models, further studies are needed to investigate ACL strength, long-term outcomes, and viability/applicability in human trials.

Stem cell therapy

The use of MSCs in orthopedic procedures has also stimulated interest in the research field. MSCs are derived from various sources, such as adipose, bone marrow, cartilage, periosteum, and muscle.[153] Their capability to differentiate into various cell types makes them a good candidate for therapeutic use, especially to improve healing. MSCs are capable of regenerating themselves, as well as developing into cells such as chondroblasts and osteoblasts, which are beneficial in the bone-healing process.[139] Kanaya et al.[154] performed a rodent study in which fluorescently tagged MSCs from the same rodent species were injected into the articular space surrounding a partially torn ACL. Results were compared to a control group where injections consisted of only buffered saline. They found that at 2 and 4 weeks after injection, the group receiving MSCs showed fluorescently tagged cells located at the partially torn ACL surface. Histologically, the group that received MSCs received a higher score, and at 4 weeks, the failure load was higher than that of the non-MSC group. In a similar rat study, Oe et al.[155] created three test groups of partially transected rat ACLs. One group received saline injections, one received cultured MSCs, and the third received fresh bone marrow cells (BMCs). They found that at 4 weeks, both the treatment groups showed cell migration to the site of healing and both appeared histologically normal. The BMC group showed more spindle cell formation, higher tensile strength, and more TGF-β in the joint space than the saline group.[140] These findings suggest that the use of fresh BMCs may improve the healing of partial ACL tears in animal models.

To our knowledge, the only existing human study that investigated BMSC injections for partial ACL tears was performed by Centeno et al.[156] in 2015. They evaluated grade 1–3 ACL tears (with grades 1 and 2 indicating partial tears) that had less than 1 cm ligament retraction. Ten patients were treated with fluoroscopically guided bone marrow concentrate PRP injections and assessed by MRI. Comparing magnetic resonance images from before and after the injection for each subject, they were able to assess ligament integrity using specific computer software and five MRI objective outcomes. Seven out of 10 patients had improved outcomes based on four out of five of their MRI measurements. Eight patients subjectively reported at least 70% improvement after the injection, and the mean improvement reported was 86.7%. Based on the findings of this study, it is possible that BMCs may be beneficial to the treatment of partial ACL tears with less than 1 cm ligament retraction, though additional human subject testing is warranted.

Future
The future of biologic augmentation in ligament reconstruction shows promise. Currently, there are

several animal studies, but few human trials, involving biologic augmentation for ACL reconstruction. More investigation of the biological treatment options, long-term effects of these treatments, and side-by-side comparisons with traditional treatment methods would provide crucial insight into the future of ACL reconstruction. To better understand the benefit of this new technology, more clinical trials are needed.

REFERENCES

1. Cooper RR, Misol S. Tendon and ligament insertion. A light and electron microscopic study. *J Bone Jt Surg Am.* 1970;52(1):1–20.
2. Cabaud HE. Biomechanics of the anterior cruciate ligament. *Clin Orthop Relat Res.* 1983;172:26–31.
3. Dodds JA, Arnoczky SP. Anatomy of the anterior cruciate ligament: a blueprint for repair and reconstruction. *Arthroscopy.* 1994;10(2):132–139.
4. Hey Groves E. Operation for repair of the crucial ligaments. *Clin Orthop Relat Res.* 1980;147:4–6.
5. Kennedy JC, Weinberg HW, Wilson AS. The anatomy and function of the anterior cruciate ligament. As determined by clinical and morphological studies. *J Bone Jt Surg Am.* 1974;56(2):223–235.
6. Last RJ. Some anatomical details of the knee joint. *J Bone Jt Surg Br.* 1948;30B(4):683–688.
7. Welsh RP. Knee joint structure and function. *Clin Orthop Relat Res.* 1980;147:7–14.
8. Girgis FG, Marshall JL, Monajem A. The cruciate ligaments of the knee joint. Anatomical, functional and experimental analysis. *Clin Orthop Relat Res.* 1975;106:216–231.
9. Butler DL, Noyes FR, Grood ES. Ligamentous restraints to anterior-posterior drawer in the human knee. A biomechanical study. *J Bone Jt Surg Am.* 1980;62(2):259–270.
10. Petersen W, Zantop T. Anatomy of the anterior cruciate ligament with regard to its two bundles. *Clin Orthop Relat Res.* 2007;454:35–47. https://doi.org/10.1097/BLO.0b013e31802b4a59.
11. Noyes FR, Butler DL, Grood ES, Zernicke RF, Hefzy MS. Biomechanical analysis of human ligament grafts used in knee-ligament repairs and reconstructions. *J Bone Jt Surg Am.* 1984;66(3):344–352.
12. Van Dommelen BA, Fowler PJ. Anatomy of the posterior cruciate ligament. A review. *Am J Sports Med.* 1989;17(1):24–29. https://doi.org/10.1177/036354658901700104.
13. Clancy WG, Shelbourne KD, Zoellner GB, Keene JS, Reider B, Rosenberg TD. Treatment of knee joint instability secondary to rupture of the posterior cruciate ligament. Report of a new procedure. *J Bone Jt Surg Am.* 1983;65(3):310–322.
14. Hughston JC, Andrews JR, Cross MJ, Moschi A. Classification of knee ligament instabilities. Part I. The medial compartment and cruciate ligaments. *J Bone Jt Surg Am.* 1976;58(2):159–172.

15. Kennedy JC, Hawkins RJ, Willis RB, Danylchuck KD. Tension studies of human knee ligaments. Yield point, ultimate failure, and disruption of the cruciate and tibial collateral ligaments. *J Bone Jt Surg Am.* 1976;58(3):350–355.

16. Hosseini Nasab SH, List R, Oberhofer K, Fucentese SF, Snedeker JG, Taylor WR. Loading patterns of the posterior cruciate ligament in the healthy knee: a systematic review. *PLoS One.* 2016;11(11):e0167106. https://doi.org/10.1371/journal.pone.0167106.

17. Brantigan OC, Voshell AF. The tibial collateral ligament: its function, its Bursae, and its relation to the medial meniscus. *J Bone Jt Surg.* 1943;25:121.

18. Sullivan D, Levy IM, Sheskier S, Torzilli PA, Warren RF. Medial restraints to anterior-posterior motion of the knee. *J Bone Jt Surg Am.* 1984;66(6):930–936.

19. Warren LA, Marshall JL, Girgis F. The prime static stabilizer of the medial side of the knee. *J Bone Jt Surg Am.* 1974;56(4):665–674.

20. Grood ES, Noyes FR, Butler DL, Suntay WJ. Ligamentous and capsular restraints preventing straight medial and lateral laxity in intact human cadaver knees. *J Bone Jt Surg Am.* 1981;63(8):1257–1269.

21. Chahla J, Moatshe G, Dean CS, Laprade RF. Posterolateral corner of the knee: current concepts. *Arch Bone Jt Surg.* 2016;97(9):97–103.

22. Chambat P, Guier C, Sonnery-Cottet B, Fayard JM, Thaunat M. The evolution of ACL reconstruction over the last fifty years. *Int Orthop.* 2013;37(2):181–186. https://doi.org/10.1007/s00264-012-1759-3.

23. Gupta R, Kapoor D, Kapoor L, et al. Immediate postoperative pain in anterior cruciate ligament reconstruction surgery with bone patellar tendon bone graft versus hamstring graft. *J Orthop Surg Res.* 2016;11(1):67. https://doi.org/10.1186/s13018-016-0399-5.

24. West RV, Harner CD. Graft selection in anterior cruciate ligament reconstruction. *J Am Acad Orthop Surg.* 2005;13(3):197–207.

25. Freedman KB, D'Amato MJ, Nedeff DD, Kaz A, Bach BR. Arthroscopic anterior cruciate ligament reconstruction: a metaanalysis comparing patellar tendon and hamstring tendon autografts. *Am J Sports Med.* 2003;31(1):2–11. https://doi.org/10.1177/03635465030310011501.

26. Aune AK, Holm I, Risberg MA, Jensen HK, Steen H. Four-strand hamstring tendon autograft compared with patellar tendon-bone autograft for anterior cruciate ligament reconstruction. A randomized study with two-year follow-up. *Am J Sports Med.* 2001;29(6):722–728. https://doi.org/10.1177/03635465010290060901.

27. Ejerhed L, Kartus J, Sernert N, Köhler K, Karlsson J. Patellar tendon or semitendinosus tendon autografts for anterior cruciate ligament reconstruction? A prospective randomized study with a two-year follow-up. *Am J Sports Med.* 2003;31(1):19–25. https://doi.org/10.1177/03635465030310011401.

28. Shaieb MD, Kan DM, Chang SK, Marumoto JM, Richardson AB. A prospective randomized comparison of patellar tendon versus semitendinosus and gracilis tendon autografts for anterior cruciate ligament reconstruction. *Am J Sports Med.* 2002;30(2):214–220. https://doi.org/10.1177/03635465020300021201.

29. Jansson KA, Linko E, Sandelin J, Harilainen A. A prospective randomized study of patellar versus hamstring tendon autografts for anterior cruciate ligament reconstruction. *Am J Sports Med.* 2003;31(1):12–18. https://doi.org/10.1177/03635465030310010501.

30. Beynnon BD, Johnson RJ, Fleming BC, et al. Anterior cruciate ligament replacement: comparison of bone-patellar tendon-bone grafts with two-strand hamstring grafts. A prospective, randomized study. *J Bone Jt Surg Am.* 2002;84-A(9):1503–1513.

31. Aglietti P, Buzzi R, D'Andria S, Zaccherotti G. Patellofemoral problems after intraarticular anterior cruciate ligament reconstruction. *Clin Orthop Relat Res.* 1993;288:195–204.

32. Hamner DL, Brown CH, Steiner ME, Hecker AT, Hayes WC. Hamstring tendon grafts for reconstruction of the anterior cruciate ligament: biomechanical evaluation of the use of multiple strands and tensioning techniques. *J Bone Jt Surg Am.* 1999;81(4):549–557.

33. Nakamura N, Horibe S, Sasaki S, et al. Evaluation of active knee flexion and hamstring strength after anterior cruciate ligament reconstruction using hamstring tendons. *Arthroscopy.* 2002;18(6):598–602.

34. Cerulli G, Placella G, Sebastiani E. ACL reconstruction: choosing the graft. *Joints.* 2013;1(1):18–24.

35. Rodeo SA, Arnoczky SP, Torzilli PA, Hidaka C, Warren RF. Tendon-healing in a bone tunnel. A biomechanical and histological study in the dog. *J Bone Jt Surg Am.* 1993;75(12):1795–1803.

36. Woo SL, Hollis JM, Adams DJ, Lyon RM, Takai S. Tensile properties of the human femur-anterior cruciate ligament-tibia complex. The effects of specimen age and orientation. *Am J Sports Med.* 1991;19(3):217–225. https://doi.org/10.1177/036354659101900303.

37. Brophy RH, Wright RW, Huston LJ, Nwosu SK. MOON Knee Group, Spindler KP. Factors associated with infection following anterior cruciate ligament reconstruction. *J Bone Jt Surg Am.* 2015;97(6):450–454. https://doi.org/10.2106/JBJS.N.00694.

38. Corry IS, Webb JM, Clingeleffer AJ, Pinczewski LA. Arthroscopic reconstruction of the anterior cruciate ligament. A comparison of patellar tendon autograft and four-strand hamstring tendon autograft. *Am J Sports Med.* 1999;27(4):444–454. https://doi.org/10.1177/03635465990270040701.

39. Shelbourne KD, Nitz P. Accelerated rehabilitation after anterior cruciate ligament reconstruction. *Am J Sports Med.* 1990;18(3):292–299. https://doi.org/10.1177/036354659001800313.

40. Marumoto JM, Mitsunaga MM, Richardson AB, Medoff RJ, Mayfield GW. Late patellar tendon ruptures after removal of the central third for anterior cruciate ligament reconstruction. A report of two cases. *Am J Sports Med.* 1996;24(5):698–701. https://doi.org/10.1177/036354659602400524.

41. Poehling-Monaghan KL, Salem H, Ross KE, et al. Long-term outcomes in anterior cruciate ligament reconstruction: a systematic review of patellar tendon versus hamstring autografts. *Orthop J Sport Med.* 2017;5(6):232596711770973. https://doi.org/10.1177/2325967117709735.

42. Samuelsen BT, Webster KE, Johnson NR, Hewett TE, Krych AJ. Hamstring autograft versus patellar tendon autograft for ACL reconstruction: is there a difference in graft failure rate? A meta-analysis of 47,613 patients. *Clin Orthop Relat Res.* 2017:1–10. https://doi.org/10.1007/s11999-017-5278-9.

43. Slone HS, Romine SE, Premkumar A, Xerogeanes JW. Quadriceps tendon autograft for anterior cruciate ligament reconstruction: a comprehensive review of current literature and systematic review of clinical results. *Arthroscopy.* 2015;31(3):541–554. https://doi.org/10.1016/j.arthro.2014.11.010.

44. Lee JK, Lee S, Lee MC. Outcomes of anatomic anterior cruciate ligament reconstruction: bone-quadriceps tendon graft versus double-bundle hamstring tendon graft. *Am J Sports Med.* 2016;44(9):2323–2329. https://doi.org/10.1177/0363546516650666.

45. Chen CH, Chen WJ, Shih CH. Arthroscopic anterior cruciate ligament reconstruction with quadriceps tendon-patellar bone autograft. *J Trauma.* 1999;46(4):678–682.

46. Fulkerson JP, Langeland R. An alternative cruciate reconstruction graft: the central quadriceps tendon. *Arthroscopy.* 1995;11(2):252–254.

47. Riaz O, Aqil A, Mannan A, et al. Quadriceps tendon-bone or patellar tendon-bone autografts when reconstructing the anterior cruciate ligament: a meta-analysis. *Clin J Sport Med.* June 2017. https://doi.org/10.1097/JSM.0000000000000451.

48. Lubowitz JH. Editorial commentary: quadriceps tendon autograft use for anterior cruciate ligament reconstruction predicted to increase. *Arthroscopy.* 2016;32(1):76–77. https://doi.org/10.1016/j.arthro.2015.11.004.

49. Geib TM, Shelton WR, Phelps RA, Clark L. Anterior cruciate ligament reconstruction using quadriceps tendon autograft: intermediate-term outcome. *Arthroscopy.* 2009;25(12):1408–1414. https://doi.org/10.1016/j.arthro.2009.06.004.

50. Shani RH, Umpierez E, Nasert M, Hiza EA, Xerogeanes J. Biomechanical comparison of quadriceps and patellar tendon grafts in anterior cruciate ligament reconstruction. *Arthroscopy.* 2016;32(1):71–75. https://doi.org/10.1016/j.arthro.2015.06.051.

51. Duchman KR, Lynch TS, Spindler KP. Graft selection in anterior cruciate ligament surgery: who gets what and why? *Clin Sports Med.* 2017;36(1):25–33. https://doi.org/10.1016/j.csm.2016.08.013.

52. Shelton WR, Treacy SH, Dukes AD, Bomboy AL. Use of allografts in knee reconstruction: II. Surgical considerations. *J Am Acad Orthop Surg.* 1998;6(3):169–175.

53. Shino K, Inoue M, Horibe S, Hamada M, Ono K. Reconstruction of the anterior cruciate ligament using allogeneic tendon. Long-term followup. *Am J Sports Med.* 1990;18(5):457–465. https://doi.org/10.1177/036354659001800502.

54. Indelicato PA, Linton RC, Huegel M. The results of fresh-frozen patellar tendon allografts for chronic anterior cruciate ligament deficiency of the knee. *Am J Sports Med.* 1992;20(2):118–121. https://doi.org/10.1177/036354659202000204.

55. Harner CD, Olson E, Irrgang JJ, Silverstein S, Fu FH, Silbey M. Allograft versus autograft anterior cruciate ligament reconstruction: 3- to 5-year outcome. *Clin Orthop Relat Res.* 1996;324:134–144.

56. Kaeding CC, Pedroza AD, Reinke EK, Huston LJ, MOON Consortium, Spindler KP. Risk factors and predictors of subsequent ACL injury in either knee after ACL reconstruction: prospective analysis of 2488 primary ACL reconstructions from the MOON cohort. *Am J Sports Med.* 2015;43(7):1583–1590. https://doi.org/10.1177/0363546515578836.

57. Kaeding CC, Pedroza AD, Reinke EK, et al. Change in anterior cruciate ligament graft choice and outcomes over time. *Arthroscopy.* 2017;33(11):2007–2014. https://doi.org/10.1016/j.arthro.2017.06.019.

58. Shelton WR, Treacy SH, Dukes AD, Bomboy AL. Use of allografts in knee reconstruction: I. Basic science aspects and current status. *J Am Acad Orthop Surg.* 1998;6(3):165–168.

59. Simonds RJ, Holmberg SD, Hurwitz RL, et al. Transmission of human immunodeficiency virus type 1 from a seronegative organ and tissue donor. *N Engl J Med.* 1992;326(11):726–732. https://doi.org/10.1056/NEJM199203123261102.

60. Paschos NK, Howell SM. Anterior cruciate ligament reconstruction: principles of treatment. *EFORT Open Rev.* 2016;1(11):398–408. https://doi.org/10.1302/2058-5241.1.160032.

61. Kaeding CC, Aros B, Pedroza A, et al. Allograft versus autograft anterior cruciate ligament reconstruction: predictors of failure from a MOON prospective longitudinal cohort. *Sports Health.* 2011;3(1):73–81. https://doi.org/10.1177/1941738110386185.

62. Kuechle DK, Pearson SE, Beach WR, et al. Allograft anterior cruciate ligament reconstruction in patients over 40 years of age. *Arthroscopy.* 2002;18(8):845–853.

63. Miller SL, Gladstone JN. Graft selection in anterior cruciate ligament reconstruction. *Orthop Clin North Am.* 2002;33(4):675–683.

64. Colombet P, Allard M, Bousquet V, de Lavigne C, Flurin P-H, Lachaud C. Anterior cruciate ligament reconstruction using four-strand semitendinosus and gracilis tendon grafts and metal interference screw fixation. *Arthroscopy.* 2002;18(3):232–237.

65. Shino K, Kawasaki T, Hirose H, Gotoh I, Inoue M, Ono K. Replacement of the anterior cruciate ligament by an allogeneic tendon graft. An experimental study in the dog. *J Bone Jt Surg Br.* 1984;66(5):672–681.

66. Jackson DW, Grood ES, Goldstein JD, et al. A comparison of patellar tendon autograft and allograft used for anterior cruciate ligament reconstruction in the goat model. *Am J Sports Med.* 1993;21(2):176–185. https://doi.org/10.1177/036354659302100203.

67. Legnani C, Ventura A, Terzaghi C, Borgo E, Albisetti W. Anterior cruciate ligament reconstruction with synthetic grafts. A review of literature. *Int Orthop*. 2010;34(4):465–471. https://doi.org/10.1007/s00264-010-0963-2.

68. Paulos LE, Rosenberg TD, Grewe SR, Tearse DS, Beck CL. The GORE-TEX anterior cruciate ligament prosthesis. A long-term followup. *Am J Sports Med*. 1992;20(3):246–252. https://doi.org/10.1177/036354659202000302.

69. Wilson WJ, Scranton Jr PE. Combined reconstruction of the anterior cruciate ligament in competitive athletes. *J Bone Jt Surg Am*. 1990;72(5):742–748.

70. Barrett GR, Line LL, Shelton WR, Manning JO, Phelps R. The Dacron ligament prosthesis in anterior cruciate ligament reconstruction. A four-year review. *Am J Sports Med*. 1993;21(3):367–373. https://doi.org/10.1177/036354659302100307.

71. Zoltan DJ, Reinecke C, Indelicato PA. Synthetic and allograft anterior cruciate ligament reconstruction. *Clin Sports Med*. 1988;7(4):773–784.

72. Kumar K, Maffulli N. The ligament augmentation device: an historical perspective. *Arthroscopy*. 1999;15(4):422–432.

73. Lavoie P, Fletcher J, Duval N. Patient satisfaction needs as related to knee stability and objective findings after ACL reconstruction using the LARS artificial ligament. *Knee*. 2000;7(3):157–163. https://doi.org/10.1016/S0968-0160(00)00039-9.

74. Jia Z, Xue C, Wang W, Liu T, Huang X, Xu W. Clinical outcomes of anterior cruciate ligament reconstruction using LARS artificial graft with an at least 7-year follow-up. *Med Baltim*. 2017;96(14):e6568. https://doi.org/10.1097/MD.0000000000006568.

75. Jia Z-Y, Zhang C, Cao S-Q, et al. Comparison of artificial graft versus autograft in anterior cruciate ligament reconstruction: a meta-analysis. *BMC Musculoskelet Disord*. 2017;18(1):309. https://doi.org/10.1186/s12891-017-1672-4.

76. Zaffagnini S, Grassi A, Marcheggiani Muccioli GM, et al. Anterior cruciate ligament reconstruction with a novel porcine xenograft: the initial Italian experience. *Joints*. 2015;3(2):85–90. https://doi.org/10.11138/jts/2015.3.2.085.

77. Cole BJ, Sayegh ET, Yanke AB, Chalmers PN, Frank RM. Fixation of soft tissue to bone: techniques and fundamentals. *J Am Acad Orthop Surg*. 2016;24(2):83–95. https://doi.org/10.5435/JAAOS-D-14-00081.

78. Chalmers P, Mall N, Yanke A, Bach BJ. Contemporary anterior cruciate ligament outcomes: does technique really matter? *Oper Tech Sports Med*. 2013:55–63.

79. Muller B, Bowman KF, Bedi A. ACL graft healing and biologics. *Clin Sports Med*. 2013;32(1):93–109. https://doi.org/10.1016/j.csm.2012.08.010.

80. Sagarriga Visconti C, Kavalkovich K, Wu J, Niyibizi C. Biochemical analysis of collagens at the ligament-bone interface reveals presence of cartilage-specific collagens. *Arch Biochem Biophys*. 1996;328(1):135–142. https://doi.org/10.1006/abbi.1996.0153.

81. Lui P, Zhang P, Chan K, Qin L. Biology and augmentation of tendon-bone insertion repair. *J Orthop Surg Res*. 2010;5:59. https://doi.org/10.1186/1749-799X-5-59.

82. Genin GM, Kent A, Birman V, et al. Functional grading of mineral and collagen in the attachment of tendon to bone. *Biophys J*. 2009;97(4):976–985. https://doi.org/10.1016/j.bpj.2009.05.043.

83. Amiel D, Frank C, Harwood F, Fronek J, Akeson W. Tendons and ligaments: a morphological and biochemical comparison. *J Orthop Res*. 1984;1(3):257–265. https://doi.org/10.1002/jor.1100010305.

84. Ćuti T, Antunović M, Marijanović I, et al. Capacity of muscle derived stem cells and pericytes to promote tendon graft integration and ligamentization following anterior cruciate ligament reconstruction. *Int Orthop*. 2017;41(6):1189–1198. https://doi.org/10.1007/s00264-017-3437-y.

85. Jackson JR, Minton JA, Ho ML, Wei N, Winkler JD. Expression of vascular endothelial growth factor in synovial fibroblasts is induced by hypoxia and interleukin 1beta. *J Rheumatol*. 1997;24(7):1253–1259.

86. Kawamura S, Ying L, Kim H-J, Dynybil C, Rodeo SA. Macrophages accumulate in the early phase of tendon-bone healing. *J Orthop Res*. 2005;23(6):1425–1432. https://doi.org/10.1016/j.orthres.2005.01.014.1100230627.

87. Kuroda R, Kurosaka M, Yoshiya S, Mizuno K. Localization of growth factors in the reconstructed anterior cruciate ligament: immunohistological study in dogs. *Knee Surg Sports Traumatol Arthrosc*. 2000;8(2):120–126. https://doi.org/10.1007/s001670050198.

88. Yoshikawa T, Tohyama H, Katsura T, et al. Effects of local administration of vascular endothelial growth factor on mechanical characteristics of the semitendinosus tendon graft after anterior cruciate ligament reconstruction in sheep. *Am J Sports Med*. 2006;34(12):1918–1925. https://doi.org/10.1177/0363546506294469.

89. Scheffler SU, Unterhauser FN, Weiler A. Graft remodeling and ligamentization after cruciate ligament reconstruction. *Knee Surg Sports Traumatol Arthrosc*. 2008;16(9):834–842. https://doi.org/10.1007/s00167-008-0560-8.

90. Florida SE, VanDusen KW, Mahalingam VD, et al. In vivo structural and cellular remodeling of engineered bone-ligament-bone constructs used for anterior cruciate ligament reconstruction in sheep. *Connect Tissue Res*. 2016;57(6):526–538. https://doi.org/10.1080/03008207.2016.1187141.

91. Kanazawa T, Soejima T, Murakami H, Inoue T, Katouda M, Nagata K. An immunohistological study of the integration at the bone-tendon interface after reconstruction of the anterior cruciate ligament in rabbits. *J Bone Jt Surg Br*. 2006;88(5):682–687. https://doi.org/10.1302/0301-620X.88B5.17198.

92. Lee BI, Kim BM, Kho DH, Kwon SW, Kim HJ, Hwang HR. Does the tibial remnant of the anterior cruciate ligament promote ligamentization? *Knee*. 2016;23(6):1133–1142. https://doi.org/10.1016/j.knee.2016.09.008.

93. Liu SH, Panossian V, Al-Shaikh R, et al. Morphology and matrix composition during early tendon to bone healing. *Clin Orthop Relat Res.* 1997;339:253–260.

94. Janssen RPA, Scheffler SU. Intra-articular remodelling of hamstring tendon grafts after anterior cruciate ligament reconstruction. *Knee Surg Sports Traumatol Arthrosc.* 2014;22(9):2102–2108. https://doi.org/10.1007/s00167-013-2634-5.

95. Amiel D, Kleiner JB, Roux RD, Harwood FL, Akeson WH. The phenomenon of "ligamentization": anterior cruciate ligament reconstruction with autogenous patellar tendon. *J Orthop Res.* 1986;4(2):162–172. https://doi.org/10.1002/jor.1100040204.

96. Rougraff BT, Shelbourne KD. Early histologic appearance of human patellar tendon autografts used for anterior cruciate ligament reconstruction. *Knee Surg Sports Traumatol Arthrosc.* 1999;7(1):9–14. https://doi.org/10.1007/s001670050113.

97. Zaffagnini S, De Pasquale V, Marchesini Reggiani L, et al. Neoligamentization process of BTPB used for ACL graft: histological evaluation from 6 months to 10 years. *Knee.* 2007;14(2):87–93. https://doi.org/10.1016/j.knee.2006.11.006.

98. Zaffagnini S, De Pasquale V, Marchesini Reggiani L, et al. Electron microscopy of the remodelling process in hamstring tendon used as ACL graft. *Knee Surg Sports Traumatol Arthrosc.* 2010;18(8):1052–1058. https://doi.org/10.1007/s00167-009-0925-7.

99. Clancy WG, Narechania RG, Rosenberg TD, Gmeiner JG, Wisnefske DD, Lange TA. Anterior and posterior cruciate ligament reconstruction in rhesus monkeys. *J Bone Jt Surg Am.* 1981;63(8):1270–1284.

100. Unterhauser FN, Bail HJ, Höher J, Haas NP, Weiler A. Endoligamentous revascularization of an anterior cruciate ligament graft. *Clin Orthop Relat Res.* 2003;414:276–288. https://doi.org/10.1097/01.blo.0000079442.64912.51.

101. Yoshikawa T, Tohyama H, Enomoto H, Matsumoto H, Toyama Y, Yasuda K. Expression of vascular endothelial growth factor and angiogenesis in patellar tendon grafts in the early phase after anterior cruciate ligament reconstruction. *Knee Surg Sports Traumatol Arthrosc.* 2006;14(9):804–810. https://doi.org/10.1007/s00167-006-0051-8.

102. Marumo K, Saito M, Yamagishi T, Fujii K. The "ligamentization" process in human anterior cruciate ligament reconstruction with autogenous patellar and hamstring tendons: a biochemical study. *Am J Sports Med.* 2005;33(8):1166–1173. https://doi.org/10.1177/0363546504271973.

103. Thomopoulos S, Williams GR, Soslowsky LJ. Tendon to bone healing: differences in biomechanical, structural, and compositional properties due to a range of activity levels. *J Biomech Eng.* 2003;125(1):106–113.

104. Nebelung W, Becker R, Urbach D, Röpke M, Roessner A. Histological findings of tendon-bone healing following anterior cruciate ligament reconstruction with hamstring grafts. *Arch Orthop Trauma Surg.* 2003;123(4):158–163. https://doi.org/10.1007/s00402-002-0463-y.

105. Roberts TT, Rosenbaum AJ. Bone grafts, bone substitutes and orthobiologics: the bridge between basic science and clinical advancements in fracture healing. *Organogenesis.* 2012;8(4):114–124. https://doi.org/10.4161/org.23306.

106. Oakes DA, Cabanela ME. Impaction bone grafting for revision hip arthroplasty: biology and clinical applications. *J Am Acad Orthop Surg.* 2006;14(11):620–628.

107. Khan SN, Cammisa FP, Sandhu HS, Diwan AD, Girardi FP, Lane JM. The biology of bone grafting. *J Am Acad Orthop Surg.* 2005;13(1):77–86.

108. Tomita F, Yasuda K, Mikami S, Sakai T, Yamazaki S, Tohyama H. Comparisons of intraosseous graft healing between the doubled flexor tendon graft and the bone-patellar tendon-bone graft in anterior cruciate ligament reconstruction. *Arthroscopy.* 2001;17(5):461–476. https://doi.org/10.1053/jars.2001.24059.

109. Di Matteo B, Loibl M, Andriolo L, et al. Biologic agents for anterior cruciate ligament healing: a systematic review. *World J Orthop.* 2016;7(9):592. https://doi.org/10.5312/wjo.v7.i9.592.

110. Vavken P, Sadoghi P, Murray MM. The effect of platelet concentrates on graft maturation and graft-bone interface healing in anterior cruciate ligament reconstruction in human patients: a systematic review of controlled trials. *Arthroscopy.* 2011;27(11):1573–1583. https://doi.org/10.1016/j.arthro.2011.06.003.

111. Del Torto M, Enea D, Panfoli N, Filardo G, Pace N, Chiusaroli M. Hamstrings anterior cruciate ligament reconstruction with and without platelet rich fibrin matrix. *Knee Surg Sports Traumatol Arthrosc.* 2015;23(12):3614–3622. https://doi.org/10.1007/s00167-014-3260-6.

112. Valentí Azcárate A, Lamo-Espinosa J, Aquerreta Beola JD, Hernandez Gonzalez M, Mora Gasque G, Valentí Nin JR. Comparison between two different platelet-rich plasma preparations and control applied during anterior cruciate ligament reconstruction. Is there any evidence to support their use? *Injury.* 2014;45(suppl 4):S36–S41. https://doi.org/10.1016/S0020-1383(14)70008-7.

113. Magnussen RA, Flanigan DC, Pedroza AD, Heinlein KA, Kaeding CC. Platelet rich plasma use in allograft ACL reconstructions: two-year clinical results of a MOON cohort study. *Knee.* 2013;20(4):277–280. https://doi.org/10.1016/j.knee.2012.12.001.

114. Darabos N, Haspl M, Moser C, Darabos A, Bartolek D, Groenemeyer D. Intraarticular application of autologous conditioned serum (ACS) reduces bone tunnel widening after ACL reconstructive surgery in a randomized controlled trial. *Knee Surg Sports Traumatol Arthrosc.* 2011;19(suppl 1):S36–S46. https://doi.org/10.1007/s00167-011-1458-4.

115. Vogrin M, Rupreht M, Crnjac A, Dinevski D, Krajnc Z, Recnik G. The effect of platelet-derived growth factors on knee stability after anterior cruciate ligament reconstruction: a prospective randomized clinical study. *Wien Klin Wochenschr.* 2010;122(suppl):91–95. https://doi.org/10.1007/s00508-010-1340-2.

116. Vadalà A, Iorio R, De Carli A, et al. Platelet-rich plasma: does it help reduce tunnel widening after ACL reconstruction? *Knee Surg Sports Traumatol Arthrosc.* 2013;21(4):824–829. https://doi.org/10.1007/s00167-012-1980-z.

117. Li F, Jia H, Yu C. ACL reconstruction in a rabbit model using irradiated Achilles allograft seeded with mesenchymal stem cells or PDGF-B gene-transfected mesenchymal stem cells. *Knee Surg Sports Traumatol Arthrosc.* 2007;15(10):1219–1227. https://doi.org/10.1007/s00167-007-0385-x.

118. CH C, Whu S, Chang C, Su C. Gene and protein expressions of bone marrow mesenchymal stem cells in a bone tunnel for tendon-bone healing. *Formos J Musculoskelet Disord.* 2011;2(3):85–93.

119. Webster KE, Feller JA, Elliott J, Hutchison A, Payne R. A comparison of bone tunnel measurements made using computed tomography and digital plain radiography after anterior cruciate ligament reconstruction. *Arthroscopy.* 2004;20(9):946–950. https://doi.org/10.1016/j.arthro.2004.06.037.

120. Fauno P, Kaalund S. Tunnel widening after hamstring anterior cruciate ligament reconstruction is influenced by the type of graft fixation used: a prospective randomized study. *Arthroscopy.* 2005;21(11):1337–1341. https://doi.org/10.1016/j.arthro.2005.08.023.

121. Silva A, Sampaio R, Pinto E. Femoral tunnel enlargement after anatomic ACL reconstruction: a biological problem? *Knee Surg Sports Traumatol Arthrosc.* 2010;18(9):1189–1194. https://doi.org/10.1007/s00167-010-1046-z.

122. Mirzatolooei F, Alamdari MT, Khalkhali HR. The impact of platelet-rich plasma on the prevention of tunnel widening in anterior cruciate ligament reconstruction using quadrupled autologous hamstring tendon: a randomised clinical trial. *Bone Jt J.* 2013;95-B(1):65–69. https://doi.org/10.1302/0301-620X.95B1.30487.

123. Starantzis KA, Mastrokalos D, Koulalis D, Papakonstantinou O, Soucacos PN, Papagelopoulos PJ. The potentially positive role of PRPs in preventing femoral tunnel widening in ACL reconstruction surgery using hamstrings: a clinical study in 51 patients. *J Sport Med (Hindawi Publ Corp).* 2014;2014:789317. https://doi.org/10.1155/2014/789317.

124. Orrego M, Larrain C, Rosales J, et al. Effects of platelet concentrate and a bone plug on the healing of hamstring tendons in a bone tunnel. *Arthroscopy.* 2008;24(12):1373–1380. https://doi.org/10.1016/j.arthro.2008.07.016.

125. Silva A, Sampaio R. Anatomic ACL reconstruction: does the platelet-rich plasma accelerate tendon healing? *Knee Surg Sports Traumatol Arthrosc.* 2009;17(6):676–682. https://doi.org/10.1007/s00167-009-0762-8.

126. Figueroa D, Melean P, Calvo R, et al. Magnetic resonance imaging evaluation of the integration and maturation of semitendinosus-gracilis graft in anterior cruciate ligament reconstruction using autologous platelet concentrate. *Arthroscopy.* 2010;26(10):1318–1325. https://doi.org/10.1016/j.arthro.2010.02.010.

127. Vogrin M, Rupreht M, Dinevski D, et al. Effects of a platelet gel on early graft revascularization after anterior cruciate ligament reconstruction: a prospective, randomized, double-blind, clinical trial. *Eur Surg Res.* 2010;45(2):77–85. https://doi.org/10.1159/000318597.

128. Rupreht M, Jevtič V, Serša I, Vogrin M, Jevšek M. Evaluation of the tibial tunnel after intraoperatively administered platelet-rich plasma gel during anterior cruciate ligament reconstruction using diffusion weighted and dynamic contrast-enhanced MRI. *J Magn Reson Imaging.* 2013;37(4):928–935. https://doi.org/10.1002/jmri.23886.

129. Guo R, Gao L, Xu B. Current evidence of adult stem cells to enhance anterior cruciate ligament treatment: a systematic review of animal trials. *Arthroscopy.* September 2017. https://doi.org/10.1016/j.arthro.2017.07.010.

130. Lim J-K, Hui J, Li L, Thambyah A, Goh J, Lee E-H. Enhancement of tendon graft osteointegration using mesenchymal stem cells in a rabbit model of anterior cruciate ligament reconstruction. *Arthroscopy.* 2004;20(9):899–910. https://doi.org/10.1016/j.arthro.2004.06.035.

131. Soon MYH, Hassan A, Hui JHP, Goh JCH, Lee EH. An analysis of soft tissue allograft anterior cruciate ligament reconstruction in a rabbit model: a short-term study of the use of mesenchymal stem cells to enhance tendon osteointegration. *Am J Sports Med.* 2007;35(6):962–971. https://doi.org/10.1177/0363546507300057.

132. Silva A, Sampaio R, Fernandes R, Pinto E. Is there a role for adult non-cultivated bone marrow stem cells in ACL reconstruction? *Knee Surg Sports Traumatol Arthrosc.* 2014;22(1):66–71. https://doi.org/10.1007/s00167-012-2279-9.

133. Seijas R, Ares O, Catala J, Alvarez-Diaz P, Cusco X, Cugat R. Magnetic resonance imaging evaluation of patellar tendon graft remodelling after anterior cruciate ligament reconstruction with or without platelet-rich plasma. *J Orthop Surg (Hong Kong).* 2013;21(1):10–14. https://doi.org/10.1177/230949901302100105.

134. Radice F, Yánez R, Gutiérrez V, Rosales J, Pinedo M, Coda S. Comparison of magnetic resonance imaging findings in anterior cruciate ligament grafts with and without autologous platelet-derived growth factors. *Arthroscopy.* 2010;26(1):50–57. https://doi.org/10.1016/j.arthro.2009.06.030.

135. Nin JRV, Gasque GM, Azcárate AV, Beola JDA, Gonzalez MH. Has platelet-rich plasma any role in anterior cruciate ligament allograft healing? *Arthroscopy.* 2009;25(11):1206–1213. https://doi.org/10.1016/j.arthro.2009.06.002.

136. Sánchez M, Anitua E, Azofra J, Prado R, Muruzabal F, Andia I. Ligamentization of tendon grafts treated with an endogenous preparation rich in growth factors: gross morphology and histology. *Arthroscopy.* 2010;26(4):470–480. https://doi.org/10.1016/j.arthro.2009.08.019.

137. Murray MM, Spindler KP, Ballard P, Welch TP, Zurakowski D, Nanney LB. Enhanced histologic repair in a central wound in the anterior cruciate ligament with a collagen-platelet-rich plasma scaffold. *J Orthop Res.* 2007;25(8):1007–1017. https://doi.org/10.1002/jor.20367.

138. Tjoumakaris FP, Donegan DJ, Sekiya JK. Partial tears of the anterior cruciate ligament: diagnosis and treatment. *Am J Orthop (Belle Mead NJ)*. 2011;40(2):92–97.

139. Dallo I, Chahla J, Mitchell JJ, Pascual-Garrido C, Feagin JA, LaPrade RF. Biologic approaches for the treatment of partial tears of the anterior cruciate ligament: a current concepts review. *Orthop J Sport Med*. 2017;5(1):2325967116681724. https://doi.org/10.1177/2325967116681724.

140. Vavken P, Fleming BC, Mastrangelo AN, Machan JT, Murray MM. Biomechanical outcomes after bioenhanced anterior cruciate ligament repair and anterior cruciate ligament reconstruction are equal in a porcine model. *Arthroscopy*. 2012;28(5):672–680. https://doi.org/10.1016/j.arthro.2011.10.008.

141. Rość D, Powierza W, Zastawna E, Drewniak W, Michalski A, Kotschy M. Post-traumatic plasminogenesis in intraarticular exudate in the knee joint. *Med Sci Monit*. 2002;8(5):CR371–CR378.

142. Vavken P, Murray MM. The potential for primary repair of the ACL. *Sports Med Arthrosc*. 2011;19(1):44–49. https://doi.org/10.1097/JSA.0b013e3182095e5d.

143. Seijas R, Ares O, Cuscó X, Alvarez P, Steinbacher G, Cugat R. Partial anterior cruciate ligament tears treated with intraligamentary plasma rich in growth factors. *World J Orthop*. 2014;5(3):373–378. https://doi.org/10.5312/wjo.v5.i3.373.

144. Bozynski CC, Stannard JP, Smith P, et al. Acute management of anterior cruciate ligament injuries using novel canine models. *J Knee Surg*. 2016;29(7):594–603. https://doi.org/10.1055/s-0035-1570115.

145. Cook JL, Smith PA, Bozynski CC, et al. Multiple injections of leukoreduced platelet rich plasma reduce pain and functional impairment in a canine model of ACL and meniscal deficiency. *J Orthop Res*. 2016;34(4):607–615. https://doi.org/10.1002/jor.23054.

146. Murray MM, Palmer M, Abreu E, Spindler KP, Zurakowski D, Fleming BC. Platelet-rich plasma alone is not sufficient to enhance suture repair of the ACL in skeletally immature animals: an in vivo study. *J Orthop Res*. 2009;27(5):639–645. https://doi.org/10.1002/jor.20796.

147. Brommer EJ, Dooijewaard G, Dijkmans BA, Breedveld FC. Depression of tissue-type plasminogen activator and enhancement of urokinase-type plasminogen activator as an expression of local inflammation. *Thromb Haemost*. 1992;68(2):180–184.

148. Dunn MG, Liesch JB, Tiku ML, Zawadsky JP. Development of fibroblast-seeded ligament analogs for ACL reconstruction. *J Biomed Mater Res*. 1995;29(11):1363–1371. https://doi.org/10.1002/jbm.820291107.

149. Murray MM, Spindler KP, Devin C, et al. Use of a collagen-platelet rich plasma scaffold to stimulate healing of a central defect in the canine ACL. *J Orthop Res*. 2006;24(4):820–830. https://doi.org/10.1002/jor.20073.

150. Murray MM, Flutie BM, Kalish LA, et al. The bridge-enhanced anterior cruciate ligament repair (BEAR) procedure. *Orthop J Sport Med*. 2016;4(11):232596711667217. https://doi.org/10.1177/2325967116672176.

151. Magarian EM, Vavken P, Connolly S a, Mastrangelo AN, Murray MM. Safety of intra-articular use of atelocollagen for enhanced tissue repair. *Open Orthop J*. 2012;6:231–238. https://doi.org/10.2174/1874325001206010231.

152. Murray MM, Forsythe B, Chen F, et al. The effect of thrombin on ACL fibroblast interactions with collagen hydrogels. *J Orthop Res*. 2006;24(3):508–515. https://doi.org/10.1002/jor.20054.

153. Fellows CR, Matta C, Zakany R, Khan IM, Mobasheri A. Adipose, bone marrow and synovial joint-derived mesenchymal stem cells for cartilage repair. *Front Genet*. 2016;7:1–20. https://doi.org/10.3389/fgene.2016.00213.

154. Kanaya A, Deie M, Adachi N, Nishimori M, Yanada S, Ochi M. Intra-articular injection of mesenchymal stromal cells in partially torn anterior cruciate ligaments in a rat model. *Arthroscopy*. 2007;23(6):610–617. https://doi.org/10.1016/j.arthro.2007.01.013.

155. Oe K, Kushida T, Okamoto N, et al. New strategies for anterior cruciate ligament partial rupture using bone marrow transplantation in rats. *Stem Cells Dev*. 2011;20(4):671–679. https://doi.org/10.1089/scd.2010.0182.

156. Centeno CJ, Pitts J, Al-Sayegh H, Freeman MD. Anterior cruciate ligament tears treated with percutaneous injection of autologous bone marrow nucleated cells: a case series. *J Pain Res*. 2015;8:437–447. https://doi.org/10.2147/JPR.S86244.

FURTHER READING

1. Amiel D, Kleiner JB, Akeson WH. The natural history of the anterior cruciate ligament autograft of patellar tendon origin. *Am J Sports Med*. 1986;14(6):449–462. https://doi.org/10.1177/036354658601400603.

2. Janssen RPA, van der Wijk J, Fiedler A, Schmidt T, Sala HAGM, Scheffler SU. Remodelling of human hamstring autografts after anterior cruciate ligament reconstruction. *Knee Surg Sports Traumatol Arthrosc*. 2011;19(8):1299–1306. https://doi.org/10.1007/s00167-011-1419-y.

3. Kleiner JB, Amiel D, Harwood FL, Akeson WH. Early histologic, metabolic, and vascular assessment of anterior cruciate ligament autografts. *J Orthop Res*. 1989;7(2):235–242. https://doi.org/10.1002/jor.1100070211.

4. Murray MM, Martin SD, Martin TL, Spector M. Histological changes in the human anterior cruciate ligament after rupture. *J Bone Jt Surg Am*. 2000;82-A(10):1387–1397.

CHAPTER 12

Treating the Subchondral Environment and Avascular Necrosis

JORGE CHAHLA, MD, PHD • ANDREAS H. GOMOLL, MD •
BERT R. MANDELBAUM, MD, DHL

INTRODUCTION

Although cartilage research has grown exponentially, basic science and clinical studies focusing on its foundation, namely the subchondral bone, have not received the same attention.[1] The subchondral bone provides mechanical and biological support for the overlying articular cartilage, and it undergoes constant adaptation in response to changes in the biomechanical environment of the joint.[1] It is noticeably involved in several chondral entities such as osteochondritis dissecans, osteoarthritis, and focal chondral defects.

Consequently, subchondral bone lesions are commonly associated with cartilage lesions. To better understand the pathology of the subchondral bone, a thorough understanding of the anatomy, morphology, and physiology of the subchondral bone and its function is required. The articular cartilage consists of 5 different zones, which can be distinguished based on the morphology and orientation of collagen fibrils.[2] In the superficial zone, the collagen fibers are tangentially oriented into tightly packed parallel laminae that radiate vertically from the calcified zone. Zone two, or intermediate zone, contains randomly oriented collagen fibrils. Zone three, which is also referred to as the radial zone, is the thickest layer with the highest amount of proteoglycans and water. The tidemark serves as the junction between the calcified and uncalcified cartilage matrix (zone 4). Finally, the zone of calcification (zone 5) serves as an anchor to a complex network of collagen fibrils (Fig. 12.1).

The definition of subchondral bone is still a subject of debate. The most accepted definition is that the subchondral plate is as a zone that divides the articular cartilage from the marrow cavity. It comprises two parts: (1) the calcified region of the articular cartilage and (2) a layer of lamellar bone.[3] The subchondral bone is located deep to the calcified layer and includes an arterial plexus that has branches to the calcified layer (Fig. 12.2). The blood flow in this zone is 3–10 times higher than that in cancellous bone.[4] Likewise, the venous systems contain a plexus of vessels that are vulnerable to compressive and shear forces. The cortical endplate contains perforations that form channels to allow communication with the basal cartilage. These channels are dynamic and change in response to compressive forces that act on the cartilage and subchondral bone.[5]

The purpose of this chapter is to review the different pathologic entities originating from the subchondral bone; define the characteristics of each; and discuss treatment indications, outcomes, and complications of different approaches for the treatment of each subchondral bone pathology.

Osteonecrosis

Spontaneous osteonecrosis of the knee (SPONK) was first described by Ahlback in 1968, in 40 patients with severe sudden onset of pain.[6] It is defined as a disease of the subchondral bone that leads to focal ischemia, with subsequent necrosis, and possible structural collapse if not addressed properly. Although the etiology is not always clearly defined (idiopathic in most of the cases), patient features as well as underlying risk factors can help classify the type of osteonecrosis (ON) and therefore guide treatment. In this regard, ON of the knee can be divided into three categories: (1) primary or SPONK, (2) secondary ON (SON), and (3) postarthroscopic ON. Irrespective of the type of ON, the treatment goals for this disease are to stop further progression and delay the onset of end-stage arthritis of the knee. Once considerable joint surface collapse has occurred or advanced osteoarthritis has developed, arthroplasty is often the most appropriate treatment option.

Biologics in Orthopaedic Surgery. https://doi.org/10.1016/B978-0-323-55140-3.00012-6

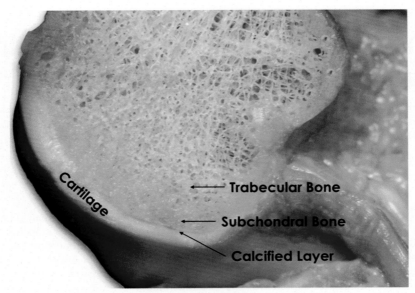

FIG. 12.1 Cadaveric dissection image of a hemicondyle as viewed from the intercondylar notch demonstrating a sagittal view of the superficial and inner layers, showing cartilage, calcified layer, and the differences between subchondral and trabecular bone.

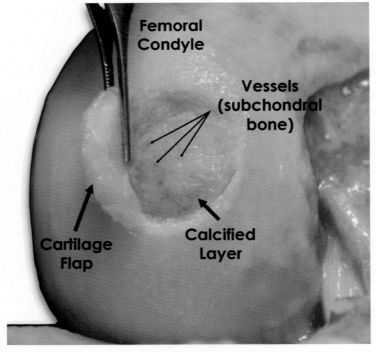

FIG. 12.2 Dissected lateral femoral condyle (right knee) demonstrating the calcified layer and the subchondral bone vessels below this layer. A cartilage flap is being retracted to demonstrate the deeper aspect of the cartilage.

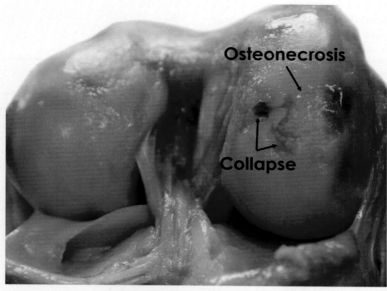

FIG. 12.3 Cadaveric dissection of a right knee demonstrating osteonecrosis of the medial femoral condyle. The black spots represent avascular areas of the cartilage that have undergone necrosis. Furthermore, collapse of the chondral surface can be seen in multiple areas of the condyle.

Spontaneous ON of the knee

SPONK classically presents in the older population with a reported incidence of 9.4% in patients older than 55 years.[7,8] It affects females three to five times more than males[9] and typically presents in the medial femoral condyle. The medial femoral condyle is typically affected in 94% of the times.[10] This can be caused because of a relatively diminished extraosseous and intraosseous blood supply to the medial femoral condyle, with apparent watershed areas making it more vulnerable to a vascular insult.[11] Despite the varying blood supply, the lateral condyle, tibial condyles, as well as the patella can also be affected.[12] Though the true incidence is not well established, it may be more prevalent than SON.

Although the precise etiology of spontaneous ON remains tenuous, various etiologies have been proposed. In ON of the hip, it is widely accepted that a vascular insult precipitates bone death. However, this has not been demonstrated in the knee as of yet. Several authors have reported that a traumatic event leads to microfractures in a debilitated subchondral bone (osteopenic) resulting in accumulated fluid in the space created by the subchondral microfractures.[13–15] The fluid accumulation results in increased intraosseous pressure and bone marrow edema, decreased blood perfusion, and eventual focal osseous ischemia.[13,14]

Although a traumatic etiology has been implicated, only a minority of patients can specifically recall an injury.[7,16] However, given the demographics of the affected patients and the high incidence of insufficiency fractures among postmenopausal women, associating an insidious precipitating event with the onset of knee pain can be challenging (Fig. 12.3).[16]

Tears involving the medial meniscus, specifically the posterior meniscal root, have been proposed as a potential etiologic factor for SPONK. Robertson et al. identified 30 consecutive patients with spontaneous ON of the medial femoral condyle. The radiographs and magnetic resonance imaging (MRI) were reviewed, and 80% of the patients were found to have a medial meniscal root tear.[17] The authors suggested that the loss of hoop stress results in an increased load in the compartment (similar to a total meniscectomized state),[18] inducing a subchondral insufficiency fracture.[17,19,20] Moreover, early detection of these lesions is crucial because knee biomechanics can be restored to a near-native state if this lesion is properly diagnosed and treated in a timely fashion, and the progression to ON and ultimately to osteoarthritis can be significantly slowed.[21,22] This theory is supported by a study demonstrating that there was a positive association between low bone mineral density and the incidence of SPONK in women older than 60 years.[23]

Clinical presentation and diagnosis. Patients with SPONK typically present with a sudden onset of medial-sided knee pain, which is not precipitated by trauma. Pain is worse at night and with weight bearing.[9] Range of motion may be somewhat limited secondary to pain or effusion, but usually not due to a mechanical reason. Focal tenderness over the medial femoral condyle is the most common finding on physical examination.[24] Ligamentous examination is usually normal in these patients. The intense pain associated with the acute phase of SPONK may last up to 6 weeks.[16,25] Patients who improve after 6 weeks typically have smaller lesions (less than 40% of the width of the femoral condyle)[26] and commonly have a satisfactory result, although mild symptoms could persist for up to a year.[25] Patients experiencing persistent symptoms even after 6 weeks are more likely to remain symptomatic. In these cases, imaging will often demonstrate a rapid progression with collapse and the development of degenerative changes.[27]

Imaging is crucial for the diagnosis of SPONK and typically includes radiographs and MRI. Initial radiographic evaluation of patients with SPONK includes weight bearing anteroposterior, flexion posteroanterior (Rosenberg), lateral, and skyline or merchant view. Radiographic findings in patients with SPONK can vary depending on the stage of the disease.[9] In early stages of the process, plain X-rays could be normal despite the presence of significant symptoms, and therefore, a high level of suspicion is necessary.[28] In later stages a radiolucent lesion with a surrounding sclerotic halo can be seen.[28] If not properly addressed, radiographs may reveal subtle flattening of the involved femoral condyle to significant subchondral collapse and secondary degenerative changes (Fig. 12.4).[29]

MRI is the gold standard for detection of incipient changes of the disease because of its high sensitivity.[16,30] T1 imaging shows a discrete low-signal area often surrounded by an area of intermediate signal intensity (structural changes can be seen in a more detailed manner). A serpiginous low-signal line is often present at the margin of the lesion, delineating the necrotic area from the adjacent area of bone marrow edema.[16,28,31] Areas affected by SPONK will demonstrate a high signal intensity in the region of the bone marrow edema with T2 imaging (more sensitivity than T1) (Fig. 12.5).[28,31,32]

Classification and prognosis. Staging of the disease constitutes the main factor when deciding which treatment algorithm to follow in each specific case. In

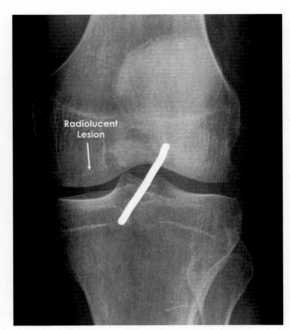

FIG. 12.4 Left knee anteroposterior radiograph demonstrating a subtle radiolucent lesion on the medial femoral condyle.

addition, size of the lesions and overall status of the joint should be considered as well. These factors also aid in predicting the clinical course and prognosis of the patient.[10] The Koshino staging system[33] takes clinical and radiographic parameters into consideration. Symptomatic patients with normal radiographic findings are classified as stage I. Stage II demonstrates the weight-bearing area with flattening and subchondral radiolucencies surrounded by osteosclerosis. Stage III demonstrates extension of the radiolucencies around the affected area and subchondral collapse. Finally, stage IV is the degenerative phase with osteosclerosis and osteophyte formation around the condyles.

Lotke et al. developed a method of determining the size of the osteonecrotic lesion on anteroposterior (AP) radiographs using a percentage of the affected femoral condyle.[24] A ratio of the width of the lesion compared with the overall width of the femoral condyle is calculated as a percentage. They reported that in patients with lesions involving 32% of the medial femoral condyle, only 6 of 23 knees required surgical management. If the lesion involved more than 50% of the medial femoral condyle, all required prosthetic arthroplasty (Fig. 12.6).[24]

Nonoperative management. As a working algorithm, it can be stated that most small lesions (typically

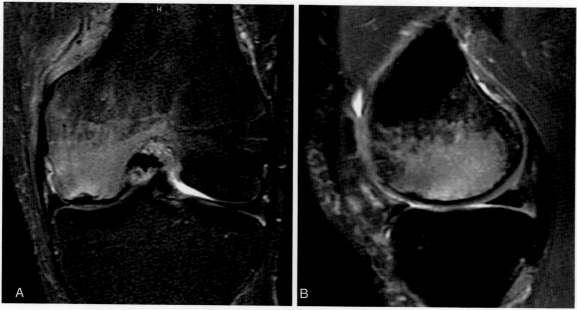

FIG. 12.5 **(A)** Coronal and **(B)** sagittal T2 MRI demonstrating a serpiginous low-signal line at the margin of the lesion (image A), delineating the necrotic area from the adjacent area of bone marrow edema.

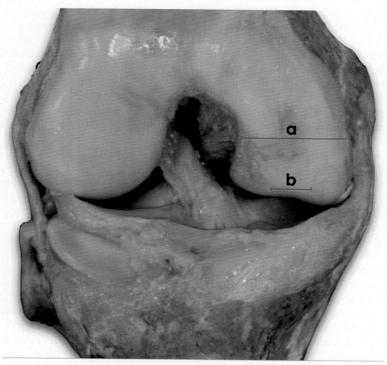

FIG. 12.6 Cadaveric representation on how the size of the osteonecrotic lesion may be determined as a percentage of the diameter of the medial femoral condyle (b/a×z100=% involvement of the medial femoral condyle).

<3.5 cm squared) can be approached with nonoperative management, whereas most large lesions (>5 cm squared) should be treated operatively to prevent progress to collapse. Medium-sized lesion (3.5–5.0 cm squared) can have an unpredictable course and should be evaluated on a case-by-case basis.[9,34]

For small lesions, protected weight bearing for 4–6 weeks constitutes the most important measure to avoid collapse, and analgesics are provided as needed.[32,35] Lotke et al. reported that 88.9% of patients with stage I disease can expect complete resolution of their symptoms after a course of conservative treatment.[24] Bisphosphonates have demonstrated a potential role in the reduction of pain and prevention of subchondral collapse associated with ON of the hip by inhibition of osteoclastic resorption of necrotic bone. Bisphosphonates bind to bone, which subsequently is resorbed by osteoclasts. Once internalized by the osteoclast, the bisphosphonate then interferes with the cellular metabolism, leading to apoptosis and ultimately inhibition of bone resorption. Jureus et al.[36] evaluated bisphosphonate use for a minimum of 6 months in 17 patients with SPONK. Although three patients progressed to subchondral collapse, they noted that 2 of the 3 patients who failed treatment ended their medication regimen prematurely.[36] Conversely, Meier et al. found no difference in pain scores and radiographic outcome measurements in those treated with bisphosphonates versus placebo in early stage SPONK.[35,37] Another nonoperative approach described in the literature is pulsed electromagnetic field therapy (PEMF). PEMF therapy has been reported to produce anti-inflammatory and bone-healing effects by decreasing the production of free radicals and stimulating osteoblasts.[38–40] A recent study reported on 28 patients who had a significant reduction in pain, size of the necrotic lesion, as well as the mean femoral bone marrow lesion's area at 6 months of follow-up.[41]

Surgical management. Patients who demonstrate radiographic evidence of a large initial, or rapidly progressing, lesion or those who have failed a trial of conservative management for at least 3 months may benefit from joint-preserving procedures or prosthetic replacement. Joint-preserving techniques such as core decompression, osteochondral allograft transplantation, and osteotomies can potentially avoid or postpone the need for joint replacement.[42] Arthroscopic debridement has a limited role in the management of SPONK because of the inability to alter the natural history of the disease. However, those with identifiable mechanical symptoms due to unstable chondral fragments or loose bodies may experience symptomatic relief.[43] A recent systematic review reported that core decompression prevented additional surgical treatment in precollapse knees with a failure rate of 10.4% and that osteochondral grafts decreased the need for additional surgery in both precollapse and postcollapse knees (Fig. 12.7).[44]

Core decompression of osteonecrotic lesions of the knee was first introduced by Jacobs el al. in 1989.[45] The reported mechanism of action is to relieve elevated intraosseous pressure and stimulate vascularity within the lesion through extra-articular drilling. Several authors have reported successful treatment using this technique in the knee.[45–47] Core decompression has been shown to slow the rate of symptomatic progression of avascular necrosis and may extend the symptom-free interval in certain patients with the hope of delaying more extensive procedures.[47] In a series of 16 patients (15 type I and 1 type II lesions), it was shown that normalization of bone marrow signal at 3-year follow-up could be obtained, along with symptomatic relief after core decompression.[46] Deie et al. treated 12 subjects with Koshino stage II or III disease with core decompression and calcium hydroxyapatite artificial bone grafting. All patients in this series reported improved knee pain and avoided total knee arthroplasty (TKA) at a mean follow-up of 25 months.[48]

Osteochondral autografting has demonstrated favorable results in patients who have progressed to subchondral collapse by restoration of the cartilage surface.[35,42,49] Duany et al. reported excellent outcomes in 9 patients who underwent osteochondral autografts for the treatment of SPONK.[42] Similarly, Tanaka et al. reported on 6 patients, who had SPONK, undergoing osteochondral autograft, in which all patients reported favorable pain relief after a mean follow-up of 28 months.[35,49]

High tibial osteotomy (HTO) is a reliable procedure to offload the affected compartment, thereby decreasing the effective intraosseous pressure within the lesion in an attempt to slow or prevent progression.[16,35,50,51] Concomitant procedures to promote healing such as core decompression and supplementation with bone substitutes or biologics can also be performed.[48,52] Koshino et al. demonstrated improved outcomes when an HTO was performed with concomitant drilling and bone grafting with an anatomical axis correction to at least 10 degrees of anatomic valgus alignment.[53]

Finally, patients who are not candidates for joint-preserving procedures or fail the treatments previously discussed can be treated with unicompartmental arthroplasty (UKA) or standard TKA. Given the high frequency of unicompartmental involvement in SPONK, UKA may

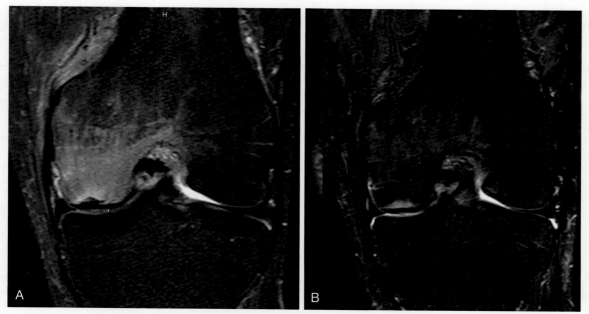

FIG. 12.7 **(A)** Coronal and **(B)** sagittal T2 MRI showing the initial imaging and progression (3 months), respectively, of a spontaneous ON treated with core decompression and bone marrow aspirate concentrate.

be an attractive option because of preservation of bone stock and functioning cruciate ligaments compared with TKA. Advocates of this treatment report a shorter rehabilitation period and less postoperative pain in patients undergoing UKA versus TKA, with less challenging future revisions options.[54] A meta-analysis of results from five reports for UKA for SPONK reported 92% good outcomes and 6% poor outcomes, with 3% of revisions in 64 knees over a mean follow-up period of 5 years.[55] However, Ritter et al. reported that patients treated for SPONK had less pain relief (82% vs. 90%) and a higher incidence of revision surgery (17% vs. 0%) than patients who underwent UKA for osteoarthritis.[56] In patients with extensive disease affecting multiple compartments, TKA may be the only alternative. Bergman and Rand evaluated patients who underwent standard TKA for SPONK and found good to excellent results in 87% of patients at 4 years. They also reported 85% implant survivorship at 5 years with revision surgery defined as the end point. However, when moderate or severe pain was used as the end point, survivorship was only 68%. They believed that the persistent pain experienced may have been due to foci of necrotic bone which support the implant.[57]

Secondary osteonecrosis
SON typically presents in patients younger than 55 years of age. Unlike SPONK, SON presents with multiple foci

of bone marrow involvement with extension into the metaphysis and diaphysis. Both condyles are usually involved,[9] and patients typically have involvement of the contralateral joint in more than 80% of cases.[9,35,55] Involvement of other joints such as the hip or proximal humerus can be seen. Therefore the clinician should have an index of suspicion regardless of the symptoms. Mont et al. demonstrated that 67% of patients with SON of the knee had disease in one or both the hips.[58]

In contrast to SPONK, numerous conditions and risk factors have been implicated in the development of SON of the knee. Corticosteroid use and alcohol abuse are the two most common associated risk factors in up to 90% of those diagnosed with SON.[9,58] Both corticosteroid use and alcohol consumption increase intraosseous adipocyte size and proliferation, leading to displacement of bone marrow.[4,9] The increase in pressure within a nonexpansile compartment leads to vascular collapse and ischemia.[59,60] Several other known risk factors for SON include caisson decompression sickness, sickle cell disease, Gaucher's disease, leukemia, myeloproliferative disorders, thrombophilia, and hypofibrinolysis. The common theme among these conditions is the underlying vaso-occlusive characteristics. Gaucher's disease, leukemia, and myeloproliferative disorders are thought to increase intraosseous pressure through bone marrow displacement. Studies have shown that patients with inherited coagulation disorders are also at high risk of SON, and it is recommended that those diagnosed early undergo pharmacologic treatment.[61,62] Liu et al. identified an autosomal dominant gene mutation in type II collagen in carrier families that developed SON.[63]

Unlike the sudden onset of pain seen with spontaneous ON, patients with SON will usually describe a gradual onset of pain over the affected area. The pain is generally localized over the femoral condyle, but in approximately 20% of cases, the tibial condyle may also be involved.[35] A thorough history should be taken to assess for associated risk factors. Initial evaluation begins with weight-bearing plain radiographs looking for any evidence of joint-space narrowing and subchondral collapse. MRI is the study of choice much as it is for SPONK because of its sensitivity in the detection of bone marrow edema, especially in the early stages of the disease. Many reactive processes can also cause bone marrow edema, and the MRI findings can be nonspecific. SON will typically show serpentine lesions with a well-demarcated border with multiple foci of involvement.[9] Bone scans have been shown to be less effective than MRI and are therefore not recommended for SON. Mont et al. reported that bone scans identified disease in only 37 of 58 patients (64%), whereas MRI detected all histopathologically confirmed lesions.[64]

Classification, operative, and nonoperative treatment. Two staging classification systems used for SON of the knee include the Koshino staging system, which was originally developed for SPONK, and the Modified Ficat and Arlet staging system. The modified Ficat system for the knee was extrapolated from the original version described for femoral head ON. Using plain radiographs, four stages are used to categorize the progression of disease based on joint-space narrowing, subchondral collapse, and trabecular pattern. Stages I and II have a normal joint space with no evidence of subchondral collapse. Stage II will display some evidence of sclerosis in the trabeculae in the subchondral region. Stage III typically demonstrates slightly narrowed joint space with subchondral collapse and a crescent sign. Stage IV has both joint-space narrowing and subchondral collapse with evidence of secondary degenerative changes.[35,65]

Unfortunately, symptomatic patients with SON will frequently require surgery, as nonsurgical management is typically recommended only for those patients who are asymptomatic.[58] To limit stress on the affected joint, nonoperative management typically involves a period of protected weight bearing and analgesics as required

for pain.[66] Unfortunately, the effectiveness of this treatment method is limited. Mont et al. reported that 19% (8 of 41) of the patients who had symptomatic lesions that were managed with observation had satisfactory outcomes at a mean follow-up of 8 years.[58]

Many of the joint-preserving techniques previously described for SPONK overlap with SON; however, the indications, effectiveness, and outcomes differ. Core decompression has demonstrated success in treating SON in cases without subchondral collapse. Woehnl and Naziri and Lee and Goodman described techniques using small-diameter (3.2 mm) percutaneous drills, using multiple passes under fluoroscopic guidance.[67] Given the diffuse involvement seen with SON, a percutaneous technique reduces morbidity and improves outcomes by reducing structural compromise of the bone and permitting immediate mobilization after surgery. Marulanda et al. reported a 92% success rate with percutaneous techniques combined with limited weight bearing for 4–6 weeks.[68]

Bone impaction grafting has also been used to restore the structural integrity and chondral continuity of the articular surface in patients with SON. The necrotic area is excised, and the defect is then reconstructed by impacting autograft or fresh frozen allograft bone to recreate the sphericity of the femoral condyle. In patients with multiple osteonecrotic lesions affecting both condyles, this alternative is unpractical.[69] Several studies have reported promising results using this technique; however, many are limited to retrospective small patient cohorts.[67,69,70] Despite this, grafting may be a useful treatment method in a young, carefully selected patient with intact articular cartilage.[7]

Standard TKA is the most appropriate surgical option in patients who have failed conservative measures and present with subchondral bone collapse (Ficat stage III and IV disease). Owing to the frequent involvement of multiple condyles, unicompartmental arthroplasty is not indicated in SON.[9,35] Mont et al. reported a 97% survival rate at mean follow-up of 9 years in patients undergoing TKA for SON. Parratte et al. demonstrated a survivorship of 96.7% at 7 years.[71] A meta-analysis looked at outcome results for patients undergoing TKA for SON and found 74% good outcomes with a 20% revision rate in 150 patients at a mean follow-up of 8 years.[72] However, when those performed before 1985 were excluded, good outcomes occurred in 97% of cases. This is likely the result of advances in surgical techniques, modern implants, improved implant fixation techniques, and better perioperative medical management.[7,72] Finally, Görtz et al.[72a] reported that osteochondral allografting is a reasonable salvage option for ON of the femoral condyles. TKA was avoided in 27 of the 28 knees at last follow-up.

Postarthroscopic ON

Postarthroscopic ON has been described after arthroscopic meniscectomy, shaver-assisted chondroplasty, anterior cruciate ligament reconstruction, and laser- or radiofrequency-assisted debridement. Although a rare condition, given the large number of arthroscopic procedures being performed each year, the reported incidence rate of postarthroscopic ON has found to be 4%.[73] Postarthroscopic ON has a predilection to affect the medial femoral condyle (82% of cases)[74]; however, the lateral femoral condyle is the second most frequently affected site.[75,76] In rare cases the medial and lateral tibial plateau as well as the patella can be affected. The epiphyseal region of the operative knee involving a single condyle is typically affected. On average, symptoms have been reported to develop at a mean time of approximately 24 weeks after surgery.[9]

The pathophysiology of ON after these procedures is not completely understood. However, several theories exist on the various etiologies of postarthroscopic ON. Pape et al. proposed that altered biomechanics and hoop stresses after meniscectomy lead to increased contact pressures and potential insufficiency fractures causing the development of ON.[8,75,77] Thermal energy or photoacoustic shock has been implicated in inciting ON of the knee. Several reports have postulated that laser- or radiofrequency-assisted arthroscopic surgery may result in ON through direct thermal injury or photoacoustic shock. Thermal damage is thought to lead to an inflammatory response causing bone edema, ischemia, and eventual necrosis. In photoacoustic shock, rapid vaporization of cellular contents and intracellular water produces an expanding gas. The expanding gas results in a shock wave that penetrates and damages subchondral bone, inciting an inflammatory response leading to necrosis.[7,78] Patients typically present with pain early in the recovery period, which is commonly mistaken as normal postoperative healing. MRI as well as AP and lateral radiographs are recommended in patients with suspected postarthroscopic ON. On T1-weighted magnetic resonance images, these lesions have an appearance similar to that of spontaneous ON of the knee, with linear foci of low signal surrounded by diffuse marrow edema adjacent to the meniscectomized compartment.[7] Initial treatment for postarthroscopic ON is with protected weight bearing and analgesics as required. Few reports of the use of joint-preserving procedures to manage postarthroscopic ON exist.

Joint-preserving surgery may be a reasonable approach in persons who have failed nonsurgical treatment; however, most of the data on outcomes are extrapolated from SPONK and SON. TKA and UKA are recommended for patients with end-stage osteoarthritis who fail nonoperative management and progress to collapse.

CONCLUSIONS

In summary, subchondral bone pathology is prevalent. Although the majority of cases are idiopathic, secondary etiologies should be investigated. A high level of suspicion is necessary to clinically identify subchondral bone disease because radiographs might fail to identify early stages of subchondral pathology. MRI is a highly sensitive and specific method for diagnosis of avascular necrosis. Although conservative treatment (protected weight bearing and analgesics) is advocated in early stages or small lesions, surgical treatment with isolated core decompression or augmented with other biological approaches, osteochondral graft transplantation, or unloading procedures such as osteotomies can be performed. Biologic approaches should be explored for focal defects in younger patients, whereas unicompartmental knee replacement is considered for more severe unicompartmental involvement. Once multiple compartments are affected and joint-space narrowing is present, TKA is indicated.

REFERENCES

1. Madry H, van Dijk CN, Mueller-Gerbl M. The basic science of the subchondral bone. *Knee Surg Sports Traumatol Arthrosc*. 2010;18:419–433.
2. Lyons TJ, McClure SF, Stoddart RW, McClure J. The normal human chondro-osseous junctional region: evidence for contact of uncalcified cartilage with subchondral bone and marrow spaces. *BMC Musculoskelet Disord*. 2006;7:52.
3. Duncan H, Jundt J, Riddle JM, Pitchford W, Christopherson T. The tibial subchondral plate. A scanning electron microscopic study. *J Bone Joint Surg Am*. 1987;69:1212–1220.
4. Imhof H, Sulzbacher I, Grampp S, Czerny C, Youssefzadeh S, Kainberger F. Subchondral bone and cartilage disease. *Invest Radiol*. 2000;35:581–588.
5. Imhof H, Breitenseher M, Kainberger F, Rand T, Trattnig S. Importance of subchondral bone to articular cartilage in health and disease. *Top Magn Reson Imaging*. 1999;10:180–192.
6. Ahlbäck S. Osteonecrosis of the knee - radiographic observations. *Calcif Tissue Res*. 1968;2:36.
7. Zywiel MG, McGrath MS, Seyler TM, Marker DR, Bonutti PM, Mont MA. Osteonecrosis of the knee: a review of three disorders. *Orthop Clin North Am*. 2009;40:193–211.
8. Pape D, Seil R, Anagnostakos K, Kohn D. Postarthroscopic osteonecrosis of the knee. *Arthroscopy*. 2007;23:428–438.

9. Mont MA, Marker DR, Zywiel MG, Carrino JA. Osteonecrosis of the knee and related conditions. *J Am Acad Orthop Surg.* 2011;19:482–494.

10. al-Rowaih A, Björkengren Å, Egund N, Lindstrand A, Wingstrand H, Thorngren KG. Size of osteonecrosis of the knee. *Clin Orthop Relat Res.* 1993;(287):68–75.

11. Reddy a S, Frederick RW. Evaluation of the intraosseous and extraosseous blood supply to the distal femoral condyles. *Am J Sports Med.* 1998;26:415–419.

12. Ohdera T, Miyagi S, Tokunaga M, Yoshimoto E, Matsuda S, Ikari H. Spontaneous osteonecrosis of the lateral femoral condyle of the knee: a report of 11 cases. *Arch Orthop Trauma Surg.* 2008;128:825–831.

13. Arnoldi CC, Lemperg K, Linderholm H. Intraosseous hypertension and pain in the knee. *J Bone Joint Surg Br.* 1975;57:360–363.

14. Kantor H. Bone marrow pressure in osteonecrosis of the femoral condyle (Ahlbäck's disease). *Arch Orthop Trauma Surg.* 1987;106:349–352.

15. Mears SC, McCarthy EF, Jones LC, Hungerford DS, Mont MA. Characterization and pathological characteristics of spontaneous osteonecrosis of the knee. *Iowa Orthop J.* 2009;29:38–42.

16. Strauss EJ, Kang R, Bush-Joseph C, Bach BR. The diagnosis and management of spontaneous and post-arthroscopy osteonecrosis of the knee. *Bull NYU Hosp Jt Dis.* 2011;69:320–330.

17. Robertson DD, Armfield DR, Towers JD, Irrgang JJ, Maloney WJ, Harner CD. Meniscal root injury and spontaneous osteonecrosis of the knee: an observation. *J Bone Joint Surg Br.* 2009;91:190–195.

18. Allaire R, Muriuki M, Gilbertson L, Harner CD. Biomechanical consequences of a tear of the posterior root of the medial meniscus. *J Bone Joint Surg Am.* 2008;90:1922–1931.

19. Muscolo DL, Costa-Paz M, Ayerza M, Makino A. Medial meniscal tears and spontaneous osteonecrosis of the knee. *Arthroscopy.* 2006;22:457–460.

20. Norman A, Baker ND. Spontaneous osteonecrosis of the knee and medial meniscal tears. *Radiology.* 1978;129:653–656.

21. Padalecki JR, Armfield DR, Towers JD, Irrgang JJ, Maloney WJ, Harner CD. Biomechanical consequences of a complete radial tear adjacent to the medial meniscus posterior root attachment site: in situ pull-out repair restores derangement of joint mechanics. *Am J Sport Med.* 2014;42:699–707.

22. Feucht MJ, Kühle J, Bode G, et al. Arthroscopic transtibial pullout repair for posterior medial meniscus root tears: a systematic review of clinical, radiographic, and second-look arthroscopic results. *Arthroscopy.* 2015;31:1808–1816.

23. Akamatsu Y, Mitsugi N, Hayashi T, Kobayashi H, Saito T. Low bone mineral density is associated with the onset of spontaneous osteonecrosis of the knee. *Acta Orthop.* 2012;83:249–255.

24. Lotke PA, Abend JA, Ecker ML. The treatment of osteonecrosis of the medial femoral condyle. *Clin Orthop Relat Res.* 1982; 109–116.

25. Lotke P, Lonner J. Spontaneous and secondary osteonecrosis of the knee. *Insa Scott.* 2006.

26. al-Rowaih A, Lindstrand A, Björkengren A, Wingstrand H, Thorngren KG. Osteonecrosis of the knee. Diagnosis and outcome in 40 patients. *Acta Orthop Scand.* 1991;62:19–23.

27. Juréus J, Lindstrand A, Geijer M, Robertsson O, Tägil M. The natural course of spontaneous osteonecrosis of the knee (SPONK): a 1- to 27-year follow-up of 40 patients. *Acta Orthop.* 2013;84:410–414.

28. Pape D, Seil R, Kohn D, Schneider G. Imaging of early stages of osteonecrosis of the knee. *Orthop Clin North Am.* 2004;35:293–303, viii.

29. Soucacos PN, Johnson EO, Soultanis K, Vekris MD, Theodorou SJ, Beris AE. Diagnosis and management of the osteonecrotic triad of the knee. *Orthop Clin North Am.* 2004;35:371–381, x.

30. Fotiadou A, Karantanas A. Acute nontraumatic adult knee pain: the role of MR imaging. *Radiol Med.* 2009;114:437–447.

31. Pollack MS, Dalinka MK, Kressel HY, Lotke PA, Spritzer CE. Magnetic resonance imaging in the evaluation of suspected osteonecrosis of the knee. *Skeletal Radiol.* 1987;16:121–127.

32. Yates PJ, Calder JD, Stranks GJ, Conn KS, Peppercorn D, Thomas NP. Early MRI diagnosis and non-surgical management of spontaneous osteonecrosis of the knee. *Knee.* 2007;14:112–116.

33. Koshino T, Okamoto R, Takamura K, Tsuchiya K. Arthroscopy in spontaneous osteonecrosis of the knee. *Orthop Clin North Am.* 1979;10(3):609–618.

34. Aglietti P, Insall JN, Buzzi R, Deschamps G. Idiopathic osteonecrosis of the knee. Aetiology, prognosis and treatment. *J Bone Joint Surg Br.* 1983;65:588–597.

35. Karim AR, Cherian JJ, Jauregui JJ, Pierce T, Mont MA. Osteonecrosis of the Knee: Review. Vol 3. 2015:1–11.

36. Jureus J, Lindstrand A, Geijer M, Roberts D, Tägil M. Treatment of spontaneous osteonecrosis of the knee (SPONK) by a bisphosphonate. *Acta Orthop.* 2012;83:511–514.

37. Meier C, Kraenzlin C, Friederich NF, et al. Effect of ibandronate on spontaneous osteonecrosis of the knee: a randomized, double-blind, placebo-controlled trial. *Osteoporos Int.* 2014;25:359–366.

38. Bassett CA, Pilla AA, Pawluk RJ. A non-operative salvage of surgically-resistant pseudarthroses and non-unions by pulsing electromagnetic fields. A preliminary report. *Clin Orthop Relat Res.* 1977:128–143.

39. De Mattei M, Caruso A, Traina GC, Pezzetti F, Baroni T, Sollazzo V. Correlation between pulsed electromagnetic fields exposure time and cell proliferation increase in human osteosarcoma cell lines and human normal osteoblast cells in vitro. *Bioelectromagnetics.* 1999;20:177–182.

40. Varani K, De Mattei M, Vincenzi F, et al. Characterization of adenosine receptors in bovine chondrocytes and fibroblast-like synoviocytes exposed to low frequency low energy pulsed electromagnetic fields. *Osteoarthritis Cartilage*. 2008;16:292–304.

41. Marcheggiani Muccioli GM, Grassi A, Setti S, et al. Conservative treatment of spontaneous osteonecrosis of the knee in the early stage: pulsed electromagnetic fields therapy. *Eur J Radiol*. 2013;82:530–537.

42. Duany NG, Zywiel MG, McGrath MS, et al. Joint-preserving surgical treatment of spontaneous osteonecrosis of the knee. *Arch Orthop Trauma Surg*. 2010;130:11–16.

43. Bedi A, Warren RF, Oh YK, et al. Restriction in hip internal rotation is associated with an increased risk of ACL injury in NFL combine athletes: a clinical and biomechanical study. *Orthop J Sport Med*. 2013;1:2325967113S00062.

44. Lieberman JR, Varthi AG, Polkowski GG. Osteonecrosis of the knee - which joint preservation procedures work? *J Arthroplasty*. 2014;29:52–56.

45. Jacobs MA, Loeb PE, Hungerford DS. Core decompression of the distal femur for avascular necrosis of the knee. *J Bone Joint Surg Br*. 1989;71:583–587.

46. Forst J, Forst R, Heller KD, Adam G. Spontaneous osteonecrosis of the femoral condyle: causal treatment by early core decompression. *Arch Orthop Trauma Surg*. 1998;117:18–22.

47. Mont MA, Tomek IM, Hungerford DS. Core decompression for avascular necrosis of the distal femur: long term followup. *Clin Orthop Relat Res*. 1997:124–130.

48. Deie M, Ochi M, Adachi N, Nishimori M, Yokota K. Artificial bone grafting [calcium hydroxyapatite ceramic with an interconnected porous structure (IP-CHA)] and core decompression for spontaneous osteonecrosis of the femoral condyle in the knee. *Knee Surg Sports Traumatol Arthrosc*. 2008;16:753–758.

49. Tanaka Y, Mima H, Yonetani Y, Shiozaki Y, Nakamura N, Horibe S. Histological evaluation of spontaneous osteonecrosis of the medial femoral condyle and short-term clinical results of osteochondral autografting: a case series. *Knee*. 2009;16:130–135.

50. Saito T, Kumagai K, Akamatsu Y, Kobayashi H, Kusayama Y. Five- to ten-year outcome following medial opening-wedge high tibial osteotomy with rigid plate fixation in combination with an artificial bone substitute. *Bone Joint J*. 2014;96-B:339–344.

51. Takeuchi R, Aratake M, Bito H, et al. Clinical results and radiographical evaluation of opening wedge high tibial osteotomy for spontaneous osteonecrosis of the knee. *Knee Surg Sports Traumatol Arthrosc*. 2009;17:361–368.

52. Hernigou P, Beaujean F. Treatment of osteonecrosis with autologous bone marrow grafting. *Clin Orthop Relat Res*. 2002:14–23. https://doi.org/10.1097/01.blo.0000038472.05771.79.

53. Koshino T. The treatment of spontaneous osteonecrosis of the knee by high tibial osteotomy with and without bone-grafting or drilling of the lesion. *J Bone Joint Surg Am*. 1982;64:47–58.

54. Springer BD, Scott RD, Thornhill TS. Conversion of failed unicompartmental knee arthroplasty to TKA. *Clin Orthop Relat Res*. 2006;446:214–220.

55. Myers TG, Cui Q, Kuskowski M, Mihalko WM, Saleh KJ. Outcomes of total and unicompartmental knee arthroplasty for secondary and spontaneous osteonecrosis of the knee. *J Bone Joint Surg Am*. 2006;88(suppl 3):76–82.

56. Ritter MA, Eizember LE, Keating EM, Faris PM. The survival of total knee arthroplasty in patients with osteonecrosis of the medial condyle. *Clin Orthop Relat Res*. 1991:108–114. https://doi.org/10.1097/00003086-199106000-00015.

57. Bergman NR, Rand JA. Total knee arthroplasty in osteonecrosis. *Clin Orthop Relat Res*. 1991:77–82.

58. Mont MA, Baumgarten KM, Rifai A, Bluemke DA, Jones LC, Hungerford DS. Atraumatic osteonecrosis of the knee. *J Bone Joint Surg Am*. 2000;82:1279–1290.

59. Lee MS, Hsieh PH, Chang YH, Chan YS, Agrawal S, Ueng SW. Elevated intraosseous pressure in the intertrochanteric region is associated with poorer results in osteonecrosis of the femoral head treated by multiple drilling. *J Bone Joint Surg Br*. 2008;90:852–857.

60. Miyanishi K, Yamamoto T, Irisa T, et al. Bone marrow fat cell enlargement and a rise in intraosseous pressure in steroid-treated rabbits with osteonecrosis. *Bone*. 2002;30:185–190.

61. Jones LC, Mont MA, Le TB, et al. Procoagulants and osteonecrosis. *J Rheumatol*. 2003;30:783–791.

62. Korompilias AV, Ortel TL, Urbaniak JR. Coagulation abnormalities in patients with hip osteonecrosis. *Orthop Clin North Am*. 2004;35:265–271, vii.

63. Liu Y-F, Chen WM, Lin YF, et al. Type II collagen gene variants and inherited osteonecrosis of the femoral head. *N Engl J Med*. 2005;352:2294–2301.

64. Mont MA, Ulrich SD, Seyler TM, et al. Bone scanning of limited value for diagnosis of symptomatic oligofocal and multifocal osteonecrosis. *J Rheumatol*. 2008;35:1629–1634.

65. Ficat RP. Idiopathic bone necrosis of the femoral head. Early diagnosis and treatment. *J Bone Joint Surg Br*. 1985;67:3–9.

66. Strauss EJ, Nho SJ, Kelly BT. Greater trochanteric pain syndrome. *Sports Med Arthrosc*. 2010;18:113–119.

67. Lee K, Goodman SB. Cell therapy for secondary osteonecrosis of the femoral condyles using the Cellect DBM system. A preliminary report. *J Arthroplasty*. 2009;24:43–48.

68. Marulanda G, Seyler TM, Sheikh NH, Mont MA. Percutaneous drilling for the treatment of secondary osteonecrosis of the knee. *J Bone Joint Surg Br*. 2006;88:740–746.

69. Rijnen WHC, Luttjeboer JS, Schreurs BW, Gardeniers JWM. Bone impaction grafting for corticosteroid-associated osteonecrosis of the knee. *J Bone Joint Surg Am*. 2006;88(suppl 3).

70. Woehnl A, Naziri QCC. Osteonecrosis of the knee. *Orthop Knowl Online J*. 2012;10.

71. Parratte S, Argenson J-NA, Dumas J, Aubaniac J-M. Unicompartmental knee arthroplasty for avascular osteonecrosis. *Clin Orthop Relat Res*. 2007;464:37–42.

72. Levine WN, Ozuna RM, Scott RD, Thornhill TS. Conversion of failed modern unicompartmental arthroplasty to total knee arthroplasty. *J Arthroplasty.* 1996;11:797–801.

72a. Görtz S, De Young AJ, Bugbee WD. Fresh osteochondral allografting for steroid-associated osteonecrosis of the femoral condyles. *Clin Orthop Relat Res.* 2010;468(5): 1269–1278. https://doi.org/10.1007/s11999-010-1250-7. Epub 2010 Feb 9.

73. Cetik O, Cift H, Comert B, Cirpar M. Risk of osteonecrosis of the femoral condyle after arthroscopic chondroplasty using radiofrequency: a prospective clinical series. *Knee Surg Sports Traumatol Arthrosc.* 2009;17:24–29.

74. Faletti C, Robba T, De Petro P. Postmeniscectomy osteonecrosis. *Arthroscopy.* 2002;18:91–94.

75. Karim AR, Cherian JJ, Jauregui JJ, Pierce T, Mont MA. Osteonecrosis of the knee: review. *Ann Transl Med.* 2015;3:6.

76. MacDessi SJ, Brophy RH, Bullough PG, Windsor RE, Sculco TP. Subchondral fracture following arthroscopic knee surgery. A Series Eight Cases. *J Bone Joint Surg Am.* 2008;90:1007–1012.

77. Mont MA, Rifai A, Baumgarten KM, Sheldon M, Hungerford DS. Total knee arthroplasty for osteonecrosis. *J Bone Joint Surg Am.* 2002;84–A:599–603.

78. Kelly BT, Warren RF. Complications of thermal energy in knee surgery - Part I. *Clin Sports Med.* 2002;21:737–751.

CHAPTER 13

Biologics in Hand Surgery

RYU YOSHIDA, MD • SAMUEL BARON, BS • CRAIG RODNER, MD•
JOEL FERREIRA, MD

BONE GRAFTS AND SUBSTITUTES

Complex fractures, nonunions, or tumor resections can leave bone defects. Autologous bone grafts are effective fillers, carrying both osteoinductive and osteoconductive properties. However, autografts require harvesting, which lead to increased operative time as well as donor site morbidities. The amount of autograft available may not be sufficient. Therefore, there is a demand for bone graft substitutes that can be readily applied.

ALLOGRAFTS

Bone allografts are widely used in hand surgery. Bones harvested from cadavers are typically freeze-dried and sometimes undergo further processing such as ethylene oxide treatment or γ-radiation for further sterilization. Allografts can also be prepared fresh or frozen, but such preparations are rarely used in hand surgery. While the osteoblasts and precursors are lost during the freeze-drying, allografts still provide favorable osteoconductive properties.

Allografts can come in several different forms such as cortical, cancellous, and corticocancellous. Cortical allografts are incorporated by creeping substitution with intramembranous ossification, while cancellous allografts are incorporated by enchondral ossification.[1]

Demineralized bone matrix (DBM) is allograft that has been decalcified, leaving organic matrix behind. The trabecular network of collagen serves as a scaffold for bone formation. The growth factors and bone morphogenic proteins (BMPs) are maintained and can help induce cells to form bone.[2] DBM does not provide mechanical strength. However, its soft consistency allows it to be placed into small defects or even be injected percutaneously.[3]

MINERAL SUBSTITUTES

Most bones are 60%–70% mineral by dry weight, with hydroxyapatite being the principal component of the mineral phase.[4] Because hydroxyapatite has an unstable crystalline structure, rapid exchange between hydroxyapatite crystals and tricalcium phosphate (TCP) takes place in vivo.[5,6] Both hydroxyapatites and TCP have been used as bone graft substitutes.

A prospective study from Germany demonstrated ingrowth and osseous integration of hydroxyapatite ceramic in augmentation of distal radius fracture fixation.[7] Ceramics are produced by "sintering" where mineral salts are heated between 700°C and 1300°C. Sintering increases the mechanical strength but slows resorption.[8]

Coralline hydroxyapatite, which is derived from marine coral, has porosity similar to cancellous bone. In a case series of 21 patients, coralline hydroxyapatite was used as a substitute for autograft to help maintain articular surface along with external fixation and K-wires. The authors reported maintenance of articular reduction in all patients and an average DASH score of 90.3.[9]

TCP comes in different forms such as blocks, granules, and powders. It was initially used in the dental field in the 1980s, but its application has been expanded since.[10] It can be used as bone void fillers by itself or as a composite graft mixed with other grafts or bone marrow aspirates[11, 12,13]. In hand surgery, there are reported case series of TCP alone as a substitute for iliac crest bone grafting. Four out of four patients had union in wrist arthrodesis for rheumatoid patients.[14] In a series of 17 patients undergoing corrective osteotomies of the distal radius, there was only one nonunion.[15]

Calcium sulfate (Ca[SO4]) is also known as plaster of Paris and has been around for centuries. It provides structural support with better compressive strength than cancellous bone. It also has osteoconductive properties.[6] The resorption of calcium sulfate is fast, with complete resorption around 13–14 weeks.[16,17] The fast resorption can be an advantage for certain applications such as using antibiotics beads; a second surgery for

Biologics in Orthopaedic Surgery. https://doi.org/10.1016/B978-0-323-55140-3.00013-8

beads removal can be avoided. However, as a bone graft substitute, calcium sulfate will only provide temporary structural strength. Jepegnanam et al. report hardware failures in two elderly patients where calcium sulfate was used as a bone graft substitute in distal radius corrective osteotomy. The authors hypothesized that the failures were due to new bone formation not occurring rapidly enough to replace the resorption of calcium sulfate.[18]

CEMENTS

Cements were developed to improve moldability of calcium phosphate and to allow better filling of defects. They are available as injectable liquid or putty that sets through isothermic reaction.[6] In a study from Austria, unstable intraarticular distal radius fracture in menopausal, osteoporotic women were treated with percutaneous pinning alone or with pin and screw construct supplemented with cement.[19] The former group was immobilized for 6 weeks, while the latter group was immobilized for 3 weeks. At 2 years, the cement group had better functional outcome, restoration of movement, and grip strength. Loss of reduction was also less frequent in the cement group. Cassidy et al. conducted a prospective randomized multicenter study with 323 distal radius fracture patients.[20] The patients were treated with closed reduction and immobilization, with or without calcium phosphate cement injection. The method of immobilization was either a cast or external fixation with or without supplemental K-wires, depending on the surgeon's preference. The group with cement augmentation had better grip strength, motion, use of hand, and social and emotional function at 6–8 weeks, but no difference was seen at 1 year.

Bone cements have been also used to fill voids after tumor removal. Enchondromas are common benign bone tumors frequently arising in hand. Several studies have reported the successful use of calcium phosphate cement [21-23] or hydroxyapatite cement [24] to fill defects after curettage of enchondromas. A biomechanical study on cadaveric enchondroma model has shown that calcium phosphate cement significantly increases strength of metacarpals.[25] Rajeh et al. also reported a series of eight patients who had calcium phosphate cement injection after curettage of enchondromas in the hand.[26] At a mean final follow-up at 16 months, 69.3% of the cement remained in the bone, with the mean pain score improving from 4.1 to 1.6. It should be noted that 2 patients with extraosseous cement leakage, with 1 patient requiring a revision surgery (Figs. 13.1 and 13.2).

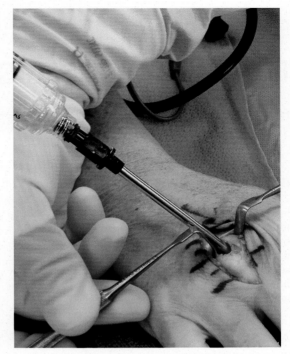

FIG. 13.1 Injection of calcium phosphate cement after curettage of metacarpal enchondroma. (Courtesy Craig Rodner MD).

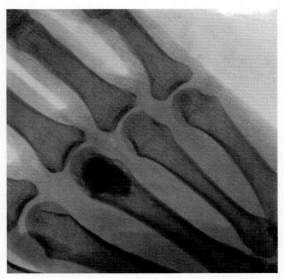

FIG. 13.2 Fluoroscopic image of the metacarpal after cement injection . (Courtesy Craig Rodner MD).

GROWTH FACTORS

Growth factors are signaling molecules that play important roles in communication between cells. While growth factors naturally exist in the body, application of exogenous growth factors to promote bone healing has received much attention.

Recombinant forms of various growth factors are currently available, including BMP-2, BMP-7, TGF-β, and platelet-derived growth factor. BMP-2 and BMP-7 belong to the bone morphogenic protein family and have been shown to stimulate bone healing. In a prospective randomized control trial, 450 patients with open tibia fractures were treated with intramedullary rod. The groups that received BMP-2 in an absorbable collagen sponge had significantly decreased risk of failure and faster fracture healing than the control group, which did not receive any BMP-2.[27] Recombinant human BMP-7, also known as osteogenic protein 1, has been used to treat tibial nonunions. In a multicenter, prospective randomized control of 122 patients undergoing intramedullary rod treatment, no difference in clinical outcomes were observed between groups treated with BMP-7 and autologous bone graft. At 9 months, 81% of the BMP-7 group and 85% of the autologous bone graft group had successful outcomes.[28]

There have been reports of BMP use in hand surgery for treatment of nonunions. Ablove et al. reported a series of four patients who underwent screw exchange supplemented with BMP-2 for treatment of scaphoid nonunion. All four patients had union.[29] Successful healing of chronic scaphoid nonunion with BMP with a single K-wire and cast immobilization has also been reported.[30]

While these studies are encouraging, it should be noted that others report less successful results. Rice et al. reported a series of 27 patients with various sites of nonunion including phalanx, carpus, distal radius, and distal ulna. Treatment with BMP-2 yielded 89% union rate. By comparing their results to published rates for nonunion repair, they concluded that BMP-2 did not improve union rates.[31] Another retrospective review case series revealed high complication rates. Brannan et al. reported six cases of revision ORIF with bone graft and BMP-2. The surgery was performed for nonunion despite previous scaphoid ORIF. Only one out of six patients healed without complications. Two patients had persistent nonunion after revision surgery. Four patients had significant heterotopic ossification, with one patient requiring revision surgery.[32]

PLATELET-RICH PLASMA

Platelet-rich plasma (PRP) is a biologic prepared from autologous blood. It contains increased concentration of platelets and growth factors compared with whole blood. PRP has received much attention for its potential benefits in various orthopaedic applications. The most extensively studied PRP application in hand surgery has been for lateral epicondylitis.

Lateral epicondylitis is a painful condition of the elbow associated with changes in the extensor carpi radialis brevis insertion.[33] Corticosteroid injections have been used traditionally, but more recent studies and metaanalyses have shown limited benefits of steroid injections.[34,35] PRP received much attention when a double-blinded randomized control trial from Netherlands demonstrated improved VAS and DASH scores compared with steroid injections at 1 and 2 year followups.[36,37] Several other trials have subsequently been performed, and recent metaanalyses have demonstrated improved long-term outcomes with PRP injections.[38,39] Others have used autologous whole blood injection, which has higher DASH scores but with more adverse effects compared with PRP, according a metaanalysis.[38]

COLLAGENASE FOR DUPUYTREN CONTRACTURES

Clostridium histolyticum collagenases (CHCs) are a group of enzymes naturally formed by the bacteria *C. histolyticum* of the Clostridium family. In 2010, CHCs were approved by the Food and Drug Administration (FDA) as the first nonsurgical treatment of Dupuytren disease under the brand name Xiaflex.

Xiaflex is a mixture of seven different enzymes (α, β, γ, δ, ε, ζ, and η), which have been assigned to one of two classes, I and II.[40] Both classes contribute to overall effectiveness of the enzymatic breakdown of collagen. Class I enzymes attack terminal domains of triple helices, whereas class II enzymes attack internal peptide bonds. Actions of both classes act synergistically to dismantle tropocollagen molecules.[41]

The proteolytic breakdown of collagen by CHC was first identified in the late 1940s.[42] Then in 1982, CHCs were first implicated for use in medical management of a connective tissue disorder, Peyronie disease.[43] Finally in 1996, CHCs were investigated as an agent to be used for enzymatic fasciotomy in the context of Dupuytren disease.[44] Many purified CHC preparations with varying strengths and specificities became available for in vivo human clinical trials. In an attempt to produce a standardized preparation, BioSpecifics Technologies Corp.

developed the CHC prep named Xiaflex, which contains a 1:1 mass ratio of class I to class II CHCs.[45] Since that time, both the U.S. FDA and European Medicines Agency have approved Xiaflex (Xiapex in Europe) specifically for treatment of Dupuytren contractures in adult patients. Xiaflex became the first approved nonsurgical treatment option available for Dupuytren disease.[46]

Xiaflex is indicated for patients with palpable cords and associated contractures. After injection into the cord, the patient undergoes manipulation 1–3 days later to straighten the digits. In a double-blinded randomized control trial, 308 patients with contractures of 20 degrees or more in metacarpophalangeal (MCP) or proximal interphalangeal (PIP) joints received up to three injections. 64% of patients achieved reduction in contracture to 0–5 degrees of full extension.[47] Common side effects of collagenase treatment include swelling, pain, bruising, and pruritis. More serious complications are rare, with rates of 1% or less, but they include tendon ruptures, skin atrophy, and complex regional pain syndrome.[47,48] Recurrences of contractures may occur and are more common in PIP joint (66% at 5 years) than MCP (39% at 5 years) joint[48].

REFERENCES

1. De Long WG, McKee M, Watson T, et al. Bone grafts and bone graft substitutes in orthopaedic trauma surgery. *J Bone Joint Surg Am.* 2007;89(3):649–658.
2. Urist MR, Silverman BF, Büring K, Dubuc FL, Rosenberg JM. The bone induction principle. *Clin Orthop Relat Res.* 1967;53:243–283.
3. Finkemeier CG. Bone-grafting and bone-graft substitutes. *J Bone Joint Surg Am.* 2002;84-A(3):454–464.
4. Boskey AL. Bone composition: relationship to bone fragility and antiosteoporotic drug effects. *Bonekey Rep.* 2013;2:447.
5. Ladd AL, Pliam NB. Bone graft substitutes in the radius and upper limb Original research article. *J Am Soc Surg Hand.* 2003;3(4):227–245.
6. Bhatt RA, Rozental TD. Bone graft substitutes. *Hand Clin.* 2012;28(4):457–468.
7. Werber KD, Brauer RB, Weiss W, Becker K. Osseous integration of bovine hydroxyapatite ceramic in metaphyseal bone defects of the distal radius. *J Hand Surg Am.* 2000;25(5):833–841.
8. Moore WR, Graves SE, Bain GI. Synthetic bone graft substitutes. *ANZ J Surg.* 2001;71(6):354–361.
9. Wolfe SW, Pike L, Slade 3rd JF, Katz LD. Augmentation of distal radius fracture fixation with coralline hydroxyapatite bone graft substitute. *J Hand Surg Am.* 1999;24(4):816–827.
10. Yao J, Ho AM. Bone graft substitutes in the treatment of distal radius and upper limb injuries. *Oper Tech Orthop.* 2009;19:77–87.
11. Szpalski M, Gunzburg R. Applications of calcium phosphate-based cancellous bone void fillers in trauma surgery. *Orthopedics.* 2002;25(suppl 5):s601–s609.
12. Erbe EM, Marx JG, Clineff TD, Bellincampi LD. Potential of an ultraporous beta-tricalcium phosphate synthetic cancellous bone void filler and bone marrow aspirate composite graft. *Eur Spine J.* 2001;10(suppl 2):S141–S146.
13. Meadows GR. Adjunctive use of ultraporous beta-tricalcium phosphate bone void filler in spinal arthrodesis. *Orthopedics.* 2002;25(suppl 5):s579–s584.
14. Nakagawa N, Saegusa Y, Abe S, et al. The effectiveness of RA wrist fusion using Beta-TCP without autogenous iliac bone grafting: a report of four cases. *Hand Surg.* 2006;11:71–75.
15. Scheer JH, Adolfsson LE. Tricalcium phosphate bone substitute in corrective osteotomy of the distal radius. *Injury.* 2009;40(3):262–267.
16. Peltier LF. The use of plaster of Paris to fill large defects in bone. A preliminary report. *Am J Surg.* 1959;97(3):311–315.
17. Kumar CY, Nalini KB, Menon J, Patro DK, Banerji BH. Calcium sulfate as bone graft substitute in the treatment of osseous bone defects, a prospective study. *J Clin Diagn Res JCDR.* 2013;7(12):2926–2928.
18. Jepegnanam TS, von Schroeder HP. Rapid resorption of calcium sulfate and hardware failure following corrective radius osteotomy: 2 case reports. *J Hand Surg Am.* 2012;37(3):477–480.
19. Zimmermann R, Gschwentner M, Pechlaner S, et al. Injectable calcium phosphate bone cement Norian SRS for the treatment of intra-articular compression fractures of the distal radius in osteoporotic women. *Arch Orthop Trauma Surg.* 2003;123:22–27.
20. Cassidy C, Jupiter JB, Cohen M, et al. Norian SRS cement compared with conventional fixation in distal radial fractures. A randomized study. *J Bone Joint Surg Am.* 2003;85-A(11):2127–2137.
21. Yasuda M, Masada K, Takeuchi E. Treatment of enchondroma of the hand with injectable calcium phosphate bone cement. *J Hand Surg Am.* 2006;31(1):98–102.
22. Kim JK, Kim NK. Curettage and calcium phosphate bone cement injection for the treatment of enchondroma of the finger. *Hand Surg.* 2012;17(1):65–70.
23. Bickels J, Wittig JC, Kollender Y, et al. Enchondromas of the hand: treatment with curettage and cemented internal fixation. *J Hand Surg Am.* 2002;27(5):870–875.
24. Joosten U, Joist A, Frebel T, Walter M, Langer M. The use of an in situ curing hydroxyapatite cement as an alternative to bone graft following removal of enchondroma of the hand. *J Hand Surg Br.* 2000;25(3):288–291.
25. Pianta TJ, Baldwin PS, Obopilwe E, Mazzocca AD, Rodner CM, Silverstein EA. A biomechanical analysis of treatment options for enchondromas of the hand. *Hand.* 2013;8(1):86–91.
26. Rajeh MA, Diaz JJ, Facca S, Matheron AS, Gouzou S, Liverneaux P. Treatment of hand enchondroma with injectable calcium phosphate cement: a series of eight cases. *Eur J Orthop Surg Traumatol.* 2017;27(2):251–254.

27. Govender S, Csimma C, Genant HK, et al. Recombinant human bone morphogenetic protein-2 for treatment of open tibial fractures: a prospective, controlled, randomized study of four hundred and fifty patients. *J Bone Joint Surg Am.* 2002;84-A(12):2123–2134.

28. Friedlaender GE1, Perry CR, Cole JD, et al. Osteogenic protein-1 (bone morphogenetic protein-7) in the treatment of tibial nonunions. *J Bone Joint Surg Am.* 2001;83-A(suppl 1(Pt 2)):S151–S158.

29. Ablove RH, Abrams SS. The use of BMP-2 and screw exchange in the treatment of scaphoid fracture non-union. *Hand Surg.* 2015;20(1):167–171.

30. Jones NF, Brown EE, Mostofi A, Vogelin E, Urist MR. Healing of a scaphoid nonunion using human bone morphogenetic protein. *J Hand Surg Am.* 2005;30(3):528–533.

31. Rice I, Lubahn JD. Use of bone morphogenetic protein-2 (rh-BMP-2) in treatment of wrist and hand nonunion with comparison to historical control groups. *J Surg Orthop Adv.* 2013;22(4):256–262.

32. Brannan PS, Gaston RG, Loeffler BJ, Lewis DR. Complications with the use of BMP-2 in scaphoid nonunion surgery. *J Hand Surg Am.* 2016;41(5):602–608.

33. Altan L, Kanat E. Conservative treatment of lateral epicondylitis: comparison of two different orthotic devices. *Clin Rheumatol.* 2008;27(8):1015–1019.

34. Olaussen M, Holmedal O, Lindbaek M, Brage S, Solvang H. Treating lateral epicondylitis with corticosteroid injections or non-electrotherapeutical physiotherapy: a systematic review. *BMJ Open.* 2013;3(10).

35. Fujihara Y, Huetteman HE, Chung TT, Shauver MJ, Chung KC. The effect of impactful papers on clinical practice in the US: corticosteroid injection for patients with lateral epicondylitis. *Plast Reconstr Surg.* 2018;141.

36. Peerbooms JC, Sluimer J, Bruijn DJ, Gosens T. Positive effect of an autologous platelet concentrate in lateral epicondylitis in a double-blind randomized controlled trial: platelet-rich plasma versus corticosteroid injection with a 1-year follow-up. *Am J Sports Med.* 2010;38(2):255–262.

37. Gosens T, Peerbooms JC, van Laar W, den Oudsten BL. Ongoing positive effect of platelet-rich plasma versus corticosteroid injection in lateral epicondylitis: a double-blind randomized controlled trial with 2-year follow-up. *Am J Sports Med.* 2011;39(6):1200–1208.

38. Arirachakaran A, Sukthuayat A, Sisayanarane T, Laoratanavoraphong S, Kanchanatawan W, Kongtharvonskul J. Platelet-rich plasma versus autologous blood versus steroid injection in lateral epicondylitis: systematic review and network meta-analysis. *J Orthop Traumatol.* 2016;17(2):101–112.

39. Chen X, Jones IA, Park C, Vangsness Jr CT. The efficacy of platelet-rich plasma on tendon and ligament healing: a systematic review and meta-analysis with bias assessment. *Am J Sports Med.* 2017.

40. Mookhtiar KA, van Wart HE. Clostridium histolyticum collagenases: a new look at some old enzymes. *Matrix Suppl.* 1992;1:116–126.

41. French MF, Mookhtiar KA, van Wart HE. Limited proteolysis of type I collagen at hyperreactive sites by Class I and Class II Clostridium histolyticum collagenases: complementary digestion patterns. *Biochemistry.* 1987;26:681–687.

42. MacLennan JD, Mandl I, Howes EL. Bacterial digestion of collagen. *J Clin Invest.* 1953;32(12):1317–1322.

43. Gelbard MK, Walsh R, Kaufman JJ. Collagenase for Peyronie's disease experimental studies. *Urol Res.* 1982;10(3):135–140.

44. Starkweather KD, Lattuga S, Hurst LC, et al. Collagenase in the treatment of Dupuytren's disease: an in vitro study. *J Hand Surg Am.* 1996;21(3):490–495.

45. Sabatino GL, Del Tito JRBJ, Bassett PJ, Tharia HA, Hitchcock AG. *Compositions and Methods for Treating Collagen-mediated Diseases.* 20070224183 US Patent; January 29, 2007.

46. FDA. XIAFLEX™ (Collagenase clostridium Histolyticum) for Injection, for Intralesional Use Initial U.S. Approval. US Food and Drug Administration; 2010. https://www.accessdata.fda.gov/drugsatfda_docs/label/2010/125338lbl.pdf.

47. Hurst LC, Badalamente MA, Hentz VR, et al. CORD I study group. injectable collagenase clostridium histolyticum for Dupuytren's contracture. *N Engl J Med.* 2009;361(10):968–979.

48. Peimer CA, Blazar P, Coleman S, Kaplan FT, Smith T, Lindau T. Dupuytren contracture recurrence following treatment with collagenase Clostridium histolyticum (CORDLESS [collagenase option for reduction of dupuytren long-term evaluation of safety study]): 5-year data. *J Hand Surg Am.* 2015;40(8):1597–1605. Epub 2015 Jun 18.

FURTHER READING

1. Geissler WB. Bone graft substitutes in the upper extremity. *Hand Clin.* 2006;22(3):329–339.

CHAPTER 14

Biologic Augmentation in Peripheral Nerve Repair

WINNIE A. PALISPIS, MD • RANJAN GUPTA, MD

INTRODUCTION

Peripheral nerve injuries remain a main source of morbidity and disability. Peripheral nerve injuries have life-altering impacts on the patients who suffer years of uncertainty while waiting for some level of recovery.[1,2] Patients may be left with devastating sensory and motor deficits such as limb numbness, dysethesias, paralysis, and neuropathic pain which renders them disabled. The management of nerve injuries is multifactorial including the location of the injury, the type of injury, the size of segmental nerve defect, the timing of injury presentation, and accompanying soft tissue injury. Nerve injuries lead to both physiological and histopathological changes to the nerve and its surrounding soft tissue, including demyelination, degeneration, remyelination, and regeneration. Despite the permissive growth environment of the peripheral nervous system (PNS), major human nerve injuries have very limited potential for spontaneous recovery. Although there has been significant amount of research addressing the molecular biology of nerve injury and numerous surgical advances detailing peripheral nerve repair, the injured limb still cannot be restored to normal function. Unfortunately, optimization of outcomes has plateaued with surgical manipulation alone as issues with the rate of regeneration, specificity of regeneration, segmental nerve defects, and degeneration of target end organ remain unaddressed by current practices.[3] Tension-free primary repair is the gold standard for peripheral nerve injuries that do not have gaps. Nerve injuries with gaps present a greater challenge for the reconstructive surgeons. Faced with this predicament, surgeons have been searching for alternative techniques to allow bridging of gaps, as well as tensionless nerve repair. The role of biologic augments in the repair of peripheral nerve injuries has long been studied in both animal models and humans to address this issue. It is, therefore, critical that we are made aware of the appropriate applications and the limitations of these tools to understand how we can promote an effective regenerative environment for damaged nerves. Adapted from our recent review,[3] we include discussions regarding microanatomy, nerve response to injury, as well as limitations of peripheral nerve regeneration, as these topics provide invaluable information to further understand the role of biologic augmentation in peripheral nerve repair and reconstruction.

MICROANATOMY

Peripheral nerves are heterogeneous composite structures that are comprised of neurons, Schwann cells (SCs), macrophages, and fibroblasts. The neuron is a polarized cell that forms the foundation of the nerve and consists of dendrites, the cell body, and a single axon. Axons project toward their sites of innervation to form synapses with their target end organs. If the axonal diameter is greater than or equal to 1 μm, each SC will wrap its plasma membrane around one single region of an axon to form myelin. SCs produce myelin to encapsulate the axon and aid in action potential transmission as myelin allows for fast and efficient conduction and propagation of an action potential down an axon. The blood supply to the nerve is a complex vascular plexus formed from anastomoses of epineural, perineural, and endoneurial plexi,[4] as well as segmental blood supply derived from a number of nutrient arteries. It is apparent that the blood supply to the nerve is fragile and may be disrupted due to trauma or tension during nerve repair. In addition, peripheral nerves have connective tissue layers to provide strength and protection to the nerve: (1) the epineurium, (2) perineurium, and (3) endoneurium. It is crucial to recognize that all surgical interventions are strictly directed at these connective tissue layers, whereas the axon and SCs must respond to injury and regenerate via their inherent biology.

Biologics in Orthopaedic Surgery. https://doi.org/10.1016/B978-0-323-55140-3.00014-X

NERVE RESPONSE TO INJURY

In contrast to chronic nerve injuries that are SC driven, acute nerve injuries are axonally mediated with Wallerian degeneration being initiated with granular disintegration of the axonal cytoskeleton. Within 48 hours after injury to the nerve, SCs break down myelin and phagocytose debris from the axon in the distal stump. Macrophages are then recruited to the area and start releasing growth factors that in turn encourage SC and fibroblast proliferation. SCs begin the reparative process by forming longitudinal bands of Bungner, which are essentially growth-promoting conduits for regenerating axons. Injection of predifferentiated SCs near injured nerves has been shown to aid remyelination in regenerating axons, reduce percent myelin debris, and improve functional recovery in rodents.[5] At the tip of the regenerating axon is the growth cone, which is composed of cellular matrix from which fingerlike projections called filopodia extrude to explore the microenvironment. Proteases are released from the growth cone to clear a path toward a target organ, which is heavily influenced by different factors. After injury, SCs upregulate neurotrophic factors nerve growth factor (NGF) and brain-derived growth factor (BDNF), as well as their corresponding receptors in the distal stumps.[6,7] This increase in expression of NGF and its low-density receptors is believed to promote extensive proliferation and migration of SCs[8] and mainly affects properties of sensory neurons. BDNF levels are also increased and are postulated to act as an anterograde trophic messenger under the influence of NGF. Ciliary neuronotrophic factor (CNTF) is a neuronotrophic factor that is believed to affect survival and regeneration of motoneurons and is found to be reduced significantly in the SCs of the distal stump, with this reduction extending to the neuromuscular junction.[9] Furthermore, there is increased retrograde axonal transport of CNTF after nerve injury.[10] Neurite-promoting factors, such as laminin and fibronectin, and matrix-forming precursors, such as fibrinogen, are all synthesized in response to nerve injury.[4]

In addition to the release of trophic factors, tubulin deacetylation is an important factor leading to decreased stability of microtubulin, which is required for axonal integrity and regeneration. Calcium-dependent activation of the histone deacetylases HDAC5 and HDAC6, in particular, leads to tubulin degeneration likely playing a role in inhibiting axonal regeneration after peripheral nerve injuries.[11,12] The interaction between axons and SCs has also emerged as an important regulator of PNS development and regeneration. Fleming et al. identified that the receptor tyrosine kinase *Ret* genetically interacts with *Er81* to control *Nrg1-Ig* in promoting the formation of Pacinian corpuscles.[13] Taken together, these factors have the potential to promote regeneration; provide signaling for cell survival, neuronal differentiation, and proliferation; and influence synaptic function.[14]

After a nerve injury, PNS neurons upregulate a number of regeneration-associated genes that may have direct role in neurite outgrowth.[15] For example, the overexpression of transcription factor Activating transcription factor 3 (ATF-3) has been shown to promote neurite outgrowth after peripheral nerve injury.[16] In their animal study, Bomze et al. concluded that growth-associated protein 43 and cytoskeleton-associated protein 23 were expressed after nerve injury and, together, were able to induce dramatic increase in the number of regenerated axons.[17] Pathways associated with increased regeneration after a nerve injury have also been identified. The ERK pathway was shown to mediate axonal elongation, with the kinases Extracellular signal regulated kinase (ERK) and Akt promoting regeneration after axonal injury.[18] After nerve injury, the cytokine interleukin-6 has been shown to work through the JAK-STAT3 pathway to overcome the inhibitory molecules and allow for axonal regeneration.[19] In addition to pathways that are involved in axonal regeneration, there are also pathways that have been associated with inhibition of axonal regeneration. The small GTPase Rho signaling pathway, for instance, has a role in cytoskeletal reorganization and cell motility. Studies have shown that activation of Rho results to collapse of growth cones, and inhibiting Rho pathway allows for contractility and promotes neurite outgrowth.[20,21]

LIMITATIONS OF PERIPHERAL NERVE REGENERATION

Despite the promise of improved functional recovery, results are still limited as detailed by these studies with all currently available techniques. Outcomes of nerve repair after a traumatic injury are commonly influenced by factors outside of the control of the surgeon such as the age of the patient, location of injury, and timing of injury presentation and nerve repair. As initially reported by Sunderland and subsequently by many others, nerve reconstruction outcomes are better with younger patients, early repairs, repairs of single function nerves, distal injuries, and short nerve grafts.[22] There are numerous challenges facing nerve repair, and optimization of outcomes has plateaued with surgical manipulations alone, offering limited capacity to effect true functional neural regeneration.

The ultimate repair and regeneration is a complex biological process that we are just beginning to understand through clinical experiences as well as animal experimental studies. Rate of regeneration, specificity of regeneration, segmental nerve deficits, and degeneration of the target end organ are challenges that need to be overcome to achieve meaningful functional recovery (Fig. 14.1).

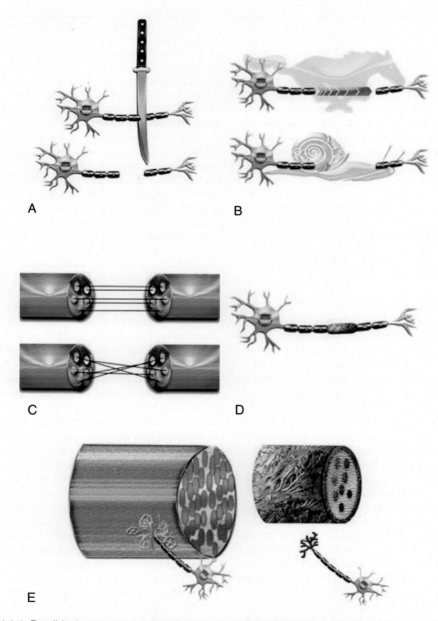

FIG. 14.1 Roadblocks to recovery after nerve injury include **(A)** the presence of a segmental nerve defect, **(B)** variable rates of regeneration, **(C)** the need for specificity of regeneration, **(D)** glial scar formation, and **(E)** the degeneration of the target end organ.

Rate of Regeneration

In adults, it is well accepted that neural regeneration occurs at a slow rate of about 1 mm per day.[23] The rate of regeneration can be monitored with a present advancing Tinel sign as it progresses from proximal to distal.[7] When a nerve is injured, the nerve must grow over substantial distances and traverse over scar and fibrous changes in its environment to reach its target. For example, a brachial plexus injury may involve distances of up to 1 m and may require up to 3 years for regenerating axons to reach the hand muscles.

Many factors can limit and influence the rate of nerve regeneration. The type of nerve injury can influence the probability of successful regeneration. A crush nerve lesion for instance has a continuous basal lamina structure that provides guidance for regenerating nerve. After axotomy, the nerve sheath discontinuity impedes reinnervation and can lead to neuroma formation. Animal studies have also shown that production of neurotrophic factors in the distal segments of a nerve gradually decreases to the point where sufficient levels are not present to support nerve growth, preventing fast regeneration.[24-27] Furthermore, this nongrowth permissive state promotes axonal retraction and "wandering axons" which is thought to prevent regeneration to the neuromuscular junction.[28,29]

Specificity of Regeneration

Axonal misdirection is believed to play a significant role in poor functional recovery after severe nerve injuries.[30] Nerve injuries induce rapid axonal sprouting so as to facilitate anterograde, target directed axonal regeneration. Moreover, the degenerating distal nerve segment has growth-promoting potential and may enhance the specificity of regeneration.[31] Quantitative retrograde labeling technique has been used to define the number of regenerating motoneurons and the specificity of their peripheral connections.[32] It has been shown that motor nerves tend to reinnervate motor pathways. Even in injured mixed sensory-motor nerves, it was observed that motor axons preferentially reinnervate motor pathways.[33] This involves recognition molecules of the L2/Human Natural Killer-1 (HNK-1) family that are detectable in ventral spinal roots and motor axons but not in dorsal root or sensory cutaneous nerves.[34] As a nerve tries to regenerate, motor axons were found to explore different pathways by sending out collateral branches. Specificity of pathway regeneration is subsequently gained by "pruning off" those collaterals that have grown into inappropriate nerve branch.[33] After injury, muscle fibers previously belonging to a specific motor unit will likely be innervated by a different motor axon. This mismatch between central commands to motor neurons and the actual distribution of muscle fibers innervated by those motor neurons contributes to unsuccessful functional recovery, as well as sensorimotor disturbances.[35] Furthermore, after injury, some axons grow in various directions and compete for innervation, which will lead to loss of prelesional innervation selectivity.[36] A study visualizing regenerating axons reported axons exposed to as many as 150 different potential distal pathways.[37] Although preferential motor reinnervation has been detailed in animals, it remains unclear as to what level this occurs in the human condition.

Segmental Nerve Defects

Intuitively, regeneration over a segmental gap is quite challenging and has been demonstrated with animal studies as epineural neurorrhaphy without a gap showed better nerve regeneration when compared with neurorrhaphy with a gap. Functional restoration after a nerve injury requires the growth of axons over the distance between the lesion and the end target. After injury, fibrosis and edema cause nerve fibers to lose their elasticity and extensibility, as well as a certain amount of retraction. If a nerve tissue is destroyed, the fascicular pattern of the proximal and distal stumps may differ in relation to the length of the defect.[38] Injury with a segmental gap precludes tension-free, end-to-end coaptation repair. There has been some disagreement regarding whether or not there is an ideal nerve defect that will allow neural regeneration and achieve functional recovery. Nerve injury repairs of short defects, between 0.5 and 5.0 mm, have been producing varying results.[39-42] Studies of segmental nerve defects have revealed the existence of a critical nerve gap length where the efficacy of conduits starts to decline. These different types of nerve conduits have been used to provide foundation for nerve regeneration to occur in nerve gaps that are less than 3 cm; however, animal models examining nerve regeneration in nerve gaps of 3 cm or more have not shown promising results.[43,44] Mackinnon and Dellon detailed that the primate peripheral nerve could regenerate across a 3-cm nerve gap when guided appropriately. They extrapolated their findings to humans with nerve gaps of 3 cm or less and demonstrated excellent recovery in 33% of the patients.[45]

Other experiments have suggested that axons should be able to align themselves in response to neurotrophic factors when allowed to grow across a conduit. This finding suggested that conduit repairs might lead to improved functional results, compared with standard end-to-end repair.[46–48] Different growth factors with different conduit luminal scaffolds such as collagen and laminin have been used. These modifications, however, did not offer substantial benefit over using autografts[49]; thus, continued investigation is being conducted to find the effective combination of scaffold, cells, and signaling factors that will yield better neural regeneration outcomes.

Degeneration of the Target End Organ

Denervation atrophy of target tissue is another important challenge that is associated with peripheral nerve repair and regeneration. Aside from the long distances that nerves need to traverse to reach their target organs, prolonged target deprivation is found to reduce the ability of motor neurons to regenerate and cause SCs to lose their growth-supportive phenotypes.[50,51] Wallerian degeneration occurs distal to the injury site, and communication is lost between the nerves and the muscles that they innervate. It has been shown in animal models that after the loss of innervation, the acetylcholine receptors located on the muscle membrane degenerate, as evidenced by decreased density and altered morphology. Furthermore, long-term denervation leads to the disassembly of the motor endplates, causing the acetylcholine receptors to redistribute throughout the muscle fiber.[52–54] The degradation of motor endplates render the target organ nonviable for the regenerating nerve despite reaching the target. There are findings that suggest that after injury, regrowth into the muscle becomes successful. However, even with successful regeneration, there is still a failure to reestablish motor function, suggesting a possible critical role of the neuromuscular junction. A recent study confirmed that regenerating fibers can reinnervate distal muscles and can reestablish structurally reformed Neuromuscular junction (NMJ) even after several weeks of denervation.[55]

The problem of end-organ atrophy is partially addressed with nerve transfer procedures as there is less time for degeneration with the shorter distance that regeneration must occur; yet, a successful nerve transfer only restores partial muscle function, and preinjury strength is not fully recovered.[56] It is then of great interest to determine if stabilization of the NMJ could potentially reduce end-organ atrophy after nerve injury. Chao et al. provided the first evidence that preservation of the NMJ after traumatic nerve injury improves functional recovery after surgical repair.[57] Matrix metalloproteinase 3 (MMP3) is the major enzyme responsible for the degradation of agrin in denervated muscles which is secreted by terminal SCs. Genetic deletion of MMP3 leads to sustained levels of agrin in denervated

muscle endplates, which in turn was able to preserve motor endplate integrity for at least 2 months after nerve degeneration.[57] Taking these into account, these data detail that it is possible to extend the optimal window beyond which destabilization of the motor endplate limits reinnervation. Pharmacological inhibition of MMP3 and local augmentation of neural agrin are a few innovations that could feasibly stabilize the NMJ and diminish end-organ atrophy after nerve injury. Moreover, the canonical Wnt/beta-catenin pathway has been implicated as a potential source of motor endplate instability after long-term denervation.[58] Therefore, targeting the Wnt/beta-catenin pathway may offer therapeutic opportunities for more effective reinnervation of endplates and subsequently improve meaningful functional recovery.

BIOLOGIC AUGMENTS IN PERIPHERAL NERVE REPAIR

Nerves that are injured do not spontaneously heal and repair themselves. The nerve continuity needs to be reestablished for the nerve to regain its function. The primary goal of nerve repair is to correctly align and approximate severed nerve segments to allow reinnervation of the target organs with hopes of achieving functional recovery. Historically, it was thought best to wait 3 weeks for the completion of the Wallerian degeneration process before nerve repair. However, studies by Fu[51] and Mackinnon[59] detail that immediate repair produced better outcomes. Major prerequisites to nerve repair include a clean wound, viable blood supply, no crush component to the injured nerve, adequate soft tissue coverage, skeletal stability, and minimal tension on the nerve repair. The current principle for a successful nerve repair is the coaptation of nerve tissue without tension and is uniformly accepted as the single most important technical factor in peripheral nerve repair.[60,61] Treatment of nerve injury continues to be a challenge as early studies detailed poor functional results after surgical repair. But with the increasing understanding of the nerve anatomy and physiology, accompanied by advances of microsurgical technology including utilization of biological augments and refinement of surgical techniques, outcomes of nerve repair have started to be promising. The challenge being posted to reconstructive surgeons today is the repair and reconstruction of long nerve gaps. The following section gives a review of the different tools that are available in our current armamentarium for improving and enhancing peripheral nerve regeneration.

AUTOGENOUS BIOLOGICAL CONDUITS

Autogenous nerve grafting provides a guided pathway composed of lamina scaffold and SCs to allow nerve regeneration. Disadvantages of autogenous nerve graft include the associated patient morbidity and poor functional outcomes, with reported postoperative strength most often only reaching grade 3.[62] Furthermore, autologous donors are usually smaller in caliber, shorter in length, and less abundant. In 1891, Bügner reported successful nerve regeneration with the use of human arterial grafts to bridge sciatic nerve gaps in dogs.[63] The use of artery as a conduit has not been implemented clinically, most likely due to lack of suitable donor vessels.

Unlike arteries, vein autografts are more available and easier to harvest. Wrede, in 1909, was the first to introduce the use of vein grafts for repairing nerve defects. In his study, he reported successful human median nerve repair using a 45-mm long vein tube.[64] Multiple animal studies have also confirmed successful nerve defect repair using vein grafts. Chui et al. reported histologic and electrophysiological evidence of nerve regeneration in 1-cm sciatic nerve gaps in rats.[65] Rice et al. used femoral vein grafts to repair sciatic nerve defects in rats and reported axonal penetration into the distal sciatic nerve segment, concluding that vein grafts are suitable conduits for nerve repair.[66] Seumatsu et al. evaluated nerve repair by vein grafting and by nerve grafting in 1-cm rat sciatic nerve defects and concluded that there was no difference in myoelectrical response between the two groups at 6 months.[67] Vein grafts have also been studied clinically. In a prospective study evaluating patients who underwent nerve repair with autogenous vein grafts and nerve grafting for symptomatic neuroma, Chiu and Strauch reported that even though superior results were found in patients in the nerve graft group, patients in the vein graft group had successful return of two-point discrimination.[68] In 1989, Walton et al. reviewed results of 22 patients with digital nerve repairs using autogenous vein grafts and reported good results for acute digital nerve repairs but poor results with delayed digital nerve repairs.[69] More recently, Rinker and Liau demonstrated equal sensory recovery after digital nerve repair (mean nerve gap of 10 mm) with autogenous vein grafts to repair with collagen conduit, with vein grafts yielding fewer complications.[70] Overall, the use of vein grafts has shown potential for nerve repair.

The main concern with the use of vein grafts is the possibility of lumen collapse, which can then impede nerve regeneration. This remained a concern even though Tseng et al. demonstrated that the vein graft remains patent during the process of nerve regeneration.[71] Efforts to limit the risk of vein collapse led to the filling of vein grafts with muscle or nerve tissue. These intraluminal additives have benefits of supplying extracellular matrix and neurotrophic factors that facilitate nerve regeneration across defects by promoting SC proliferation, migration, and axonal growth cone guidance.[72–74]

Veins that are interposed with neuronal tissue have shown to produce meaningful recovery results in ulnar, median, superficial radial, and digital defects of 2.5–4.5 cm.[75,76]

The use of skeletal muscle for nerve repair was prompted by the early observation that skeletal muscle fibers have a basal lamina oriented in a longitudinal fashion resembling endoneurial tubes of degenerating nerves.[72,77] Potential skeletal muscle fiber donor sites are numerous; however, there is a risk that nerve fibers can grow out of the muscle tissue during nerve regeneration.[78] Both fresh and denatured muscles have been used in studies. Glasby et al. used degenerated muscle grafts to repair a 30-mm nerve gap in adult marmosets and reported successful regeneration.[79] Pereira et al. used denatured muscle grafts for reconstruction of digital nerve defects between 15 and 28 mm and reported better results than nerve grafting.[80] However, not every study reported positive results. Raganovic et al. reported worse quality of recovery in patients with radial nerve defects repaired with denatured muscle grafts compared with outcomes of nerve graft repair.[81]

Another biologic conduit that has been studied for nerve repair is the tendon autograft because of its collagen content and ECM components. Using a rat model, Brandt et al. suggested that tendon grafts can be used as nerve conduits to bridge 10- and 15-mm gap defects.[82,83] Even though the aforementioned studies show tendons as a feasible neural gap conduit because of the lack of clinical studies, it is still uncertain if tendon autografts are useful in human nerve repair.

NONAUTOGENOUS BIOLOGICAL CONDUITS

Nerve allografts have been studied as a potential alternative for nerve repair. Nerve allografts provide a readily available tissue source for nerve reconstruction. The first clinical results from the use of nerve allografts dated back in 1885 reported poor clinical outcomes.[84] Multiple early studies on nerve allografts suggested that the likely cause of clinical failure is immune rejection, which can lead to scarring and fibrosis and eventually act as a mechanical barrier for regenerating fibers.[85,86]

The advent of host immunosuppression allowed for nerve allografts to be a possible reconstruction alternative for nerve repair. Techniques such as administration of concurrent immunosuppressants[87] and pretreatment with radiation and lyophilization have been used to combat the problem of immunogenicity.[88] The allograft is believed to serve as a temporary scaffold for regenerating host nerve fibers. As regeneration proceeds, the donor determinants within the allograft are slowly replaced by host components.[89] Mackinnon et al. applied the concept of allografting with immunosuppression clinically in patients with large peripheral nerve gaps. In this study, return of motor and sensory function was observed, and only 1 patient experienced rejection secondary to subtherapeutic immunosuppression.[90]

Decellularized nerve allografts (DCAs) were developed in efforts to completely eliminate the need for immunosuppression as it imposes harmful side effects. In DCAs, human nervous tissues are processed to render the grafts nonimmunogenic, hence precluding the need for immune modulation but at the same time retaining the physical macrostructure that facilitates nerve regeneration.[91] In DCAs, host SCs are considered the driving force for regeneration as they migrate from neighboring nerve stumps and create the neurosupportive environment to encourage axonal regeneration.[92] While processed nerve allografts are acellular, they are able to revascularize and repopulate with host cells, thus providing an environment that is conducive for regeneration.[93] Methods of nerve decellularization include freeze thawing, irradiation, detergent processing, enzyme digestion, and cold preservation. AxoGen is currently the only commercially available allograft that is approved by the Food and Drug Administration (FDA) for clinical use. The propriety preparation of AxoGen allografts is a combination of detergent processing, enzyme digestion to remove axonal growth inhibition by chondroitin sulfate proteoglycans, and gamma irradiation.[92,94] The decellularization process alters the molecular and structural properties of the nerve, and the specific method of preparing the acellular nerve allografts can actually affect the overall quality of regeneration. Moore and colleagues experimented with rat nerves that were processed using different methods of decellularization to bridge a 14-mm nerve defect in an animal model. In their study, they showed that allografts processed with detergent had similar performance to autografts, whereas allografts prepared by either cold preservation or AxoGen processing showed inferior nerve regeneration in comparison to autografts.[94] It was theorized that the detergent processing

allowed retention of growth factors released from the ECM. Yet, Whitlock et al., via a rat sciatic model, showed that regeneration across gaps of 14 and 28 mm using AxoGen allografts was inferior to autografts.[95] Guisti et al. evaluated return of motor function in rats with 10-mm sciatic nerve defects treated with autografts, DCAs, and collagen conduits. They concluded that processed allografts were overall inferior to autografts but resulted in better motor function than those that were treated with collagen conduits.[96]

There have also been studies looking at the efficacy of nerve allografts in humans. In 2009, Karabekmez and colleagues reported the first study to examine the short-term clinical nerve function recovery after nerve repair with AxoGen nerve allograft. In this study, they concluded that DCAs are capable of adequate sensory repair in nerve defects up to 30 mm without infection or rejection.[91] Brooks et al. published results from the first multicenter trial on the Avance (AxoGen) processed allograft. The study was based on a total of 76 peripheral nerve defect injuries (5–50 mm) which included 49 sensory, 18 mixed, and 9 motor nerves. They reported 87% meaningful sensory and motor recovery based on the Mackinnon grading system.[97] Guo et al. evaluated digital nerve repair using DCAs in 5 patients with an average defect of 23 mm. They reported S3+ or better sensation in all subjects and an average two-point discrimination of 6 mm at 13-month follow-up.[98] In 2015, Rinker and colleagues reported on 37 short-gap sensory repairs using DCAs after which 92% of subjects showed meaningful recovery.[99] Cho et al. demonstrated recovery of M3 or better motor function in 75% of median nerve repairs and 66% of ulnar nerve repairs.[93] The use of DCA in repair of long nerve gap was also documented. Fleming et al. confirm return of motor and sensory function in a patient who underwent DCA ulnar nerve repair for a 70-mm nerve defect.[13] Multiple studies have shown that decellularized nerve allografts seem to provide promising results; however, not all outcomes of studies have shown such promise. Cho et al. reported that 2 of their subjects reported no functional recovery. Of note, one injury is a 491-day-old median nerve injury, and the other was a high-energy blast injury to the ulnar nerve.[93] Berrocal and colleagues reported a case of failure of DCA repair after a high-energy fracture of the distal ulna, highlighting the importance of nerve diameter and length of defect in successful repair.[100]

Consistently, attempts of functional recovery over larger nerve gaps >30 mm have been more difficult to achieve. In 2013, using an animal model, a study looked at SC senescence in acellular nerve allografts during nerve repair. Interestingly, they observed high evidence of cellular senescence in DNAs with gaps >60 mm.[101] Clinical length limitations in DCAs have been debated. AxoGen's Avance is supplied in lengths between 15 and 70 mm, with internal diameters between 1 and 5 mm.

Critical analysis of data presented previously revealed that the best results were in digital nerves, i.e., pure sensory nerves with limited gap. Although some authors concluded that the processed nerve allografts could be effectively used in nerve gaps of 5–50 cm in length,[93] this claim has not been widely accepted in clinical practice. The upper limit for clinical use of DCAs is not yet fully established and is most often used when the magnitude of nerve injuries exceed the capacity of donor autografts.

SYNTHETIC CONDUITS

Synthetic conduits work by encasing the distal and proximal ends of the nerve within a tube, allowing for macroalignment for the nerve. Fibrin matrix then forms between the nerve ends that can support cellular migration between the nerve endings. As cells start to invade the cable, band of Büngner form within the disorganized matrix to allow for neurite outgrowth. This mechanism depends on the volumetric output from the nerve stumps.[102] The earliest success with synthetic conduits was observed back in 1898 by Merle et al., who bridged nerve defects with silicone polymer nerve guides.[103] Lundborg and colleagues then published several reports illustrating the feasibility of silicone conduits for nerve repair and reconstruction.[104–106] Moreover, a study by Braga-Silva reported effective late repair with silicone tubes in peripheral nerve injuries with gaps of up to 30 mm.[107] Despite the early promising results, the nonresorbable nature of the silicone tube caused permanent fibrotic encapsulation of the implant with subsequent chronic nerve compression. In fact, these tubes have been used by many investigators to create Chronic Nerve Compression (CNC) injuries in animal models. This critical limitation led to the development of absorbable synthetic conduits that will allow diffusion of oxygen and micronutrients across the outer walls and into the matrix. There are 3 types of synthetic conduits that are FDA approved, each made from different biomaterials: (1) polyglycolic acid (PGA), (2) collagen type I, and (3) caprolactone. The use of these conduits is currently limited to defects of 3 cm or smaller; however, with the advent of bioengineering, there is a potential for these conduits to be an option for larger nerve defects. Of the FDA-approved nerve conduits, the collagen-based NeuraGen and the PGA-based NeuroTube conduits have the most encouraging clinical data to date.[108]

Polyglycolic Acid

PGA is a commonly used suture material and was the first material used to construct nerve conduits when the limitations of silicone tubes were observed. It has excellent mechanical properties and is rapidly degraded into lactic acid. PGA conduits have yielded positive outcomes in both sensory and motor recovery in segmental nerve defects. Animal studies showed early support for PGA tubes as good alternatives to nerve grafts. Dellon et al. described histologic and electrophysiologic evidence of regeneration that is achieved after PGA conduit repair of a 30-mm ulnar nerve gap in monkeys and concluded that there is no significant difference when compared with repair with sural nerve graft.[109] Matsumoto et al. reported successful regeneration across an 80-mm nerve gap in dog peroneal nerve with the use of a PGA conduit.[110] PGA conduits also were used in human nerve reconstruction. Mackinnon and Dellon reported a case series of 15 secondary reconstructions of digital nerve defects 30 mm or smaller and reported 86% meaning recovery.[45] Weber and colleagues reported on the first randomized prospective multicenter evaluation of the first commercially available PGA conduit, NeuroTube, for digital nerve repair. NeuroTube was approved by the FDA in 1999 for human use in the United States. The study concluded that in nerve defects of less than 40 mm, NeuroTube provided significantly better return of sensory function than direct suture repair.[48] Efforts to extend the use of PGA to larger nerve defects and motor nerves were undertaken by Rosson et al., who bridged median nerve defects (15–40 mm) and reported meaningful recovery in all patients.[111] Subsequent studies comparing PGA to other methods of nerve repair found PGA to perform equally, if not better. For example, Battison and colleagues compared PGA nerve repair to nerve repair with autogenous vein grafts filled with muscle. In this series of 17 patients with 19 digital nerve injuries repaired using NeuroTube conduits across 10–40 mm nerve gaps showed positive results and no differences in functional recovery between the 2 cohorts.[112] In 2011, Rinker et al. compared PGA conduits and autogenous vein grafts for both short (<10 mm) and long (>10 mm) digital nerve defects and found no difference in meaningful recovery between the two groups.[70] A documented disadvantage of the NeuroTube is the extrusion of the conduit even in healthy-looking tissues. Weber et al. reported 46 cases of PGA conduit implantation, 3 of which got extruded.[48] Duncan and colleagues reported on a patient with a radial digital nerve that was bridged with PGA conduit, who, on postoperative week 4, was found to have extrusion of the conduit through the wound. They mentioned that the cause for this complication was not very clear, but the properties of the PGA conduit and the patient's own immunological properties are some factors to consider.[113]

Collagen Conduits

Collagen conduits are made from purified type 1 collagen derived from bovine flexor tendons. Collagen is the major component of the ECM and is believed to facilitate adhesion and enhance cell proliferation.[114] The utilization of collagen conduits in nerve reconstruction has been demonstrated both in animal and human studies. Archibald et al. demonstrated the feasibility of collagen nerve guides in regeneration of a 5-mm nerve gap in nonhuman primates.[115] Using rat models, Keilhoff et al. tested collagen type I/III tubes as potential nerve guides and reported that collagen can serve as template to ensure nerve regeneration through nerve defects.[116]

NeuraGen was commercially available in 2001 and has been examined by numerous investigators. Clinical studies evaluating the efficacy of collagen conduits have demonstrated favorable outcomes in defects of 20 mm or less. Ashley et al. used NeuroGen as graft material in five patients with obstetrical brachial plexus palsy. Collagen tubes were used to repair nerve gaps smaller than 20 mm. They reported that four out of the five patients made good functional recovery, being able to dress and feed themselves at 2-year follow-up.[117] In a retrospective study, Bushnell et al. followed up 12 patients with repair of digital injury using NeuroGen bovine collagen nerve tube and reported effective restoration of digital nerve function in the early postoperative period.[118] Lohmeyer and colleagues found that collagen conduits provided consistent functional recovery in nerve gaps that are less than 15 mm. No functional recovery was seen in gaps that are greater than 15 mm.[119] Wangensteen et al., in a retrospective review, reported an overall 35% recovery of quantitative nerve function in nerve defects of 2.5–20 mm and 31% going on revision surgery.[120] In 2011, Taras et al. reported a 73% meaningful recovery in 5–15 mm digital nerve lacerations repaired with NeuroGen.[121]

Several investigators have studied collagen conduit repair in comparison to other methods of nerve repair. In a rat model comparing NeuraGen to Avance (AxoGen allograft), NeuroGen produced inferior results in rat model across 14- and 28-mm gaps.[95] Boeckstyns et al. evaluated and compared repair of acute lacerations of

mixed sensory-motor nerves in 43 patients using collagen tube versus traditional neurorrhaphy. The study concluded that the use of collagen conduit produces sensory and motor functional recovery that is equivalent to direct suture in nerve gaps that were 6 mm or less.[122]

There are documented studies that show failed collagen conduits in mixed nerve repair and digital nerve repairs.[43,123] Liodaki and colleagues reported cases of poor regeneration in 4 patients with unsuccessful implantation of NeuraGen conduit. Evidence of scarring and fibrosis was observed with the conduit and the surrounding tissue bed. Moreover, histologic assessment found neuromas and evidence of foreign body reaction.[123] Other collagen conduits are available in the market; however, there are limited clinical or preclinical data available for NeuroWrap, NeuroFlex, NeuroMatrix, and NeuroMend. As such, it is challenging to draw any conclusions about their clinical utility.

Poly D, L Lactide-co-epsilon-caprolactone Conduits (PCL)

PCL nerve guides are the most recent FDA-approved synthetic conduits. These conduits have the advantage of being transparent in nature allowing good visualization of nerve stumps within the chamber. The PCL material degrades into small particles over a period of time until it is fully resorbed. Its crystalline structure remains impermeable to fluid longer than PGA and collagen conduits.[124] The material itself, however, is very rigid, which renders PCL conduits more difficult to handle in the clinical setting. Efforts to assess the efficacy of PCL conduits for nerve repair have yielded mixed outcomes, and the use of NeuroLac in the clinical setting has been less encouraging. Preclinical data in rat models with a 10-mm sciatic nerve defect using NeuroLac suggested favorable motor recovery comparable to autografts.[125] Bertleff et al. evaluated digital nerve repair of a 20-mm or less nerve gap in 21 nerve lesions. They concluded that recovery results in the PCL group are comparable to those obtained after end-to-end repair.[126] Studies by Meek et al.[127] on digital nerve repair in the foot and Hernandez Cortez et al.[128] on a digital nerve gap in the thumb demonstrated no meaningful recovery when PCL conduits were used. Hernandez Cortez reported that failure of the implant was accompanied by histological evidence of biomaterial fragments and foreign body reactions.[128] Moreover, Chiriac et al., in 2012, analyzed a series of 28 nerve repairs of the upper extremity with PCL conduits and reported only a 25% meaningful recovery with complications such as neuroma formation and fistularization of the conduit into the joint.[129] With conflicting results presented previously, the efficacy of PCL conduits for clinical use remains largely unclear.

EXOGENOUS AGENTS

The addition of exogenous neurotrophic factors in peripheral nerve injury has garnered attention in the past few years.[130] Presently, there are no clinically available pharmacological treatments for nerve injury; however, there are several small molecules, peptides, hormones, and growth factors that have been studied and have been suggested as potential candidates to improve nerve regeneration. The addition of factors such as NGF, BDNF, and Human ciliary neurotrophic factor (CTNF) in conduits used for nerve repair shows to enhance axonal outgrowth and improve remyelination and speed of axonal regeneration.[131,132] Derby et al. reported positive effects on neuronal regeneration in rat sciatic models of 10- and 15-mm defects when NGF was added to silicone chambers.[131] In 1999, Ho and colleagues evaluated if BNDF and CNTF in collagen tubules can successfully achieve functional recovery in rat sciatic nerve defect model. They concluded that BDNF and CTNF can be covalently linked to collagen tubules to allow regeneration and that cotreatment with both BDNF and CTNF produced the best functional recovery in their model.[132] Another animal model reported that rat tibial nerves (of 8-mm gap) reconstructed with fibroblast growth factor within a silicone conduit had 30% more regenerating axons than autografts.[133] Walter et al. evaluated the effects of recombinant FGF on conduit bridging a 15-mm nerve gap. They reported functional motor recovery and increased muscle action potential in the Fibroblast growth factor (FGF) group compared to the control group.[134] Wang et al. also experimented on rat sciatic nerve model and documented enhanced peripheral nerve regeneration when using PCL tubes containing FGF to repair 15-mm nerve gaps.[135] GDNF is another neurotrophic factor secreted by SCs after nerve injury which is known to improve neuronal survival and outgrowth. Fine and colleagues used a rat model and demonstrated enhanced motor and sensory neuronal regeneration across a 15-mm synthetic nerve tube with NGF and GDNF inclusion.[136] Lee et al. used heparin-containing delivery system to slow the diffusion of NGF from a fibrin matrix in a conduit bridging a 13-mm gap in rats. The study revealed a dose-dependent effect of NGF on nerve regeneration and that the total number of nerve fibers was similar to that of isografts.[137] Marquardt et al. used scaffolding containing GDNF and tetracycline-inducible GDNF

overexpressing SCs to repair a 30-mm defect in a rat model. In this study, GDNF was delivered in a well-controlled manner both spatially and temporally. Results showed enhanced axonal regeneration which in turn resulted in increased gastrocnemius and tibialis anterior muscle mass.[138] Glial growth factor is a trophic factor specific for SCs and plays an important role in the interaction between SCs and neurons and is theorized to increase SC motility and proliferation.[139] Using a rabbit common peroneal nerve transection model, Mohanna et al. demonstrated a progressive increase in SC number and axonal regeneration when glial growth factor is applied into polyhydroxybutyrate conduits bridging nerve gaps of 20–40 mm.[140] Vascular endothelial growth factor (VEGF),[141] Leukemia inhibitory factor (LIF),[142] and PDGF[143] are other examples of neurotrophic factors that have demonstrated some efficacy in peripheral nerve repair but are used less.

Additional agents have been investigated to help improve outcomes in peripheral nerve repair. Betamethasone was studied to assess its effect on peripheral nerve regeneration and functional recovery after sciatic nerve transection and repair of a 10-mm defect in rat models. Functional study confirmed faster recovery of regenerated axons in the betamethasone group.[144] Thyroid hormone (T3) was also investigated as a possible agent to enhance regeneration. In their rat animal study, Papakostas and colleagues observed the effects of T3 hormone on peripheral nerve regeneration as it was injected into silicone tubes to bridge nerve gaps. They reported accelerated return of sensory function without significant effect on motor nerve recovery.[145] Vitamin E and pyrroloquinoline (PQQ) were studied using a rat sciatic nerve transection model and it was found that the combination of the two provides better functional recovery of nerve regeneration than Vitamin E or PQQ solely.[146]

More recently, local rapamycin has been studied in a model of rat sciatic nerve defect of 15 mm. It was found that rapamycin is able to reduce secondary nerve injury and promote regeneration of peripheral nerve.[147] Around the same year, Shahraki et al. reported on the effects of tacrolimus (FK506) on nerve regeneration in a rat sciatic nerve model. In this study, they concluded that the administration of FK506 could accelerate functional recovery of the sciatic nerve after nerve allografting.[148] Despite positive results in animal studies of nerve repair, these agents have not been widely used due to mixed and limited demonstrable efficacy in humans as well as the possible adverse effects of the drugs. There are a few human studies however that included tacrolimus as an essential part of the immunosuppression protocol. FK506 has been reported as an agent used for immunosuppression in cases of human upper extremity transplantation. Martin et al. in 2005 demonstrated successful autoreplantation of a proximal arm with 1-year treatment of oral tacrolimus.[149] Authors reported electromyographical improvements in the ulnar and median nerve distribution. In another study, Schuind et al. reported return of intrinsic muscle function as well as a two-point discrimination of 6 mm at the thumb and index finger after a hand transplant with tacrolimus as part of their immunosuppression protocol.[150] In 2011, 9 years after hand transplant, authors report that the patient is able to go back to work.[151] Focusing more on nerve repair, Phan and Schuind looked to investigate the effects of FK506 on axonal regeneration after nerve suture or autograft repair. In their study which included 5 patients with nerve transection, they concluded that FK506 did not demonstrate evidence that it enhances nerve regeneration, stating that the timing and duration of tacrolimus treatment may not have been optimal.[152] The aforementioned human studies mentioned no major side effects of tacrolimus during the duration of treatment.

In general, these factors mentioned previously are either injected directly into nerve conduits or embedded within a hydrogel and can be used on their own or in combination with each other. For the future, continued research should focus on the importance of neurotrophic factor dose response and understand how possible combinations of these factors can be used to create optimal scaffold designs for nerve regeneration.

SC TRANSPLANTATION

SCs, as discussed previously, play an important role in mediating nerve regeneration. Thus, SCs seem to hold the most promise in nerve restoration. SCs have been seeded onto synthetic conduits to enrich the regenerative environment and improve regeneration during nerve repair and reconstruction. In most experimental studies published so far, significant improvement in morphological and functional recovery have been observed. Strauch and colleagues reported excellent nerve regeneration through a 60-mm venous nerve conduits seeded with autologous SCs in their animal model.[153] Furthermore, another animal study by Hoben et al. reported the addition of SCs in acellular nerve allografts improves peripheral nerve regeneration in 20-mm nerve defects.[154] One of the initial concerns with using SCs for nerve repair is that the process of culturing SCs can take a long time. There are now novel techniques available that address this challenge, yielding SC cultures in a shorter period of time (about 2 weeks).[155]

An SC–stem cell cocultured system has also been studied in the animal models of 15-mm nerve defect. In this study, Dai et al. suggested that when incorporated to nerve conduits, sciatic nerve repair with the SC–stem cell coculture resulted in functional recovery, as evaluated by the walking track, functional gait, nerve conduction velocity (NCV), and histological analysis.[156] More recently, Xu and his colleagues also described an SC–stem cell coculture system in their animal model used to seed scaffolds to bridge 10-mm nerve defect in rats and reported regenerative results that are equal to that of autologous nerve grafts but superior to those repaired with plain nerve scaffold.[157] Although there are many studies reporting the benefits of SCs in animal models, clinical trials have not been reported to date. The University of Stanford investigated use of cultured SCs for peripheral nerve injuries of short and long gaps; however, no clinical data from the study have been documented in the literature.[158]

More recently, Levi et al. published the first human experience of using autologous SCs grown from sciatic nerve and sural nerve graft. SCs were seeded onto sural nerve graft to repair sciatic nerve defect of 7.5 cm. After repair, the patient had evidence of sensory and motor recovery distal to the repair.[159] This seminal work supports the possibility of cellular therapy to improve functional neural recovery. We predict that the recent advances in stem cell biology will continue to offer clinical use of SC-enriched conduits because there is an overwhelming evidence that SCs are able to be derived from stem cells.[160]

STEM CELLS TRANSPLANTATION

Recent availability of stem cells has prompted investigation on seeding stem cells to synthetic conduits for nerve regeneration. The success of regeneration will require close interaction between neuronal and non-neuronal supporting cells. Current research has focused on stem cells as they have the potential to differentiate into supporting cells that can guide peripheral nerve regeneration. Stem cells have been shown to differentiate into glial fibrillary acidic protein–positive SC to support myelination,[161] as well as differentiate into fibroblasts capable to producing neurotrophic factors.[162] Multiple types of stem cells have been used including embryonic, mesenchymal, somatic stem cells, neural crest stem cells, and adipose-derived stem cells (ADSCs).

Embryonic stem cells are self-replicating totipotent stem cells derived from early human embryo stage. This fact, unfortunately, limits their availability and subjects these cells to regulatory restrictions. Embryonic stem cells were shown to have the potential to differentiate into Schwann-like cells that express an SC phenotype. These Schwann-like cells were also shown to wrap around axons suggesting the process of myelination.[163] Cui et al. investigated the use of embryonic stem cells injected within a conduit in rat sciatic nerve across a 10-mm gap. They reported 64% of myelinated axons compared with 7% in autografts.[164] Transplantation of embryonic stem cells improves nerve repair and functional recovery after severe sciatic nerve axotomy in rats.[164] Ethical concerns with the use of embryonic stem cells as well as their tendency to form teratomas and immunologic rejection have most likely limited their clinical use in nerve repair.[165]

Induced pluripotent stem cells (iPSCs) are somatic cells that have been genetically manipulated to express a certain phenotype and behavior.[166] iPSCs have been formed from both mouse and human dermal fibroblasts.[167] An animal study that used nerve conduits coated with these pluripotent stem cells in combination with FGF resulted in improvements in regeneration; however, results were subordinate to autograft outcomes.[168] In 2014, Uemura and colleagues used mouse iPSCs in a polylactic acid conduit to bridge a 5-mm gap in mouse sciatic nerves. Based on their histological and functional data, they reported that the addition of iPSCs resulted in significantly enhanced axonal regeneration and myelination, as well as enhanced sensory and motor regeneration at all time points.[169] The process of retroviral silencing occurs when somatic cells transform to the pluripotent state, allowing them to stop expressing the viral transgenes. When this happens, fully reprogrammed iPSCs are achieved and can be labeled superior iPS cells. The timing as to when they undergo retroviral silencing affects the quality of stability of the iPS cells, which in turn can be seen as a disadvantage to their use in nerve repair.[170]

ADSCs were first discovered and defined as mesenchymal stem cells isolated from processed lipoaspirate in 2001.[171] ADSCs are thought to have neurotrophic properties, have the ability to differentiate into multiple lineages, and are shown to form many structures resembling the adult PNS.[172] The fact that ADSCs can be readily obtained using liposuction techniques and can be rapidly cultured without significant morbidity making it one of the most exploited cells in peripheral nerve repair.[173] Wei and colleagues reported that exogenous ADSCs produced similar regenerative outcomes as exogenous SCs in a conduit when used in a 10-mm rat sciatic nerve model.[174] Just recently, Klein et al., also using a 10-mm sciatic nerve rat model, demonstrated

that nerve repair with ADSC-seeded NeuraGen conduit significantly improves motor and sensory nerve regeneration. Moreover, the ADSC-seeded conduits presented a more organized axon arrangement than NeuraGen conduits alone.[175] ADSCs were also used in combination with fibrin glue (FG) to repair nerve defects in rats. Authors concluded that the use of ADSCs in a fibrin matrix can enhance regeneration and angiogenesis after primary coaptation.[176] Some investigators had suggested that ADSC can promote repair by differentiating into SCs and secreting neurotrophic and angiogenic factors.[177] On the other hand, some investigators reported that ADCSs do not differentiate into SCs or SC-like cell; however, they still are able to promote peripheral nerve regeneration that is comparable to that of SCs.[178] Undifferentiated ADSCs were shown to secrete neurotrophic factors such as NGF, BDNF, and GDNF, supporting their role in myelinating regenerating axons, however, in lesser quantity than ADSCs that do differentiate into SCs.[179] Whether ADSCs differentiate into SCs or not, we can at least conclude that the beneficial effects that ADSCs offer in peripheral nerve regeneration are not entirely dependent on the ability to differentiate into SCs but are enhanced by SC differentiation. This is important to note as it has been reported that differentiated ADSCs do rapidly dedifferentiate back into their stem cell–like characteristics with withdrawal of stimulating medium.[180]

Neural crest cells emerge from the dorsal aspect of the neural tube during early vertebrate development. These cells have been of interest because of its multipotency and ability to generate a remarkably number of differentiated cell types. Peripheral nerves, melanocytes, thymus, adrenal glands, and SCs are a few of the derivatives of neural crest cell.[181] Neural crest cells can be harvested from the skin and derived from human fibroblasts, embryonic stem cells, and pluripotent stem cells.[182-184] Using their rat animal model, Lin et al. constructed xenografts seeded with neurons and SCs that were induced from rat hair follicle neural crest stem cells to bridge and repair 10-mm-long nerve defects. They reported that neurons derived from the neural crest stem cells were able to survive up to 52 weeks after transplantation. Moreover, they observed that the treated group had a greater number of regenerated axons than the untreated xenograft.[185] During the same year, Amoh and his colleagues demonstrated that pluripotent hair follicles from human scalp can differentiate into glial fibrillary acidic protein–positive SCs. According to the authors, these stem cells are able to result in greater axonal growth and greater muscle contraction in their rat model.[161] In 2012, Liard et al.

attempted the transplantation of adult neural stem cells inside venous grafts to bridge a 30-mm femoral nerve gap in pigs and demonstrated that the cells that survived inside the graft all displayed a neuronal phenotype, were well distributed along the severed nerve, and were able to activate intrinsic SC activity.[186] Ni et al. used xenogeneic mouse undifferentiated neural crest stem cells in a conduit to bridge a 15-mm sciatic nerve gap in rats and reported outstanding functional and histological improvement.[187] In 2015, Grimoldi and colleagues reported possibly the only clinical use of neural crest stem cells for peripheral nerve repair. In this study, authors used collagen conduit seeded with autologous skin-derived stem cells that included neural crest cells in a young patient after a knife-stabbing accident. They were able to conclude that the use of these stem cells was able to demonstrate regeneration across gaps; however, the motor function recovery remained poor after a 3-year follow-up period.[188]

Bone marrow stem cells (BMSCs) differentiate into neural lineages including neurons and SC-like cells.[189] As they differentiate into SC-like cells, they express trophic factors such as NGF, BDNF, GDNF, and Myelin basic protein (MBP) to improve neural regeneration[162]; however, the beneficial effects of MBSCs on nerve regeneration are not entirely dependent on differentiation into SCs. For instance, in their study, Ceuvas et al. reported functional recovery of rats treated with BMSCs, even though only 5% of BMSCs expressed SC-like phenotypes. In another rat study, Chen and colleagues used silicone conduits with stromal cells to repair 15-mm nerve gaps and showed beneficial effects of these BMSCs on quantity of axons, muscle mass, functional recovery despite not detecting any SCs within the conduit.[162] Mohammadi et al. evaluated the effects of undifferentiated BMSCs seeded in an inside-out vein graft in repairing a 10-mm rat sciatic nerve defect. They reported increased number and an increased diameter of regenerating axons compared with those that were found in vein grafting alone.[190] In 2014, Sakar et al. also evaluated undifferentiated BMSCs in rat sciatic nerve model of 10-mm gap. In this study, BMSCs were seeded in poly(3-hydroxybutyrate-co-3-hydroxyhexanoate) (PHB-HHx) conduit. They concluded that nerve regeneration is better with the combination of BMSCs and PHBHHx rather than PHBHHx alone and that functional outcomes reached the same statistical treatment when compared with autografting.[191] BMSCs that are differentiated into SCs or SC-like cells have also been documented to have positive results in nerve repair and regeneration. Wakao et al. observed that BMSCs differentiated to SC-like cells in a collagen conduit for the repair of monkey median nerve defect. This study showed histological, behavioral, and electrophysiological improvements of up to 1 year.[192] Ladak et al. studied differentiated BMSCs in cocultures and in collagen nerve guides. They found that BMSCs that are differentiated to SC-like cells have positive effect on neurite outgrowth; however, this effect did not translate into significant functional reinnervation as evidenced by their EMG and muscle mass measurements.[193] BMSCs that differentiate into SC-like cells when used with acellular nerve grafts have shown improvements in rat sciatic nerve regeneration over undifferentiated BMSCs and shown results comparable to autograft repair.[194] In addition, the effects of BMSCs in nerve regeneration can be dose dependent, with better improvements in nerve defects treated with high dose of cells versus low dose.[195] When looking at current literature, BMSC regenerative outcomes are at most just similar to outcomes of autograft repairs.

Amniotic fluid mesenchymal stem cells (AF-MSCs) are shown to have the potential to differentiate into neuronal cells, which in turn can develop into SC-like cells.[196] This presents as a promising tool for nerve repair as it can be readily obtained from discarded amniotic fluid used in prenatal diagnosis and by less invasive methods. AF-MSCs are believed to be an encouraging alternative to BMSCs as AF-MSCs were shown to have higher proliferative capacity and are able to secrete higher levels of BDGF and NGF in culture medium than BMSCs.[197] The effects of human AF-MSCs have been investigated in tibia fracture healing[198] and tendon healing[199] in rabbit models. Animal studies have investigated the use of AF-MSCs in nerve repair with successful results. In a rat sciatic nerve transection model repaired with epineural suture, injection of human amniotic fluid around the repair site resulted in less scar formation and faster functional recovery than nerve repair injected with saline.[200] The adjunct use of AF-MSCs has also shown beneficial effects in peripheral nerve regeneration in animal crush model.[201] Still, more research needs to be carried out to fully understand the full capacity of AF-MSCs and its potential benefit in human nerve repair and reconstruction.

FIBRIN

FG is another tool of interest in nerve repair and reconstruction. FG has been used clinically for decades in peripheral nerve repair, with the major role of maximizing the competency of surgical repair.[202] FG has been used as a conduit, a luminal filler, and a scaffold in nerve repair.[202,203] Nerve repair with FG has been reported to decrease fibrosis, nerve scarring, and inflammation as it introduces minimal trauma to nerve fascicles.[203] Even though literature search reveals studies that show FG has the potential to inhibit nerve regeneration, there are studies that show favorable outcomes with the utilization of FG in nerve repair. Nishimura et al. looked at mechanical resistance of nerve repair using FG and conventional suture postoperatively in their rat animal model in which they concluded that resistance is equivalent for the two types of repair 2- and 4-week postoperative repairs.[204] Ornelas and colleagues compared FG repair with conventional epineurial suture repair in their rat nerve transection model and reported faster recovery of NCV and faster return to baseline functional performance in the FG cohort.[205] In a subsequent study, the authors also reported that nerve repair with FG produced less inflammatory response and had better fiber alignment histology than nerves repaired with microsuture technique.[206] FG has also been used as an adjunct to repair of nerve defects. Rafijah et al. reported no significant difference in axonal regeneration and functional recovery in rats with a 10-mm nerve defect repaired with 4 different techniques including collagen conduits with FB, conduit without FB, autograft, and autograft with FB. This study demonstrated that FB does not impede nerve regeneration and suggests that FB is a useful adjunct to segmental nerve repair.[207] Recently, Childe et al. in his cadaveric study looked at the role of FG on digital nerve repair. They have demonstrated that the addition of FG adds to the tensile strength of conduit-assisted digital nerve repairs and that the use of FG may allow for fewer suture placement at the coaptation site. Sameem et al. mentioned one human study during their systematic review of FG for peripheral nerve repair, which reported comparable results of FG repair to standard suture technique for nerve anastomoses, with the advantage of faster operative time.[203] Even with the positive results demonstrated previously, further research is recommended to further determine FG's sufficiency for improving nerve regeneration in the clinical setting.

NERVE TISSUE ENGINEERING AND STRUCTURAL MODULATION

Recent advances in nanotechnology and tissue engineering have been exploited in regenerative medicine and neural defect repairs. Nerve tissue engineering refers to the development and design of biocompatible constructs that will allow for and support tissue regeneration.[208] The ideal properties that need to be considered when designing scaffolds are biocompatibility, biodegradability, porosity, and the mechanical properties that will closely mimic the ECM.

Two bioengineered grafts that have been successful in human and animal studies of nerve repair are the nerve/vein and muscle/vein combined grafts. The utilization of nerve/vein grafts evaluated in human study was determined to be a feasible alternative repair mechanism for nerve defects between 20 and 45 mm.[76] Superior functional and histological outcomes have also been demonstrated with combined vein-muscle conduits, with limitations to gaps of 2 cm or smaller.[73] In 2003, Geuna et al. studied SC activity in muscle-vein combined conduits used to bridge 10-mm nerve defect in rat models. Their results demonstrated continued cell proliferation within a growth-supportive graft environment.[209] More recently, Mohammadi et al. reported that muscle-vein graft used to repair 10-mm nerve defect in rats resulted in better functional recovery and effective nerve regeneration than muscle grafts alone. In the clinical world, Manoli et al. conducted a retrospective study comparing regeneration results after digital nerve reconstruction using nerve autografts, direct suture, or muscle-vein conduits. In 53 total digital nerve injuries with defects ranging from 1 to 6 cm, no statistically significant difference between 3 groups was found.[210]

The application of nanofibers internal scaffold and surface micropatterning are some techniques that when used properly can have the potential to mimic the ECM topography and thus help with cell signaling and interaction as well as nutrient support.[211] In 2004, Yang et al. reported that neural stem cells can attach and differentiate on a nanofiber polylactic scaffold, with the scaffold acting to support neurite outgrowth.[212] Mesenchymal stem cells were also found to be able to differentiate into neuronal cells on nanofibrous scaffolds.[213] A few animal studies on nanofiber scaffold and their role in nerve regeneration have reported positive outcomes. Jin and colleagues, when evaluating nerve regeneration across 10 mm rat sciatic nerve gap using polylactic nanofiber conduit, reported functional recovery that is comparable to the autograft group.[214] Zhan et al. investigated outcomes of using a nanofiber conduit made of blood vessels to repair a 10-mm nerve defect. They concluded that the nanofiber scaffold is able to promote regeneration in their sciatic nerve injury model.[215]

Electrospinning is a technique used to fabricate and imprint micropatterns on a matrix with the goal of creating a greater area-to-volume surface for scaffolds. This in turn allows for maximum adsorption of molecules and superior SC attachment.[216,217]

The advent of 3D printing technology is another area of interest as it is theorized to help toward advancing tissue regeneration after peripheral nerve injury. 3D printing allows the creation of a scaffold with internal cues and spatial gradients of factors to allow guided and targeted regeneration of mixes sensory and motor nerves.[218,219] 3D printing has also been used in conjunction with computed microtomography to demonstrate and replicate the internal structure of acellular nerve allografts.[220]

LOOKING FORWARD TO THE FUTURE

The ultimate goal of peripheral nerve repair is to restore normal function to enable a fruitful and productive lifestyle. Even with the numerous studies and the advancement in nerve repair techniques, we are still in the process of gaining complete understanding of the complex biological process of regeneration. Based on our literature review, it is well recognized that there is still much room for improvement in terms of regeneration outcome. Tensionless end-to-end repair continues to be the gold standard for nerve repair. Nerve conduits and allografts are alternatives that allow orthopedic surgeons to avoid autograft-associated morbidities. Although there have been some preclinical data to support the use of a variety of nerve conduits, allografts, cells, and growth factor additives, the lack of well-designed, randomized control trials make it very difficult for us to compare these techniques to one another and to standard repair methods. For simple, short defects, clinical data suggest the effectiveness of biological conduits. Complex injuries such as those with large defects and injuries involving mixed sensory and motor nerves present a different challenge to reconstructive surgeons. Many have investigated the use of growth factors and neurotrophins inside conduits; however, they have not been introduced to the clinical settings. Stem cell and SC transplant studies have also shown promising results in animal models of nerve repair and some human studies. The long-term effects of these factors, as well as the many undifferentiated, differentiated, and dedifferentiated cells presented in this review remain to be determined. More research should also focus on understanding the complex interactions between growth cones and different molecules, so as to be able to determine correct concentration of molecules and the most effective combination of nerve conduits and guidance factors to enable faster and more accurate regeneration. As technology advances, more techniques have been presented to assist with specificity of nerve regeneration toward their target organs. Tissue engineering adds the benefit of being able to allow alterations in the properties of synthetic conduits such as porosity, topography, biocompatibility, and mechanical strength of the material. The evidence shows that manufactured conduits and allografts, as well as the nanofiber internal scaffolds, are tools that can definitely be included in the nerve regeneration armamentarium. Synergistic effects on nerve regeneration by a combination of the methods listed previously should also be considered as this may further improve functional recovery after peripheral nerve injury. Although conclusions have been drawn using data gathered from animal studies, these results should be interpreted with caution because as we already are aware, animals can achieve histological and functional recovery that are unreachable by humans. For example, rodent nerves can spontaneously regenerate across a 5-cm nerve defect, whereas a human transected nerve needs to be surgically repaired for recovery to occur.[95] As with all nerve repairs, may it be simple or complex, with autografts or allografts, factors such as chronicity of injury, adequacy of debridement, characteristic of the wound bed, location of injury, amount of tension, and overall health of the patient need to be taken into consideration as we deliberate our plan of attack for nerve reconstruction. Advances in laboratory and translational research will no doubt continue to shape our current clinical practices and will prepare surgeons to take on the challenge to revolutionize and refine the approach to nerve repair and reconstruction.

REFERENCES

1. Grinsell D, Keating CP. Peripheral nerve reconstruction after injury: a review of clinical and experimental therapies. *Biomed Res Int.* 2014;2014:1–13. https://doi.org/10.1155/2014/698256.
2. Kang JR, Zamorano DP, Gupta R. Limb salvage with major nerve injury: current management and future directions. *J Am Acad Orthop Surg.* 2011;19(suppl 1):S28–S34.
3. Palispis WA, Gupta R. Surgical repair in humans after traumatic nerve injury provides limited functional neural regeneration in adults. *Exp Neurol.* 2017;290:106–114. https://doi.org/10.1016/j.expneurol.2017.01.009.
4. Yegiyants S, Dayicioglu D, Kardashian G, et al. Traumatic peripheral nerve injury: a wartime review. *J Craniofac Surg.* 2010;21(4):998–1001. https://doi.org/10.1097/SCS.0b013e3181e17aef.
5. Khuong HT, Kumar R, Senjaya F, et al. Skin derived precursor Schwann cells improve behavioral recovery for acute and delayed nerve repair. *Exp Neurol.* 2014;254:168–179. https://doi.org/10.1016/j.expneurol.2014.01.002.
6. Stoll G, Müller HW. Nerve injury, axonal degeneration and neural regeneration: basic insights. *Brain Pathol.* 1999;9(2):313–325. https://doi.org/10.1111/j.1750-3639.1999.tb00229.x.
7. Flores AJ, Lavernia CJ, Owens PW. Anatomy and physiology of peripheral nerve injury and repair. *Am J Orthop (Belle Mead NJ).* 2000;29(3):167–173.

8. Anton ES, Weskamp G, Reichardt LF, et al. Nerve growth factor and its low-affinity receptor promote Schwann cell migration. *Proc Natl Acad Sci USA.* 1994;91(7):2795–2799. https://doi.org/10.1073/pnas.91.7.2795.

9. Hiruma S, Shimizu T, Huruta T, et al. Ciliary neurotrophic factor immunoreactivity in rat intramuscular nerve during reinnervation through a silicone tube after severing of the rat sciatic nerve. *Exp Mol Pathol.* 1997;64(1):23–30. https://doi.org/10.1006/exmp.1997.2206.

10. Curtis R, Adryan KM, Zhu Y, et al. Retrograde axonal transport of ciliary neurotrophic factor is increased by peripheral nerve injury. *Nature.* 1993;365(6443):253–255. https://doi.org/10.1038/365253a0.

11. Cho Y, Cavalli V. HDAC5 is a novel injury-regulated tubulin deacetylase controlling axon regeneration. *EMBO J.* 2012;31(14):3063–3078. https://doi.org/10.1038/emboj.2012.160.

12. Rivieccio M a, Brochier C, Willis DE, et al. HDAC6 is a target for protection and regeneration following injury in the nervous system. *Proc Natl Acad Sci USA.* 2009;106(46):19599–19604. https://doi.org/10.1073/pnas.0907935106.

13. Fleming ME, Bharmal H, Valerio I. Regenerative medicine applications in combat casualty care. *Regen Med.* 2014;9(2):179–190. https://doi.org/10.2217/rme.13.96.

14. Rummler LS, Gupta R. Peripheral nerve repair: a review. *Curr Opin Orthop.* 2004;15(4):215–219.

15. Chandran V, Coppola G, Nawabi H, et al. A systems-level analysis of the peripheral nerve intrinsic axonal growth program. *Neuron.* 2016;89(5):956–970. https://doi.org/10.1016/j.neuron.2016.01.034.

16. Seijffers R, Allchorne AJ, Woolf CJ. The transcription factor ATF-3 promotes neurite outgrowth. *Mol Cell Neurosci.* 2006;32(1–2):143–154. https://doi.org/10.1016/j.mcn.2006.03.005.

17. Bomze HM, Bulsara KR, Iskandar BJ, et al. Spinal axon regeneration evoked by replacing two growth cone proteins in adult neurons. *Nat Neurosci.* 2001;4(1):38–43. https://doi.org/10.1038/82881.

18. Chierzi S, Ratto GM, Verma P, et al. The ability of axons to regenerate their growth cones depends on axonal type and age, and is regulated by calcium, cAMP and ERK. *Eur J Neurosci.* 2005;21(8):2051–2062. https://doi.org/10.1111/j.1460-9568.2005.04066.x.

19. Cao Z, Gao Y, Bryson JB, et al. The cytokine interleukin-6 is sufficient but not necessary to mimic the peripheral conditioning lesion effect on axonal growth. *J Neurosci.* 2006;26(20):5565–5573. https://doi.org/10.1523/JNEUROSCI.0815-06.2006.

20. Jalink K, Van Corven EJ, Hengeveld T, et al. Inhibition of lysophosphatidate- and thrombin-induced neurite retraction and neuronal cell rounding by ADP ribosylation of the small GTP-binding protein Rho. *J Cell Biol.* 1994;126(3):801–810. https://doi.org/10.1083/jcb.126.3.801.

21. Wahl S, Barth H, Ciossek T, et al. Ephrin-A5 induces collapse of growth cones by activating Rho and Rho kinase. *J Cell Biol.* 2000;149(2):263–270. https://doi.org/10.1083/jcb.149.2.263.

22. Lee SK, Wolfe SW. Peripheral nerve injury and repair. *J Am Acad Orthop Surg.* 2000;8:243–252. https://doi.org/10.1097/00006534-198804000-00086.

23. Sulaiman W, Gordon T. Neurobiology of peripheral nerve injury, regeneration, and functional recovery: from bench top research to bedside application. *Ochsner J.* 2013;13(1):100–108. https://doi.org/10.1043/1524-5012-13.1.100.

24. Eggers R, Tannemaat MR, Ehlert EM, et al. A spatiotemporal analysis of motoneuron survival, axonal regeneration and neurotrophic factor expression after lumbar ventral root avulsion and implantation. *Exp Neurol.* 2010;223(1):207–220. https://doi.org/10.1016/j.expneurol.2009.07.021.

25. Fu SY, Gordon T. The cellular and molecular basis of peripheral nerve regeneration. *Mol Neurobiol.* 1997;14(1–2):67–116. https://doi.org/10.1007/BF02740621.

26. Höke A, Redett R, Hameed H, et al. Schwann cells express motor and sensory phenotypes that regulate axon regeneration. *J Neurosci.* 2006;26(38):9646–9655. https://doi.org/10.1523/JNEUROSCI.1620-06.2006.

27. Höke A, Gordon T, Zochodne DW, et al. A decline in glial cell-line-derived neurotrophic factor expression is associated with impaired regeneration after long-term Schwann cell denervation. *Exp Neurol.* 2002;173(1):77–85. https://doi.org/10.1006/exnr.2001.7826.

28. Gordon T, Chan KM, Sulaiman OAR, et al. Accelerating axon growth to overcome limitations in functional recovery after peripheral nerve injury. *Neurosurgery.* 2009;65(suppl 4):A132–A144. https://doi.org/10.1227/01.NEU.0000335650.09473.D3.

29. Luo L, O'Leary DDM. Axon retraction and degeneration in development and disease. *Annu Rev Neurosci.* 2005;28:127–156. https://doi.org/10.1146/annurev.neuro.28.061604.135632.

30. de Alant JDV, Senjaya F, Ivanovic A, et al. The impact of motor axon misdirection and attrition on behavioral deficit following experimental nerve injuries. *PLoS One.* 2013;8(11):e82546. https://doi.org/10.1371/journal.pone.0082546.

31. Brushart TM, Gerber J, Kessens P, et al. Contributions of pathway and neuron to preferential motor reinnervation. *J Neurosci.* 1998;18(21):8674–8681.

32. O'Daly A, Rohde C, Brushart T. The topographic specificity of muscle reinnervation predicts function. *Eur J Neurosci.* 2016;43(3):443–450. https://doi.org/10.1111/ejn.13058.

33. Brushart TM. Motor axons preferentially reinnervate motor pathways. *J Neurosci.* 1993;13(6):2730–2738.

34. Martini R, Schachner M, Brushart TM. The L2/HNK-1 carbohydrate is preferentially expressed by previously motor axon-associated Schwann cells in reinnervated peripheral nerves. *J Neurosci.* 1994;14(11 Pt 2):7180–7191.

35. Monti RJ, Roy RR, Reggie Edgerton V. Role of motor unit structure in defining function. *Muscle Nerve*. 2001;24(7):848–866. https://doi.org/10.1002/mus.1083.

36. Valls-Sole J, Castillo CD, Casanova-Molla J, et al. Clinical consequences of reinnervation disorders after focal peripheral nerve lesions. *Clin Neurophysiol*. 2011;122(2):219–228. https://doi.org/10.1016/j.clinph.2010.06.024.

37. Witzel C, Rohde C, Brushart TM. Pathway sampling by regenerating peripheral axons. *J Comp Neurol*. 2005;485(3):183–190. https://doi.org/10.1002/cne.20436.

38. Millesi H. The nerve gap. Theory and clinical practice. *Hand Clin*. 1986;2(4):651–663.

39. Brushart TM. Preferential motor reinnervation: a sequential double-labeling study. *Restor Neurol Neurosci*. 1990;1(3):281–287. https://doi.org/B344361407737614 [pii]\r10.3233/RNN-1990-13416.

40. Hasegawa J, Shibata M, Takahashi H. Nerve coaptation studies with and without a gap in rabbits. *J Hand Surg Am*. 1996;21(2):259–265.

41. Heijke GC, Klopper PJ, Dutrieux RP. Vein graft conduits versus conventional suturing in peripheral nerve reconstructions. *Microsurgery*. 1993;14(9):584–588.

42. Scherman P, Lundborg G, Kanje M, et al. Sutures alone are sufficient to support regeneration across a gap in the continuity of the sciatic nerve in rats. *Scand J Plast Reconstr Surg Hand Surg*. 2000;34(1):1–8.

43. Moore AM, Kasukurthi R, Magill CK, et al. Limitations of conduits in peripheral nerve repairs. *Hand*. 2009;4(2):180–186. https://doi.org/10.1007/s11552-008-9158-3.

44. Kim PD, Hayes A, Amin F, et al. Collagen nerve protector in rat sciatic nerve repair: a morphometric and histological analysis. *Microsurgery*. 2010;30:392–396. https://doi.org/10.1002/micr.

45. Mackinnon S, Dellon A. Clinical nerve reconstruction with a bioabsorbable polyglycolic acid tube. *Plast Reconstr Surg*. 1990:419–424. https://doi.org/10.1097/00006534-199003000-00015.

46. Brushart TME, Seiler IVWA. Selective reinnervation of distal motor stumps by peripheral motor axons. *Exp Neurol*. 1987;97(2):289–300. https://doi.org/10.1016/0014-4886(87)90090-2.

47. Seckel BR, Ryan SE, Gagne RG, et al. Target-specific nerve regeneration through a nerve guide in the rat. *Plast Reconstr Surg*. 1986;78(6):793–800.

48. Weber RA, Breidenbach WC, Brown RE, et al. A randomized prospective study of polyglycolic acid conduits for digital nerve reconstruction in humans. *Plast Reconstr Surg*. 2000;106(5):1036–1038. https://doi.org/10.1097/00006534-200109150-00056.

49. Pfister BJ, Gordon T, Loverde JR, et al. Biomedical engineering strategies for peripheral nerve repair: surgical applications, state of the art, and future challenges. *Crit Rev Biomed Eng*. 2011;39(2):81–124. https://doi.org/2809b9b432c80c2c, https://doi.org/0fb500fc3eef5342[pii].

50. Furey MJ, Midha R, Xu Q-G, et al. Prolonged target deprivation reduces the capacity of injured motoneurons to regenerate. *Neurosurgery*. 2007;60(4):723–732-3. https://doi.org/10.1227/01.NEU.0000255412.63184.CC.

51. Fu SY, Gordon T. Contributing factors to poor functional recovery after delayed nerve repair: prolonged denervation. *J Neurosci*. 1995;15(5 Pt 2):3886–3895.

52. Frank E, Gautvik K, Sommerschild H. Cholinergic receptors at denervated mammalian motor end-plates. *Acta Physiol Scand*. 1975;95(1):66–76. https://doi.org/10.1111/j.1748-1716.1975.tb10026.x.

53. Hartzell HC, Fambrough DM. Acetylcholine receptors. Distribution and extrajunctional density in rat diaphragm after denervation correlated with acetylcholine sensitivity. *J Gen Physiol*. 1972;60(3):248–262. https://doi.org/10.1085/jgp.60.3.248.

54. Steinbach JH. Neuromuscular junctions and alpha-bungarotoxin-binding sites in denervated and contralateral cat skeletal muscles. *J Physiol*. 1981;313:513–528.

55. Sakuma M, Gorski G, Sheu S-H, et al. Lack of motor recovery after prolonged denervation of the neuromuscular junction is not due to regenerative failure. *Eur J Neurosci*. 2016;43(3):451–462. https://doi.org/10.1111/ejn.13059.

56. Noaman HH, Shiha AE, Bahm J. Oberlin's ulnar nerve transfer to the biceps motor nerve in obstetric brachial plexus palsy: indications, and good and bad results. *Microsurgery*. 2004;24(3):182–187. https://doi.org/10.1002/micr.20037.

57. Chao T, Frump D, Lin M, et al. Matrix metalloproteinase 3 deletion preserves denervated motor endplates after traumatic nerve injury. *Ann Neurol*. 2013;73(2):210–223. https://doi.org/10.1002/ana.23781.

58. Kurimoto S, Jung J, Tapadia M, et al. Activation of the Wnt/β-catenin signaling cascade after traumatic nerve injury. *Neuroscience*. 2015;294:101–108. https://doi.org/10.1016/j.neuroscience.2015.02.049.

59. Mackinnon S. New directions in peripheral nerve surgery. *Ann Plast Surg*. 1989;22(3):257–273.

60. Millesi H. Peripheral nerve repair: terminology, questions, and facts. *J Reconstr Microsurg*. 1985;2:21–31. https://doi.org/10.1055/s-2007-1007042.

61. McDonald DS, Bell MS. Peripheral nerve gap repair facilitated by a dynamic tension device. *Can J Plast Surg*. 2010;18(1):e17–e19.

62. Kim DH, Han K, Tiel RL, et al. Surgical outcomes of 654 ulnar nerve lesions. *J Neurosurg*. 2003;98(5):993–1004. https://doi.org/10.3171/jns.2003.98.5.0993.

63. Bügner O. Degenerations-und regeneration-vorgange am nerven nach verletzungen. *Beitr Pathol Anat*. 1891;10:312–393.

64. Wrede L. Uberbruckung eines nervendefektes mittels seidennhat und lebenden venenstuckes. *Dtsch Med Wochenschr*. 1909;35:1125.

65. Chiu DT, Janecka I, Krizek TJ, et al. Autogenous vein graft as a conduit for nerve regeneration. *Surgery*. 1982;91(2):226–233.

66. Rice DH, Berstein FD. The Use Autogenous Vein Nerve Grafting. *Otolaryngol Head Neck Surg*. 1984;92(5):410–412.

67. Suematsu N, Atsuta Y, Hirayama T. Vein graft for repair of peripheral nerve gap. *J Reconstr Microsurg.* 1988;4(4):313–318. https://doi.org/10.1055/s-2007-1006937.

68. Chiu DT, Strauch B. A prospective clinical evaluation of autogenous vein grafts used as a nerve conduit for distal sensory nerve defects of 3 cm or less. *Plast Reconstr Surg.* 1990;86(5):928–934.

69. Walton RL, Brown RE, Matory WE, et al. Autogenous vein graft repair of digital nerve defects in the finger: a retrospective clinical study. *Plast Reconstr Surg.* 1989;84(6):944–949-2.

70. Rinker B, Liau JY. A prospective randomized study comparing woven polyglycolic acid and autogenous vein conduits for reconstruction of digital nerve gaps. *J Hand Surg Am.* 2011;36(5):775–781. https://doi.org/10.1016/j.jhsa.2011.01.030.

71. Tseng CY, Hu G, Ambron RT, et al. Histologic analysis of Schwann cell migration and peripheral nerve regeneration in the autogenous venous nerve conduit (AVNC). *J Reconstr Microsurg.* 2003;19(5):331–339. https://doi.org/10.1055/s-2003-42502.

72. Lundborg G, Dahlin L, Danielsen N, et al. Trophism, tropism, and specificity in nerve regeneration. *J Reconstr Microsurg.* 1994;10(5):345–354. https://doi.org/10.1055/s-2007-1006604.

73. Brunelli GA, Battiston B, Vigasio A, et al. Bridging nerve defects with combined skeletal muscle and vein conduits. *Microsurgery.* 1993;14(4):247–251. https://doi.org/10.1002/micr.1920140407.

74. Fawcett JW, Keynes RJ. Muscle basal lamina: a new graft material for peripheral nerve repair. *J Neurosurg.* 1986;65(3):354–363. https://doi.org/10.3171/jns.1986.65.3.0354.

75. Tang JB. Group fascicular vein grafts with interposition of nerve slices for long ulnar nerve defects: report of three cases. *Microsurgery.* 1993;14(6):404–408. https://doi.org/10.1002/micr.1920140611.

76. Tang JB. Vein conduits with interposition of nerve tissue for peripheral nerve defects. *J Reconstr Microsurg.* 1995;11(1):21–26. https://doi.org/10.1055/s-2007-1006506.

77. Edgar D, Timpl R, Thoenen H. The heparin-binding domain of laminin is responsible for its effects on neurite outgrowth and neuronal survival. *EMBO J.* 1984;3(7):1463–1468.

78. Meek MF, Varejao AS, Geuna S. Use of skeletal muscle tissue in peripheral nerve repair: review of the literature. *Tissue Eng.* 2004;10(7–8):1027–1036. https://doi.org/10.1089/1076327041887655.

79. Glasby MA, Gschmeissner SE, Huang CLH, et al. Degenerated muscle grafts used for peripheral nerve repair in primates. *J Hand Surg Am.* 1986;11(3):347–351. https://doi.org/10.1016/0266-7681(86)90155-5.

80. Pereira JH, Bowden REM, Gattuso JM, et al. Comparison of results of repair of digital nerves by denatured muscle grafts and end-to-end sutures. *J Hand Surg Am.* 1991;16(5):519–523. https://doi.org/10.1016/0266-7681(91)90107-Y.

81. Roganovic Z, Ilic S, Savic M. Radial nerve repair using an autologous denatured muscle graft: comparison with outcomes of nerve graft repair. *Acta Neurochir (Wien).* 2007;149(10):1033–1038. https://doi.org/10.1007/s00701-007-1269-z.

82. Brandt J, Dahlin LB, Lundborg G. Autologous tendons used as grafts for bridging peripheral nerve defects. *J Hand Surg Br.* 1999;24(3):284–290. https://doi.org/10.1054/jhsb.1999.0074.

83. Brandt J, Dahlin LB, Kanje M, et al. Functional recovery in a tendon autograft used to bridge a peripheral nerve defect. *Scand J Plast Reconstr Surg Hand Surg.* 2002;36(1):2–8. https://doi.org/10.1080/028443102753478309.

84. Rinker B, Vyas KS. Clinical applications of autografts, conduits, and allografts in repair of nerve defects in the hand: current guidelines. *Clin Plast Surg.* 2014;41(3):533–550. https://doi.org/10.1016/j.cps.2014.03.006.

85. Zalewski AA, Silvers WK. An evaluation of nerve repair with nerve allografts in normal and immunologically tolerant rats. *J Neurosurg.* 1980;52(4):557–563. https://doi.org/10.3171/jns.1980.52.4.0557.

86. Levinthal R, Brown WJ, Rand RW. Fascicular nerve allograft evaluation. Part 2: comparison with whole-nerve allograft by light microscopy. *J Neurosurg.* 1978;48(3):428–433. https://doi.org/10.3171/jns.1978.48.3.0428.

87. Sosa I, Reyes O, Kuffler DP. Immunosuppressants: neuroprotection and promoting neurological recovery following peripheral nerve and spinal cord lesions. *Exp Neurol.* 2005;195(1):7–15. https://doi.org/10.1016/j.expneurol.2005.04.016.

88. Myckatyn TM, Mackinnon SE. A review of research endeavors to optimize peripheral nerve reconstruction. *Neurol Res.* 2004;26(2):124–138. https://doi.org/10.1179/016164104225013743.

89. Midha R, Mackinnon SE, Becker LE. The fate of Schwann cells in peripheral nerve allografts. *J Neuropathol Exp Neurol.* 1994;53(3):316–322.

90. Mackinnon SE, Doolabh VB, Novak CB, et al. Clinical outcome following nerve allograft transplantation. *Plast Reconstr Surg.* 2001;107(6):1419–1429. https://doi.org/10.1097/00006534-200105000-00016.

91. Karabekmez FE, Duymaz A, Moran SL. Early clinical outcomes with the use of decellularized nerve allograft for repair of sensory defects within the hand. *Hand.* 2009;4(3):245–249. https://doi.org/10.1007/s11552-009-9195-6.

92. Tang P, Chauhan A. Decellular nerve allografts. *J Am Acad Orthop Surg.* 2015;23(11):641–647. https://doi.org/10.5435/JAAOS-D-14-00373.

93. Cho MS, Rinker BD, Weber RV, et al. Functional outcome following nerve repair in the upper extremity using processed nerve allograft. *J Hand Surg Am.* 2012;37(11):2340–2349. https://doi.org/10.1016/j.jhsa.2012.08.028.

94. Moore AM, MacEwan M, Santosa KB, et al. Acellular nerve allografts in peripheral nerve regeneration: a comparative study. *Muscle Nerve.* 2011;44(2):221–234. https://doi.org/10.1002/mus.22033.

95. Whitlock EL, Tuffaha SH, Luciano JP, et al. Processed allografts and type I collagen conduits for repair of peripheral nerve gaps. *Muscle Nerve.* 2009;39(6):787–799. https://doi.org/10.1002/mus.21220.

96. Giusti G, Willems WF, Kremer T, et al. Return of motor function after segmental nerve loss in a rat model: comparison of autogenous nerve graft, collagen conduit, and processed allograft (AxoGen). *J Bone Jt Surg Am.* 2012;94(5):410–417. https://doi.org/10.2106/JBJS.K.00253.

97. Brooks DN, Weber RV, Chao JD, et al. Processed nerve allografts for peripheral nerve reconstruction: a multicenter study of utilization and outcomes in sensory, mixed, and motor nerve reconstructions. *Microsurgery.* 2012;32(1):1–14. https://doi.org/10.1002/micr.20975.

98. Guo Y, Chen G, Tian G, et al. Sensory recovery following decellularized nerve allograft transplantation for digital nerve repair. *J Plast Surg Hand Surg.* 2013:1–3. https://doi.org/10.3109/2000656X.2013.778862.

99. Rinker BD, Ingari JV, Greenberg JA, et al. Outcomes of short-gap sensory nerve injuries reconstructed with processed nerve allografts from a multicenter registry study. *J Reconstr Microsurg.* 2015;31(5):384–390. https://doi.org/10.1055/s-0035-1549160.

100. Berrocal YA, Almeida VW, Levi AD. Limitations of nerve repair of segmental defects using acellular conduits. *J Neurosurg.* 2013;119(3):733–738. https://doi.org/10.3171/2013.4.JNS121938.

101. Saheb-Al-Zamani M, Yan Y, Farber SJ, et al. Limited regeneration in long acellular nerve allografts is associated with increased Schwann cell senescence. *Exp Neurol.* 2013;247:165–177. https://doi.org/10.1016/j.expneurol.2013.04.011.

102. Dahlin LB, Lundborg G. Use of tubes in peripheral nerve repair. *Neurosurg Clin N Am.* 2001;12(2):341–352.

103. Merle M, Lee Dellon A, Campbell JN, et al. Complications from silicon-polymer intubation of nerves. *Microsurgery.* 1989;10(2):130–133. https://doi.org/10.1002/micr.1920100213.

104. Lundborg G, Rosén B, Dahlin L, et al. Tubular repair of the median or ulnar nerve in the human forearm: a 5-year follow - up. *J Hand Surg Am.* 2004;29 B(2):100–107. https://doi.org/10.1016/j.jhsb.2003.09.018.

105. Lundborg G, Rosen B, Dahlin L, et al. Tubular versus conventional repair of median and ulnar nerves in the human forearm: early results from a prospective, randomized, clinical study. *J Hand Surg Am.* 1997;22(1):99–106. https://doi.org/10.1016/S0363-5023(05)80188-1.

106. Lundborg G, Dahlin L, Danielsen N. Ulnar nerve repair by the silicone chamber technique. Case report. *Scand J Plast Reconstr Surg Hand Surg.* 1991;25(1):79–82. https://doi.org/10.3109/02844319109034927.

107. Braga-Silva J. The use of silicone tubing in the late repair of the median and ulnar nerves in the forearm. *J Hand Surg J Br Soc Surg Hand.* 1999;24(6):703–706. https://doi.org/10.1054/jhsb.1999.0276.

108. Jones S, Eisenberg HM, Jia X. Advances and future applications of augmented peripheral nerve regeneration. *Int J Mol Sci.* 2016;17(9). https://doi.org/10.3390/ijms17091494.

109. Dellon AL, Mackinnon SE. An alternative to the classical nerve graft for the management of the short nerve gap. *Plast Reconstr Surg.* 1988;82(5):849–856.

110. Matsumoto K, Ohnishi K, Kiyotani T, et al. Peripheral nerve regeneration across an 80-mm gap bridged by a polyglycolic acid (PGA)-collagen tube filled with laminin-coated collagen fibers: a histological and electrophysiological evaluation of regenerated nerves. *Brain Res.* 2000;868(2):315–328. https://doi.org/10.1016/S0006-8993(00)02207-1.

111. Rosson GD, Williams EH, Dellon AL. Motor nerve regeneration across a conduit. *Microsurgery.* 2009;29(2):107–114. https://doi.org/10.1002/micr.20580.

112. Battiston B, Geuna S, Ferrero M, et al. Nerve repair by means of tubulization: literature review and personal clinical experience comparing biological and synthetic conduits for sensory nerve repair. *Microsurgery.* 2005;25(4):258–267. https://doi.org/10.1002/micr.20127.

113. Duncan SFM, Kakinoki R, Rizzo M, et al. Extrusion of a NeuroTube: a case report. *Ochsner J.* 2015;15(2):191–192.

114. Kitahara AK, Suzuki Y, Qi P, et al. Facial nerve repair using a collagen conduit in cats. *Scand J Plast Reconstr Surg Hand Surg.* 1999;33(2):187–193. https://doi.org/10.1080/02844319950159442.

115. Archibald SJ, Shefner J, Krarup C, et al. Monkey median nerve repaired by nerve graft or collagen nerve guide tube. *J Neurosci.* 1995;15(5 Pt 2):4109–4123.

116. Keilhoff G, Stang F, Wolf G, et al. Bio-compatibility of type I/III collagen matrix for peripheral nerve reconstruction. *Biomaterials.* 2003;24(16):2779–2787. https://doi.org/10.1016/S0142-9612(03)00084-X.

117. Ashley WW, Weatherly T, Park TS. Collagen nerve guides for surgical repair of brachial plexus birth injury. *J Neurosurg.* 2006;105(suppl 6):452–456. https://doi.org/10.3171/ped.2006.105.6.452.

118. Bushnell BD, McWilliams AD, Whitener GB, et al. Early clinical experience with collagen nerve tubes in digital nerve repair. *J Hand Surg Am.* 2008;33(7):1081–1087. https://doi.org/10.1016/j.jhsa.2008.03.015.

119. Lohmeyer JA, Sommer B, Siemers F, et al. Nerve injuries of the upper extremity-expected outcome and clinical examination. *Plast Surg Nurs.* 2009;29(2):85–88. https://doi.org/10.1097/01.PSN.0000356867.18220.73.

120. Wangensteen KJ, Kalliainen LK. Collagen tube conduits in peripheral nerve repair: a retrospective analysis. *Hand (NY).* 2010;5(3):273–277. https://doi.org/10.1007/s11552-009-9245-0.

121. Taras JS, Jacoby SM, Lincoski CJ. Reconstruction of digital nerves with collagen conduits. *J Hand Surg Am.* 2011;36(9):1441–1446. https://doi.org/10.1016/j.jhsa.2011.06.009.

122. Boeckstyns MEH, Sørensen AI, Viñeta JF, et al. Collagen conduit versus microsurgical neurorrhaphy: 2-year follow-up of a prospective, blinded clinical and electrophysiological multicenter randomized, controlled trial. *J Hand Surg Am.* 2013;38(12):2405–2411. https://doi.org/10.1016/j.jhsa.2013.09.038.

123. Liodaki E, Bos I, Lohmeyer JA, et al. Removal of collagen nerve conduits (NeuraGen) after unsuccessful implantation: focus on histological findings. *J Reconstr Microsurg.* 2013;29(8):517–521. https://doi.org/10.1055/s-0033-1348033.

124. Siemionow M, Bozkurt M, Zor F. Regeneration and repair of peripheral nerves with different biomaterials: review. *Microsurgery.* 2010;30(7):574–588. https://doi.org/10.1002/micr.20799.

125. Shin RH, Friedrich PF, Crum BA, et al. Treatment of a segmental nerve defect in the rat with use of bioabsorbable synthetic nerve conduits: a comparison of commercially available conduits. *J Bone Jt Surg Am.* 2009;91(9):2194–2204. https://doi.org/10.2106/JBJS.H.01301.

126. Bertleff MJOE, Meek MF, Nicolai JPA. A prospective clinical evaluation of biodegradable Neurolac nerve guides for sensory nerve repair in the hand. *J Hand Surg Am.* 2005;30(3):513–518. https://doi.org/10.1016/j.jhsa.2004.12.009.

127. Meek MF, Nicolai JPA, Robinson PH. Secondary digital nerve repair in the foot with resorbable p(DLLA-??-CL) nerve conduits. *J Reconstr Microsurg.* 2006;22(3):149–151. https://doi.org/10.1055/s-2006-939959.

128. Hernández-Cortés P, Juan G, Cámara M, et al. Failed digital nerve reconstruction by foreign body reaction to Neurolac nerve conduit. *Microsurgery.* 2010;30(5):414–416. https://doi.org/10.1002/micr.20730.

129. Chiriac S, Facca S, Diaconu M, et al. Experience of using the bioresorbable copolyester poly(DL-lactide-e-caprolactone) nerve conduit guide NeurolacTM for nerve repair in peripheral nerve defects: report on a series of 28 lesions. *J Hand Surg Eur.* 2011;37(4):342–349. https://doi.org/10.1177/1753193411422226.

130. Faroni A, Mobasseri SA, Kingham PJ, et al. Peripheral nerve regeneration: experimental strategies and future perspectives. *Adv Drug Deliv Rev.* 2015;82:160–167. https://doi.org/10.1016/j.addr.2014.11.010.

131. Derby A, Engleman VW, Frierdich GE, et al. Nerve growth factor facilitates regeneration across nerve gaps: morphological and behavioral studies in rat sciatic nerve. *Exp Neurol.* 1993;119(2):176–191. https://doi.org/10.1006/exnr.1993.1019.

132. Ho PR, Coan GM, Cheng ET, et al. Repair with collagen tubules linked with brain-derived neurotrophic factor and ciliary neurotrophic factor in a rat sciatic nerve injury model. *Arch Otolaryngol Head Neck Surg.* 1998;124(7):761–766.

133. Hirakawa CK, Grecco MAS, dos Santos oão BG, et al. Estudo comparativo da ação do fator de crescimento de fibroblastos e fragmentos de nervo na regeneração de nervo tibial em ratos. *Acta Ortopédica Bras.*

2007;15(2):114–117. https://doi.org/10.1590/S1413-78522007000200012.

134. Walter MA, Kurouglu R, Caulfield JB, et al. Enhanced peripheral nerve regeneration by acidic fibroblast growth factor. *Lymphokine Cytokine Res.* 1993;12(3):135–141.

135. Wang S, Cai Q, Hou J, et al. Acceleration effect of basic fibroblast growth factor on the regeneration of peripheral nerve through a 15-mm gap. *J Biomed Mater Res A.* 2003;66(3):522–531. https://doi.org/10.1002/jbm.a.10008.

136. Fine EG, Decosterd I, Papaloïzos M, et al. GDNF and NGF released by synthetic guidance channels support sciatic nerve regeneration across a long gap. *Eur J Neurosci.* 2002;15(4):589–601. https://doi.org/10.1046/j.1460-9568.2002.01892.x.

137. Lee AC, Yu VM, Lowe JB, et al. Controlled release of nerve growth factor enhances sciatic nerve regeneration. *Exp Neurol.* 2003;184(1):295–303. https://doi.org/10.1016/S0014-4886(03)00258-9.

138. Marquardt LM, Ee X, Iyer N, et al. Finely tuned temporal and spatial delivery of GDNF promotes enhanced nerve regeneration in a long nerve defect model. *Tissue Eng A.* 2015;21(23–24):2852–2864. https://doi.org/10.1089/ten.tea.2015.0311.

139. Mahanthappa NK, Anton ES, Matthew WD. Glial growth factor 2, a soluble neuregulin, directly increases Schwann cell motility and indirectly promotes neurite outgrowth. *J Neurosci.* 1996;16(15):4673–4683.

140. Mohanna PN, Young RC, Wiberg M, et al. A composite pol-hydroxybutyrate-glial growth factor conduit for long nerve gap repairs. *J Anat.* 2003;203(6):553–565. https://doi.org/10.1046/j.1469-7580.2003.00243.x.

141. Hobson MI, Green CJ, Terenghi G. VEGF enhances intraneural angiogenesis and improves nerve regeneration after axotomy. *J Anat.* 2000;197(Pt 4):591–605. https://doi.org/10.1046/j.1469-7580.2000.19740591.x.

142. Hart AM, Wiberg M, Terenghi G. Exogenous leukaemia inhibitory factor enhances nerve regeneration after late secondary repair using a bioartificial nerve conduit. *Br J Plast Surg.* 2003;56(5):444–450. https://doi.org/10.1016/S0007-1226(03)00134-6.

143. Wells MR, Kraus K, Batter DK, et al. Gel matrix vehicles for growth factor application in nerve gap injuries repaired with tubes: a comparison of biomatrix, collagen, and methylcellulose. *Exp Neurol.* 1997;146(2):395–402. https://doi.org/10.1006/exnr.1997.6543.

144. Mohammadi R, Amini K, Eskafian H. Betamethasone-enhanced vein graft conduit accelerates functional recovery in the rat sciatic nerve gap. *J Oral Maxillofac Surg.* 2013;71(4):786–792. https://doi.org/10.1016/j.joms.2012.08.009.

145. Papakostas I, Mourouzis I, Mourouzis K, et al. Functional effects of local thyroid hormone administration after sciatic nerve injury in rats. *Microsurgery.* 2009;29(1):35–41. https://doi.org/10.1002/micr.20546.

146. Azizi A, Azizi S, Heshmatian B, et al. Improvement of functional recovery of transected peripheral nerve by means of chitosan grafts filled with vitamin E, pyrroloquinoline quinone and their combination. *Int J Surg*. 2014;12(1):76–82. https://doi.org/10.1016/j.ijsu.2013.10.002.

147. Ding T, Zhu C, Yin JB, et al. Slow-releasing rapamycin-coated bionic peripheral nerve scaffold promotes the regeneration of rat sciatic nerve after injury. *Life Sci*. 2014;122:92–99. https://doi.org/10.1016/j.lfs.2014.12.005.

148. Shahraki M, Mohammadi R, Najafpour A. Influence of tacrolimus (FK506) on nerve regeneration using allografts: a rat sciatic nerve model. *J Oral Maxillofac Surg*. 2015;73(7):1438.e1–e9. https://doi.org/10.1016/j.joms.2015.03.032.

149. Martin D, Pinsolle V, Merville P, et al. First case in the world of autoreplantation of a limb associated with oral administration of an immunosupressant agent (FK 506-Tacrolimus). *Ann Chir Plast Esthet*. 2005;50(4):257–263. https://doi.org/10.1016/j.anplas.2005.02.001.

150. Schuind F, Van Holder C, Mouraux D, et al. The first Belgian hand transplantation-37 month term results. *J Hand Surg Am*. 2006;31(4):371–376. https://doi.org/10.1016/j.jhsb.2006.01.003.

151. Schuind F, Van Holder C, Mouraux D, et al. The first Belgian hand transplantation case. Nine years follow-up. *Rev Med Brux*. 2011;32(suppl 6):S66–S70.

152. Phan DQD, Schuind F. Tolerance and effects of FK506 (tacrolimus) on nerve regeneration: a pilot study. *J Hand Surg Eur*. 2012;37:537–543. https://doi.org/10.1177/1753193411427826.

153. Strauch B, Rodriguez DM, Diaz J, et al. Autologous Schwann cells drive regeneration through a 6-cm autogenous venous nerve conduit. *J Reconstr Microsurg*. 2001;17(8):589–595. https://doi.org/10.1055/s-2001-18812.

154. Hoben G, Yan Y, Iyer N, et al. Comparison of acellular nerve allograft modification with schwann cells or VEGF. *Hand*. 2015;10(3):396–402. https://doi.org/10.1007/s11552-014-9720-0.

155. Dilwali S, Patel PB, Roberts DS, et al. Primary culture of human Schwann and schwannoma cells: improved and simplified protocol. *Hear Res*. 2014;315:25–33. https://doi.org/10.1016/j.heares.2014.05.006.

156. Dai LG, Huang GS, Hsu SH. Sciatic nerve regeneration by cocultured schwann cells and stem cells on microporous nerve conduits. *Cell Transpl*. 2013;22(11):2029–2039. https://doi.org/10.3727/096368912X658953.

157. Xu Y, Zhang Z, Chen X, et al. A silk fibroin/collagen nerve scaffold seeded with a co-culture of schwann cells and adipose-derived stem cells for sciatic nerve regeneration. *PLoS One*. 2016;11(1). https://doi.org/10.1371/journal.pone.0147184.

158. Sullivan R, Dailey T, Duncan K, et al. Peripheral nerve injury: stem cell therapy and peripheral nerve transfer. *Int J Mol Sci*. 2016;17(12). https://doi.org/10.3390/ijms17122101.

159. Levi AD, Burks SS, Anderson KD, et al. The use of autologous Schwann cells to supplement sciatic nerve repair with a large gap - first in human experience. *Cell Transpl*. 2015;305:1–26. https://doi.org/10.3727/096368915X690198.

160. Dezawa M, Takahashi I, Esaki M, et al. Sciatic nerve regeneration in rats induced by transplantation of in vitro differentiated bone-marrow stromal cells. *Eur J Neurosci*. 2001;14(11):1771–1776. https://doi.org/10.1046/j.0953-816X.2001.01814.x.

161. Amoh Y, Kanoh M, Niiyama S, et al. Human hair follicle pluripotent stem (hfPS) cells promote regeneration of peripheral-nerve injury: an advantageous alternative to ES and iPS cells. *J Cell Biochem*. 2009;107(5):1016–1020. https://doi.org/10.1002/jcb.22204.

162. Chen CJ, Ou YC, Liao SL, et al. Transplantation of bone marrow stromal cells for peripheral nerve repair. *Exp Neurol*. 2007;204(1):443–453. https://doi.org/10.1016/j.expneurol.2006.12.004.

163. Ziegler L, Grigoryan S, Yang IH, et al. Efficient generation of schwann cells from human embryonic stem cell-derived neurospheres. *Stem Cell Rev*. 2011;7(2):394–403. https://doi.org/10.1007/s12015-010-9198-2.

164. Cui L, Jiang J, Wei L, et al. Transplantation of embryonic stem cells improves nerve repair and functional recovery after severe sciatic nerve axotomy in rats. *Stem Cells*. 2008;26(5):1356–1365. https://doi.org/10.1634/stemcells.2007-0333.

165. Nelakanti RV, Kooreman NG, Wu JC. Teratoma formation: a tool for monitoring pluripotency in stem cell research. *Curr Protoc Stem Cell Biol*. 2015;2015:4a.8.1–4a.8.17. https://doi.org/10.1002/9780470151808.sc04a08s32.

166. Papp B, Plath K. Epigenetics of reprogramming to induced pluripotency. *Cell*. 2013;152(6):1324–1343. https://doi.org/10.1016/j.cell.2013.02.043.

167. Nakagawa M, Koyanagi M, Tanabe K, et al. Generation of induced pluripotent stem cells without Myc from mouse and human fibroblasts. *Nat Biotechnol*. 2008;26(1):101–106. https://doi.org/10.1038/nbt1374.

168. Ikeda M, Uemura T, Takamatsu K, et al. Acceleration of peripheral nerve regeneration using nerve conduits in combination with induced pluripotent stem cell technology and a basic fibroblast growth factor drug delivery system. *J Biomed Mater Res A*. 2014;102(5):1370–1378. https://doi.org/10.1002/jbm.a.34816.

169. Uemura T, Ikeda M, Takamatsu K, et al. Long-term efficacy and safety outcomes of transplantation of induced pluripotent stem cell-derived neurospheres with bioabsorbable nerve conduits for peripheral nerve regeneration in mice. *Cells Tissues Organs*. 2014;200(1):78–91. https://doi.org/10.1159/000370322.

170. Okada M, Yoneda Y. The timing of retroviral silencing correlates with the quality of induced pluripotent stem cell lines. *Biochim Biophys Acta Gen Subj*. 2011;1810(2):226–235. https://doi.org/10.1016/j.bbagen.2010.10.004.

171. Zuk PA, Zhu M, Mizuno H, et al. Multilineage cells from human adipose tissue: implications for cell-based therapies. *Tissue Eng.* 2001;7(2):211–228. https://doi.org/10.1089/107632701300062859.

172. Zack-Williams SD, Butler PE, Kalaskar DM. Current progress in use of adipose derived stem cells in peripheral nerve regeneration. *World J Stem Cells.* 2015;7(1):51–64. https://doi.org/10.4252/wjsc.v7.i1.51.

173. He X, Ao Q, Wei Y, et al. Transplantation of miRNA-34a overexpressing adipose-derived stem cell enhances rat nerve regeneration. *Wound Repair Regen.* 2016;24(3):542–550. https://doi.org/10.1111/wrr.12427.

174. Wei Y, Gong K, Zheng Z, et al. Chitosan/silk fibroin-based tissue-engineered graft seeded with adipose-derived stem cells enhances nerve regeneration in a rat model. *J Mater Sci Mater Med.* 2011;22(8):1947–1964. https://doi.org/10.1007/s10856-011-4370-z.

175. Klein SM, Vykoukal J, Li D-P, et al. Peripheral motor and sensory nerve conduction following transplantation of undifferentiated autologous adipose tissue-derived stem cells in a biodegradable U.S. Food and drug administration-approved nerve conduit. *Plast Reconstr Surg.* 2016;138(1):132–139. https://doi.org/10.1097/PRS.0000000000002291.

176. Reichenberger MA, Mueller W, Hartmann J, et al. ADSCs in a fibrin matrix enhance nerve regeneration after epineural suturing in a rat model. *Microsurgery.* 2016;36(6):491–500. https://doi.org/10.1002/micr.30018.

177. Kingham PJ, Kalbermatten DF, Mahay D, et al. Adipose-derived stem cells differentiate into a Schwann cell phenotype and promote neurite outgrowth in vitro. *Exp Neurol.* 2007;207(2):267–274. https://doi.org/S0014-4886(07)00257-9 [pii]\r10.1016/j.expneurol.2007.06.029.

178. Sowa Y, Kishida T, Imura T, et al. Adipose-derived stem cells promote peripheral nerve regeneration in vivo without differentiation into schwann-like lineage. *Plast Reconstr Surg.* 2016;137(2):318e–330e. https://doi.org/10.1097/01.prs.0000475762.86580.36.

179. Tomita K, Madura T, Sakai Y, et al. Glial differentiation of human adipose-derived stem cells: implications for cell-based transplantation therapy. *Neuroscience.* 2013;236:55–65. https://doi.org/10.1016/j.neuroscience.2012.12.066.

180. Faroni A, Smith RJP, Lu L, et al. Human Schwann-like cells derived from adipose-derived mesenchymal stem cells rapidly de-differentiate in the absence of stimulating medium. *Eur J Neurosci.* 2016;43(3):417–430. https://doi.org/10.1111/ejn.13055.

181. Shyamala K, Yanduri S, Girish H, et al. Neural crest: the fourth germ layer. *J Oral Maxillofac Pathol.* 2015;19(2):221. https://doi.org/10.4103/0973-029X.164536.

182. Lee G, Chambers SM, Tomishima MJ, et al. Derivation of neural crest cells from human pluripotent stem cells. *Nat Protoc.* 2010;5(4):688–701. https://doi.org/10.1038/nprot.2010.35.

183. Kim YJ, Lim H, Li Z, et al. Generation of multipotent induced neural crest by direct reprogramming of human postnatal fibroblasts with a single transcription factor. *Cell Stem Cell.* 2014;15(4):497–506. https://doi.org/10.1016/j.stem.2014.07.013.

184. Lee G, Kim H, Elkabetz Y, et al. Isolation and directed differentiation of neural crest stem cells derived from human embryonic stem cells. *Nat Biotechnol.* 2007;25(12). https://doi.org/10.1038/nbt1365.

185. Lin H, Liu F, Zhang C, et al. Pluripotent hair follicle neural crest stem-cell-derived neurons and schwann cells functionally repair sciatic nerves in rats. *Mol Neurobiol.* 2009;40(3):216–223. https://doi.org/10.1007/s12035-009-8082-z.

186. Liard O, Segura S, Sagui E, et al. Adult-brain-derived neural stem cells grafting into a vein bridge increases postlesional recovery and regeneration in a peripheral nerve of adult pig. *Stem Cells Int.* 2012. https://doi.org/10.1155/2012/128732.

187. Ni H-C, Tseng T-C, Chen J-R, et al. Fabrication of bioactive conduits containing the fibroblast growth factor 1 and neural stem cells for peripheral nerve regeneration across a 15 mm critical gap. *Biofabrication.* 2013;5(3):35010. https://doi.org/10.1088/1758-5082/5/3/035010.

188. Grimoldi N, Colleoni F, Tiberio F, et al. Stem cell salvage of injured peripheral nerve. *Cell Transpl.* 2015;24(2):213–222. https://doi.org/10.3727/096368913X675700.

189. Lin W, Chen X, Wang X, et al. Adult rat bone marrow stromal cells differentiate into Schwann cell-like cells in vitro. *In Vitro Cell Dev Biol Anim.* 2008;44(1–2):31–40. https://doi.org/10.1007/s11626-007-9064-y.

190. Mohammadi R, Azizi S, Delirezh N, et al. The use of undifferentiated bone marrow stromal cells for sciatic nerve regeneration in rats. *Int J Oral Maxillofac Surg.* 2012;41(5):650–656. https://doi.org/10.1016/j.ijom.2011.10.028.

191. Sakar M, Korkusuz P, Demirbilek M, et al. The effect of poly(3-hydroxybutyrate-co-3-hydroxyhexanoate) (PHB-HHx) and human mesenchymal stem cell (hMSC) on axonal regeneration in experimental sciatic nerve damage. *Int J Neurosci.* 2014;124(9). https://doi.org/10.3109/00207454.2013.876636.

192. Wakao S, Hayashi T, Kitada M, et al. Long-term observation of auto-cell transplantation in non-human primate reveals safety and efficiency of bone marrow stromal cell-derived Schwann cells in peripheral nerve regeneration. *Exp Neurol.* 2010;223(2):537–547. https://doi.org/10.1016/j.expneurol.2010.01.022.

193. Ladak A, Olson J, Tredget EEE, et al. Differentiation of mesenchymal stem cells to support peripheral nerve regeneration in a rat model. *Exp Neurol.* 2011;228(2):242–252. https://doi.org/10.1016/j.expneurol.2011.01.013.

194. Fan L, Yu Z, Li J, et al. Schwann-like cells seeded in acellular nerve grafts improve nerve regeneration. *BMC Musculoskelet Disord.* 2014;15(1):165. https://doi.org/10.1186/1471-2474-15-165.

195. Raheja A, Suri V, Suri A, et al. Dose-dependent facilitation of peripheral nerve regeneration by bone marrow-derived mononuclear cells: a randomized controlled study. Laboratory investigation. *J Neurosurg.* 2012;117(6):1170–1181. https://doi.org/10.3171/2012.8.JNS111446.

196. Tsai MS, Lee JL, Chang YJ, et al. Isolation of human multipotent mesenchymal stem cells from second-trimester amniotic fluid using a novel two-stage culture protocol. *Hum Reprod.* 2004;19(6):1450–1456. https://doi.org/10.1093/humrep/deh279.

197. Yan Z-J, Hu Y-Q, Zhang H-T, et al. Comparison of the neural differentiation potential of human mesenchymal stem cells from amniotic fluid and adult bone marrow. *Cell Mol Neurobiol.* 2013;33:465–475. https://doi.org/10.1007/s10571-013-9922-y.

198. Kerimoğlu S, Livaoğlu M, Sönmez B, et al. Effects of human amniotic fluid on fracture healing in rat tibia. *J Surg Res.* 2009;152(2):281–287. https://doi.org/10.1016/j.jss.2008.02.028.

199. Özgenel GY, Şamli B, Özcan M. Effects of human amniotic fluid on peritendinous adhesion formation and tendon healing after flexor tendon surgery in rabbits. *J Hand Surg Am.* 2001;26(2):332–339. https://doi.org/10.1053/jhsu.2001.22524.

200. Ozgenel GY, Filiz G. Effects of human amniotic fluid on peripheral nerve scarring and regeneration in rats. *J Neurosurg.* 2003;98(2):371–377. https://doi.org/10.3171/jns.2003.98.2.0371.

201. Pan H-C, Chen C-J, Cheng F-C, et al. Combination of G-CSF administration and human amniotic fluid mesenchymal stem cell transplantation promotes peripheral nerve regeneration. *Neurochem Res.* 2008;34(3):518–527. https://doi.org/10.1007/s11064-008-9815-5.

202. Bhatnagar D, Bushman JS, Sanjeeva Murthy N, et al. Fibrin glue as a stabilization strategy in peripheral nerve repair when using porous nerve guidance conduits. *J Mater Sci Mater Med.* 2017;28. https://doi.org/10.1007/s10856-017-5889-4.

203. Sameem M, Wood TJ, Bain JR. A systematic review on the use of fibrin glue for peripheral nerve repair. *Plast Reconstr Surg.* 2011;127(6):2381–2390. https://doi.org/10.1097/PRS.0b013e3182131cf5.

204. Nishimura MT, Mazzer N, Barbieri CH, et al. Mechanical resistance of peripheral nerve repair with biological glue and with conventional suture at different postoperative times. *J Reconstr Microsurg.* 2008;24(5):327–332. https://doi.org/10.1055/s-2008-1080535.

205. Ornelas L, Padilla L, Di Silvio M, et al. Fibrin glue: an alternative technique for nerve coaptation - Part I. Wave amplitude, conduction velocity, and plantar-length factors. *J Reconstr Microsurg.* 2006;22(2):119–122. https://doi.org/10.1055/s-2006-932506.

206. Ornelas L, Padilla L, Di Silvio M, et al. Fibrin glue: an alternative technique for nerve coaptation - Part II. Nerve regeneration and histomorphometric assessment. *J Reconstr Microsurg.* 2006;22(2):123–128. https://doi.org/10.1055/s-2006-932507.

207. Rafijah G, Bowen AJ, Dolores C, et al. The effects of adjuvant fibrin sealant on the surgical repair of segmental nerve defects in an animal model. *J Hand Surg Am.* 2013;38(5):847–855. https://doi.org/10.1016/j.jhsa.2013.01.044.

208. Subramanian A, Krishnan U, Sethuraman S. Development of biomaterial scaffold for nerve tissue engineering: biomaterial mediated neural regeneration. *J Biomed Sci.* 2009;16(1):108. https://doi.org/10.1186/1423-0127-16-108.

209. Geuna S, Raimondo S, Nicolino S, et al. Schwann-cell proliferatin in muscle-vein combined conduits for bridging rat sciatic nerve defects. *J Reconstr Microsurg.* 2003;19(2):119–123. https://doi.org/10.1055/s-2003-37818.

210. Manoli T, Schulz L, Stahl S, et al. Evaluation of sensory recovery after reconstruction of digital nerves of the hand using muscle-in-vein conduits in comparison to nerve suture or nerve autografting. *Microsurgery.* 2014;34(8):608–615. https://doi.org/10.1002/micr.22302.

211. Xie J, Li X, Xia Y. Putting electrospun nanofibers to work for biomedical research. *Macromol Rapid Commun.* 2008;29(22):1775–1792. https://doi.org/10.1002/marc.200800381.

212. Yang F, Murugan R, Ramakrishna S, et al. Fabrication of nano-structured porous PLLA scaffold intended for nerve tissue engineering. *Biomaterials.* 2004;25(10):1891–1900. https://doi.org/10.1016/j.biomaterials.2003.08.062.

213. Prabhakaran MP, Venugopal JR, Ramakrishna S. Mesenchymal stem cell differentiation to neuronal cells on electrospun nanofibrous substrates for nerve tissue engineering. *Biomaterials.* 2009;30(28):4996–5003. https://doi.org/10.1016/j.biomaterials.2009.05.057.

214. Jin J, Park M, Rengarajan A, et al. Functional motor recovery after peripheral nerve repair with an aligned nanofiber tubular conduit in a rat model. *Regen Med.* 2012;7(6):799–806. https://doi.org/10.2217/rme.12.87.

215. Zhan X, Gao M, Jiang Y, et al. Nanofiber scaffolds facilitate functional regeneration of peripheral nerve injury. *Nanomed Nanotechnol Biol Med.* 2013;9(3):305–315. https://doi.org/10.1016/j.nano.2012.08.009.

216. Chew SY, Mi R, Hoke A, et al. Aligned protein-polymer composite fibers enhance nerve regeneration: a potential tissue-engineering platform. *Adv Funct Mater.* 2007;17(8):1288–1296. https://doi.org/10.1002/adfm.200600441.

217. Beachley V, Wen X. Polymer nanofibrous structures: fabrication, biofunctionalization, and cell interactions. *Prog Polym Sci.* 2010;35(7):868–892. https://doi.org/10.1016/j.progpolymsci.2010.03.003.

218. Johnson BN, Lancaster KZ, Zhen G, et al. 3D printed anatomical nerve regeneration pathways. *Adv Funct Mater.* 2015;25(39):6205–6217. https://doi.org/10.1002/adfm.201501760.

219. Johnson BN, Mcalpine MC. From print to patient: 3D-printed personalized nerve regeneration. *Beyond Cell.* August 2016:28–31.

220. Zhu S, Zhu Q, Liu X, et al. Three-dimensional reconstruction of the microstructure of human acellular nerve allograft. *Sci Rep.* 2016;6:30694. https://doi.org/10.1038/srep30694.

CHAPTER 15

Biologics in Spinal Fusion

HARDEEP SINGH, MD • ISAAC L. MOSS, MD

INTRODUCTION

As the medical community has developed a greater understanding of the critical steps necessary for tissue healing, biologics, both natural and synthesized, have become an important adjunct to many orthopedic procedures. Much research is underway to devise biologic strategies to repair or prevent many pathologies of the vertebral column. However, currently the most widely used application for biologics in spinal surgeries is to improve the success of spinal fusion. Spinal fusion procedures are performed for a variety of reasons including degenerative conditions, deformity, trauma, and tumors.[1–3] There are estimates of up to 200,000 fusion procedures performed in the United States annually.[3] According to a retrospective cohort study, rates of lumbar spine fusion alone have increased upward of 220% from 1990 to 2001.[4] The goal of spinal fusion surgery is to augment or restore spinal stability by achieving solid bony union between two or more vertebral motion segments. Fusion procedures generally provide temporary mechanical support with implants and initiate the biological process necessary for osseous growth and eventual long-term stability.[2] Failure of this process, referred to as a pseudoarthrosis, can result in persistent pain, loss of deformity correction, and eventual mechanical failure of the fusion construct.[2]

The biology of spinal fusion is a complex process with steps similar to what occurs in natural bone fracture healing. However, in the case of fusion, the goal is to achieve bone growth in an environment not originally developed for this purpose, i.e., the disc space or the intertransverse space. Therefore modification of the biologic microenvironment is necessary to stimulate the bone growth process. This augmentation is often achieved with combination of enhanced mechanical stability with metallic or polymeric implants and the addition of graft material and biologic agents that function through osteoconductive, osteoinductive, and/or osteogenic mechanisms.[5] (Fig. 15.1) These three essential mechanisms are necessary for the integration of the graft material and host bone.[6] Biologic agents with osteoconductive properties provide a structural scaffold

or framework that is conducive to cellular growth and tissue formation. Osteoinductive agents facilitate the recruitment of immature cells and stimulate their transformation into bone-forming cells that can effect de novo bone formation. Finally, osteogenic materials contain live bone-forming cells that can be implanted for bone regeneration. In addition, an adequate vascular supply to allow for the migration of stem cells and nutrients to the fusion site is of paramount importance for successful fusion to occur.[7] Furthermore, the environment required needs to be a low-strain environment with mechanical stability to prevent excessive strain and adverse effects on the bone formation process. Osteogenic signals, such as growth factors, are needed for the stem cells to proliferate, recruit, and differentiate in a conducive microenvironment for new bone formation.[7] The end product is replacement of the grafted bone with a new bone matrix that can endure the physiologic loads applied to the spine during normal activities of daily living.[2]

Despite our improved understanding of the mechanisms underlying bone healing and modern surgical techniques and technologies, failure of spine fusion is not uncommon with rates of up to 17% in primary fusion surgeries performed in adult populations.[8] Augmentation with biologics provides an additional strategy to limit the rate of pseudoarthrosis by acting to alter the environment and making it more conducive for osteogenesis.[1]

BONE GRAFTING

Use of bone grafts to augment healing is one of the most common adjuncts to many orthopedic procedures, with greater than 500,000 grafting procedures performed annually in the United States.[6] The rationale for the use of bone graft is to stimulate bone healing by osteoconduction and, depending on the type of graft used, potentially provide osteogenic and/or osteoinductive properties.[6] Bone grafting options can be divided into autograft, allograft, and synthetic grafts. A variety of graft types and material are available; however, the ideal graft should have

Biologics in Orthopaedic Surgery. https://doi.org/10.1016/B978-0-323-55140-3.00015-1

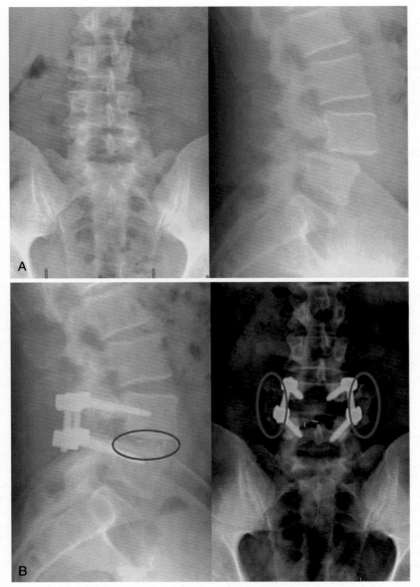

FIG. 15.1 Pre-operative (A) and post-operative (B) radiographs of the lumbar spine of a patient who underwent spinal fusion for L4-5 spondylolisthesis using metallic (pedicle screws and polymeric (interbody device) implants as well as local autograft and allograft demineralized bone matrix to achieve reduction of the spondylolisthesis and successful bony fusion (encircled in red).

low immunogenicity, have desirable biologic activity, bioresorbability, and bioconductivty, and be cost-effective.[9]

Autograft Bone

Autograft is considered the gold standard as it provides all three essential properties (osteogenic, osteoconductive, and osteoinductive) required for new bone formation and is easily integrated in the host bone. Autografts are divided into three types: cancellous, cortical, and vascularized cortical grafts. Cancellous grafts provide an abundance of cells for bone regeneration, whereas cortical grafts provide enhanced mechanical and structural integrity.

Iliac crest is one of the most frequently used and favored bone graft harvest sites. The site is easily accessible and provides a graft with excellent bone quality and quantity. Iliac crest bone graft possesses all three essential properties needed for bone regeneration.[1] Studies have demonstrated fusion rates as high as 93% with the use of iliac crest bone graft.[1] However, donor site morbidity including infection, chronic pain, scarring, and propagation of a fracture at harvest site, can occur with complications ranging from 10% to 39%.[1,9–11] To avoid the complications of donor site morbidity, local bone autograft can be obtained from various sites such as the spinous processes, lamina, and facet joints, often removed during spinal canal decompression at the time of fusion surgery. Obtaining local bone graft avoids the complications of another site surgery and reduces surgical time as no additional surgical exposure time is required.[12] Fusion rates are as high as 80% with the use of local graft, and in some studies it has been quoted to be equivalent to iliac crest bone graft.[10,13]

Cancellous grafts are the most common autografts used and provide excellent osteoconductivity allowing for bone growth. Harvesting cortical and/or corticocancellous grafts results in greater morbidity due to the increased surgical exposure required; however, these grafts provide the advantage of immediate load sharing secondary to their structural integrity.[7] As demonstrated by Enneking et al., cortical bone grafts lose significant strength around 6 weeks secondary to bone remodeling; however, they recover by about 1 year.[14] The use of vascularized cortical bone grafts can counteract the loss of strength secondary to remodeling as a vascular pedicle is anastomosed to the graft at the fusion site, thus providing vascular supply needed for osteointegration. Use of a vascularized cortical graft is beneficial for bridging large bony defects; however, there is a significant increase in the operative time and is a very technically demanding procedure requiring larger surgical exposure and potential for increased donor site morbidity. Thus it is not a technique often used in spinal surgery.[7,15]

Allograft Bone

Allogenic bone graft, harvested from another human, is another common adjuvant to spinal fusion. Use of an allograft is advantageous as it avoids the complications of donor site morbidity, readily available, and able to provide bone graft in varying forms and large quantity.[1] Although all allografts have osteoconductive properties, the osteoinductivity of various grafts is highly dependent on preparation and sterilization techniques.[7] Allografts, however, have an inherent weakness in that they are costly and tend to have a slower osteointegration rate, increased resorption, and infection risk as compared to autografts.[7,16] Allografts can be broadly categorized into fresh or processed, with fresh allografts being transplanted immediately after procurement and processed allografts being generally treated and then stored to be available for transplantation at a later time point. The form of allograft used can be dependent on the function or application anticipated for the graft.[16] Immunogenicity is a concern while using allograft as cell surface antigens present on the allograft can entice an adverse immune response and result in rejection. The immunogenicity of the graft can be tailored during allograft processing via immunosuppression, histocompatibility matching, freeze-drying, or fresh-freezing. The freeze-dried allografts are the least immunogenic, and fresh vascularized composite grafts are the most immunogenic.[16]

Bone graft extenders are a form of allografts that are used as viable substitutes, with the most common being demineralized bone matrix (DBM).[3,16–18] DBM is prepared via an elaborate process involving harvesting and cleaning of cortical bone that is subsequently ground and demineralized through acid extraction, generating a noncollagenous proteinaceous product with varying levels of osteoinductive cytokines.[16] When present, these cytokines are released during the demineralization process and act on various cellular cascades to promote bone repair and regeneration.[16] The DBM can be combined and modified with various different carriers depending on its application and is commercially available in powder, granule, putty, gel, or chips form. DBM is one of the least immunogenic allografts, and studies have shown induction of new bone formation in animal fusion models.[16–19]

Cellular Allograft

In recent years, processed cellularized allografts have come to market in an effort to increase the efficacy of allograft bone. These products are processed to remove immunogenic cells while retaining mesenchymal stem cells within a demineralized matrix and are designed to simulate human autograft bone and promote bone regeneration while avoiding the complications associated with harvesting autograft.[20] The cellular allografts have the three essential properties (osteogenic, osteoconductive, and osteoinductive) needed for bone regeneration as they contain mesenchymal stem cells, DBM, and cancellous bone. Osteocel Plus (Nuvasive, San Diego, CA), a minimally modified human allograft, is one of the most well-studied products in this category and has been demonstrated to contain viable cells capable of self-renewal and multipotential differentiation.[20-22] Tomeh et al. conducted a radiographic and clinical outcome study in patients who had an extreme lateral interbody fusion with Osteocel Plus and demonstrated a 90.2% complete interbody fusion with the remaining 9.8% being partially consolidated and progression toward fusion.[21] Ammerman et al. conducted a retrospective chart review on patients undergoing a minimally invasive transformational lumbar interbody fusion with Osteocel Plus and demonstrated that 91.3% of the patients were able to achieve bony arthrodesis by 12 months.[20]

Trinity Evolution (Orthofix, Lewisville, TX) is another cellular allograft designed as an alternative to autograft. It contains supraphysiologic concentrations of mesenchymal stem cells in a cancellous bone matrix and a demineralized bone component. It had been studied with positive results demonstrated in the foot and ankle surgery.[23] Bio4 (Stryker, Mahwah, NJ) is another cellular allograft that is angiogenic in addition to being osteoconductive, osteoinductive, and osteogenic. It contains mesenchymal stem cells, osteoprogenitor cells, osteoblasts, and osteoinductive and angiogenic growth factors, making it a theoretically attractive choice for an allograft;[24] however, clinical efficacy has not yet been demonstrated in the literature.

SYNTHETIC GRAFTS
Ceramics
Ceramic compounds are an often-used substitute for both autogeneic and allogeneic bone graft and have several properties that promote osteogenesis. These products are categorized into three types: sintered, replamiform, and collagen mesh.[7] Sintered ceramics are synthetic porous compounds made of hydroxyapatite. Although the ability to mass produce synthetic sintered ceramics is advantageous, these compounds do not have the interconnectivity seen in trabecular bone. Conversely, replamiform ceramics, made from sea coral, have more structural similarity to bone.[7] All ceramics serve an osteoinductive role allowing for bone repair and regeneration.[25] They do not generate an inflammatory response; however, ceramics may lead to formation of a seroma secondary to a nonimmune inflammatory response.[26] Yuan et al. investigated the osteogenic potential of porous ceramic materials and demonstrated that after implantation in a large bone defect in sheep, the porous ceramic materials led to equally efficient bone repair as autologous bone graft.[25]

Bioactive Glass
Bioactive glasses are another alternative to autografts which have gained significant interest in recent years. In particular, bioactive glass 45S5 and Bioglass were composed of 46.1 mol% SiO_2, 24.4 mol% Na_2O, 26.9 mol% CaO, and 2.6 mol% P_2O_5.[27,28] This is now sold and known as PerioGlas (Novabone, Alachua, FL). It is osteoconductive with significant initial mechanical strength as compared to other grafts types.[6] When first created by Hench, it was found to form a strong bond with bone.[28] lharreborde et al. investigated bioactive glass in a comparative study with iliac crest bone graft as a bone graft substitute for the treatment of idiopathic scoliosis. The study demonstrated that bioactive glass was indeed as effective as iliac crest bone graft in achieving fusion and maintaining correction, thus, being a viable bone graft alternative for spinal fusion.[9] Bioactive glass has also been combined with ceramics, in products such as Vitoss BA (Stryker, Mawah, NJ), to take advantage of the favorable properties of both materials.

GROWTH FACTORS
Growth factors have been among the most extensively studied biologics in spine surgery to promote successful fusion and prevention of a pseudoarthrosis. Of particular interest, bone morphogenetic proteins (BMPs) have been studied at length in spine fusion due to their substantial osteoinductive properties.[7] BMPs were initially discovered by Marshall Urist in 1965. They belong to the transforming growth factor β (TGF-β) superfamily and play an important role in postnatal bone development. BMPs are important in recruiting mesenchymal stem cells and stimulating their differentiation into osteoblasts. BMPs act upon cell membrane receptors to activate various intracellular signaling cascades resulting in target gene expression and ultimately bone matrix formation.[2,29,30]

Concentrations of BMPs and BMP receptors are upregulated and play a vital role in fracture healing and bone formation.[31-34] Studies of the use of BMPs for spinal fusion have shown excellent fusion rates and have been marketed as a stand-alone product to promote the proliferation of mesenchymal stem cells and formation of osteoprogenitor cells, resulting in bone remodeling and formation.[35] Recombinant BMP-2 (rhBMP-2), marketed as INFUSE (Medtronic, Minneapolis, Mn), has been approved by the FDA for use in anterior lumbar interbody spine fusions; however, it has been widely used in an off-label capacity for a variety of other spinal fusion techniques.[36,37] In its current formulation, a supraphysiologic

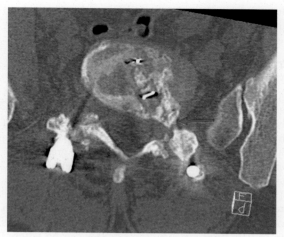

FIG. 15.2 Axial computed tomography image of the L5-S1 disc space following a fusion procedure augmented with BMP-2 (Infuse, Medtronic, Mn). Overgrowth of bone into the neural foramen (red arrow), one of the potential complication of this biologic therapy, is evident and can lead to persistent radicular leg pain from nerve root compression.

extremely high loading dose of rhBMP-2 is required for bone formation, which can result in variety of adverse side effects. The nature of these side effects could not be predicted initially as rhBMP-2 acted on a number of different physiological pathways leading to a wide variety of adverse events including tissue reaction, osteolysis, ectopic bone formation, bony overgrowth, systemic toxicity, and inflammation.[2,37] Although initial clinical studies demonstrated the positive effects of rhBMP-2 on inducing bone formation, study design biases were later discovered which brought several safety concerns to the forefront.[37] The studies were industry funded and shared similar findings with regards to safety, reporting a very low risk of adverse events.[37] This perceived absence of a significant incidence of complications led to a widespread use of rhBMP-2 for spine arthrodesis, rising from use in 0.7% of spinal fusions after its FDA approval in 2002 to 25% in 2006 in the United States.[38] After the widespread use of both on-label and off-label applications, a wide array of complications were seen (Fig. 15.2) and led to investigations of original studies reporting minimal complications. These complications included neck and soft tissue swelling, injury to neurological structures, dysphagia requiring intubation, antiinflammatories, tracheostomy, and additional surgeries.[37]

Carragee et al. conducted a systematic review evaluating the safety concerns with the use of rhBMP-2 in spine surgery.[37] The use of rhBMP-2 was investigated in posterolateral lumbar fusion, and Boden et al. demonstrated

greater leg pain, inferior early functional outcome scores, and wound complications in the rhBMP-2 group versus iliac crest bone graft.[37] Review of the Scoliosis Research Society database by Williams et al. revealed a 500% higher rate of wound complication and epidural hematoma with the use of rhBMP-2 and posterior approach.[39] Vaidya et al. revealed a significant graft subsidence rate in patients undergoing Anterior lumbar interbody fusion (ALIF) with rhBMP-2.[40] Carragee et al. demonstrated greater subsidence and higher rate of reoperation in patients with use of rhBMP-2 with interbody fusion versus allograft.[41] Other studies demonstrated retrograde ejaculation rates of 5%–7% in male patients undergoing ALIF surgery with rhBMP-2, rates which were greater than those in the original published studies.[42–44] Osteolytic defects associated with the use of rhBMP-2 are common and have led to bone loss, implant migration, and kyphosis secondary to bone collapse.[45,46] Incidence as high as 56% has been demonstrated with very low resolution at long-term follow-up.[44,45] Use of BMPs and their association with development of neoplasms has been questioned and studied at length. Thawani et al. performed a review of the literature on BMPs and neoplasms in which there was no definitive association noted between the use of BMPs and promotion of neoplasm.[47] Even though there was no definitive association, they did recommend practicing caution against widespread use.[47]

The high-dose rhBMP-2 formulation (AMPLIFY, Medtronic) used for posterolateral fusion in lumbar spine was initially noted to have no adverse events. However, a recent FDA Executive Summary revealed major back pain and leg pain in the AMPLIFY group at 4 and 8 weeks after surgery, and as a result, the product is not commercially available.[37] Despite the identified risks, rhBMP is still currently in use as an adjunct to spinal fusion, especially in patients with physiology which may reduce their chance of successful fusion. Most surgeons will limit the use to the lowest dose possible as this may reduce the risk of complications; however, data to support this hypothesis are not currently available.

IMPLANT OPTIMIZATION

Metallic and polymeric implants are routinely used in spinal fusion procedures to provide initial vertebral stability and/or correct deformity while bony fusion occurs. Traditionally,[48] spinal implants were designed as biologically inert objects, serving only a mechanical role. Recently, research has focused on the modification of both the surface and structure of spinal implants in an effort to add biologic activity to their mechanical properties. Optimization of these implants is critical as they serve as carrier vehicles to augment the fusion process. Interbody devices are mechanical devices placed in the intervertebral disc space to support restore disc height after degeneration and promote osteogenesis and osteointegration during the fusion process. These devices are often filled with bone graft, graft substitute, or biologics and are commonly used for a variety of spinal pathologies.[49] The implant interface or surface texture and implant topography are principal factors in promoting formation of a fusion mass.[49] Studies have revealed that titanium alloy implants have a stimulatory effect on osteoblastic differentiation, generation of osteoid, and its mineralization[49] and thus have become an increasingly popular material of choice for interbody devices. Surface texture of implants has been recognized as an important factor in the modulation of cellular function during bone formation. Studies have demonstrated an increased production of growth factors and cytokines when cells interact with rough surface along with cell modulation, leading to improved osteogenesis when compared to smooth surface.[50,51] Boyan et al. examined the effects of surface roughness on the proliferation, differentiation, and matrix production by osteoblast-like cells and demonstrated increased cell proliferation and increased production of prostaglandin E2 and transforming growth factor beta 1 (TGF-β1) on rougher surfaces as compared to smooth ones.[51] There are currently several implants on the market which have been specifically designed to take advantage of the effect of microsurface and nanosurface topography modification. The clinical effects of these strategies on success of spinal fusion are still undetermined.

MESECHYMAL STEM CELLS

Tissue engineering and bone regeneration is another biological alternative to bone graft. Mesenchymal stem cells (MSCs) are pluripotent cells with the ability to give rise to various tissues and have been increasingly studied for their potential use in biologics for spine fusion. They are readily available in the human body and can be isolated from bone marrow, fat, and muscle.[52] They represent a potential untapped source for bone regeneration and tissue engineering. Various signaling pathways can be activated to differentiate the MSCs toward a specific lineage. MSCs can be loaded into various scaffolds and implanted into areas of bone defects to allow for bone engineering. Peterson et al. demonstrated the ability of BMP-2–producing human adipose-derived MSCs to heal a critically sized femoral defect in a nude rat model.[53] Although it has immense potential in the future, mesenchymal stem technology is still largely in the development stage without proven clinical efficacy.

THE FUTURE OF BIOLOGICS FOR SPINE SURGERY

A clinical need for additional biological bone graft extenders is needed, and various bioactive factors are being studied. Small molecules (SMs) are a type of bioactive factor with osteoinductive properties being investigated for their application as bone graft extenders. SMs have a low molecular weight, typically 1 kDa, significantly smaller than large recombinant proteins. Their small size allows them to evade an immune response, have a greater bioavailability, diffuse through cellular membranes, and act on various cellular cascades to initiate bone regeneration.[2,54] SMs can be tailored toward a specific application, provide a cheap reliable alternative to current bone grafting options, and avoid the complications associated with autograft harvesting. Montgomery et al. investigated oxysterol (Oxy133) and demonstrated induction of osteogenesis via its action on sonic hedgehog signaling pathway in an in vitro model and spine fusion in an in vivo rat model.[55] Sintuu et al. investigated proteolytic fragments of spp24, a BMP-binding protein, and demonstrated promotion of BMP activity in an in vivo rat spinal fusion model.[56] Bone morphogenetic protein–binding protein was demonstrated to improve the efficacy of BMP-2 in a rodent spine fusion model resulting in early fusion.[57]

The delivery of SMs to specific sites in the body is being investigated to isolate their desired function and avoid undesirable systemic side effects. Carrier vehicles loaded with SMs have been investigated to provide a controlled release of the SMs for a sustained bioavailability. Hydrogels, composed of a hydrophilic polymers, are among the most widely studied carriers with excellent biocompatibility and provide a three-dimensional scaffold for cell and tissue regeneration. Bioactive molecules and growth factors can be loaded into hydrogels that can be fabricated with a variety of properties to control the release characteristics of the SMs and optimize their efficacy.[2]

Scaffolds fabricated from nanofibers are another attractive carrier vehicle for the localized delivery of SMs. Nanofiber scaffolds can be manufactured with a three-dimensional structure similar to the extracellular matrix with a very high surface-to-volume ratio. Nanofiber scaffolds are fabricated through an electrospinning process and can also be preloaded with various molecules or drugs.[2] Similarly, microspheres are engineered spheres with the molecules or drugs encapsulated within them. Their size and porosity are tailored for the desired release characteristics and application.[58] Research in SMs is increasing as they provide a viable alternative as bone graft extenders while avoiding the morbidities associated with autograft harvest, cost of allograft, and adverse events with use of growth factors and recombinant proteins.

A more recently studied class of biologics is using small peptides, specifically P-15. It is a synthetic 15-amino acid polypeptide with the capability of activating various cellular cascades leading to bone formation by mimicking the cell-binding domain of type I collagen.[48,59] P-15 acts to promote cellular migration and proliferation and differentiation of osteoblasts. P-15 is available in a product called i-FACTOR Bone Graft (Cerapedics, Inc., Westminister, CO). i-FACTOR is P-15 adsorbed onto an organic bone mineral and delivered in a hydrogel carrier. Arnold et al. investigated the safety and efficacy of i-FACTOR and compared it to local autograft in single-level Anterior cervical discectomy and fusion (ACDF). At their 1-year follow-up, patients receiving i-FACTOR had demonstrated a fusion rate of 88.97% versus 85.82% in the autograft group, significant improvement in Neck Disability Index (NDI), high neurological success rate, and no difference in adverse events.[48] The study demonstrated that i-FACTOR met the FDA criteria for noninferiority as compared to autografts.

BIOLOGICS FOR INTERVERTEBRAL DISC REGENERATION

Spinal fusion is an end-stage therapy that alleviates the symptoms of disc degeneration by eliminating motion at the effected segment. Although this is clinically effective, it does not correct the underlying pathological process. Many investigators are working to elucidate the biologic mechanisms leading to disc degeneration and develop disease-modifying treatments to halt or reverse the degenerative process and serve as an alternative to spinal fusion. Disc degeneration occurs with age as various cellular changes take place with regard to cell type, density, cellular senescence, and cell death. Degeneration is thought to begin in the nucleus pulposus at the center of the Intervertebral disc (IVD), a tissue with extremely low cell density and very limited capacity for self-repair. With aging, the vascular supply and cell density with the nucleus diminish further, resulting in an alteration in matrix homeostasis toward catabolism. This starts a cascade of events leading to degeneration of the entire spinal motion segment. Various treatment strategies have been investigated to limit disc degeneration and attempt to regenerate disc tissue. Biological therapy with injection of bioactive factors

directly into the intervertebral disc has been investigated to prevent further degeneration. These include injection of growth factors, proteins, gene therapy, stem cells, anticatabolic agents, mitogens, morphogens, and intracellular regulators.[60-64]

MSCs can be harvested from bone marrow, fat, or muscle and injected into the disc for regeneration.[65] Henriksson et al. demonstrated survival of MSCs after implantation into a porcine model for at least 6 months along with expression of collagen IIA, IIB, versican, aggrecan, and Sox9, indicating differentiation of cells into disc-like cells.[66] Orozco et al. demonstrated an improvement in pain and disability in 10 patients with injection of autologous expanded bone marrow mesenchymal stem cells into the nucleus pulposus.[67] Stem cells from healthy discs can be harvested, expanded ex vivo, and implanted into degenerative discs with the hopes of regenerating the disc. However, this requires aspiration of cells from a healthy disc which may injure the healthy disc resulting in degeneration.[60] An increase in proteoglycan synthesis was seen in the nucleus pulposus after injection of growth factor TGF-β1 into intervertebral discs.[64] Injection of osteogenic protein-1 and TGF-β into the intervertebral discs of rabbits led to an increase in the disc height and increased proteoglycan content at 2, 4, and 8 weeks, as demonstrated by An et al.[68] Similarly, treatment with platelet-derived growth factor (PDGF) has been demonstrated to decrease disc cell apoptosis and slow the degenerative process in both in vitro and in vivo studies[69,70] (Fig. 15.3). Gene therapy was demonstrated to be an effective modality by Nishida et al. in which a human TGF-β1 adenoviral vector was used to transduce a rabbit IVD resulting in a 30-fold increase in its production and increased proteoglycan synthesis.[71]

CONCLUSION

Biology of spinal fusion is a complex process that is evoked during the treatment of patients with degenerative conditions, spine deformity, trauma, and tumor. With increasing rates of spinal fusion procedures being performed annually in the United States, it is important to prevent pseudoarthrosis—failure of the bone formation process. The biology of spinal fusion is complex and occurs via three essential mechanisms including osteoconduction, osteoinduction, and osteogenesis. To prevent pseudoarthrosis, the biologic environment can be augmented with various bioactive factors. Grafting including autografts, allografts, and synthetic bone grafts which have been used to augment the fusion process for bone regeneration. Despite being the gold

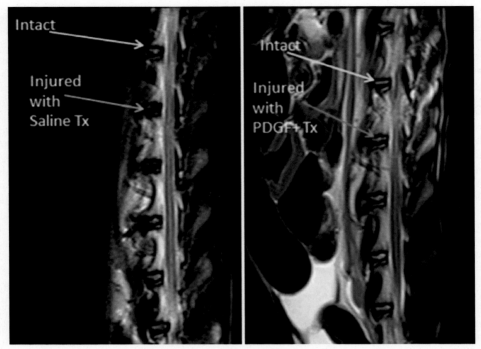

FIG. 15.3 Sagittal magnetic resonance images of rabbit lumbar spine demonstrating preservation of disc architecture and hydration when treated with PDGF (green arrow), as compared to an injured but untreated disc (blue arrow).

standard, autografts are associated with many comorbidities. Allografts provide an alternative to autografts; however, they are costly, with slower osteointegration rate, increased resorption, and higher infection risk as compared with autografts. Growth factors are used to promote the fusion process; however, they have been associated with various controversies. Increased focus is needed in optimizing graft choices, various implants, growth factors, proteins, MSCs, and SMs. Ultimately, biologic therapies for the IVD will be used to prevent progression of the degenerative process and the associated debilitating symptoms, obviating the need for the current widely used end-stage treatment options.

REFERENCES

1. Kannan A, Dodwad S-NM, Hsu WK. Biologics in spine arthrodesis. *Clin Spine Surg.* 2015;28(5):163–170.
2. Singh H, Karukonda T, Presciutti S. The use of small molecules to aid with spinal fusion. *Semin Spine Surg.* 2016;28(4):255–262.
3. Boden SD. Overview of the biology of lumbar spine fusion and principles for selecting a bone graft substitute. *Spine (Phila Pa 1976).* 2002;27(16 suppl 1):S26–S31.
4. Deyo RA, et al. United States trends in lumbar fusion surgery for degenerative conditions. *Spine (Phila Pa 1976).* 2005;30(12):1441–1445; discussion 1446-7.
5. Leach JK, Mooney DJ. Bone engineering by controlled delivery of osteoinductive molecules and cells. *Expert Opin Biol Ther.* 2004;4(7):1015–1027.
6. Giannoudis PV, Dinopoulos H, Tsiridis E. Bone substitutes: an update. *Injury.* 2005;36(3):S20–S27.
7. Vaccaro AR, et al. Bone grafting alternatives in spinal surgery. *Spine J.* 2002;2(3):206–215.
8. Kim YJ, et al. Pseudarthrosis in primary fusions for adult idiopathic scoliosis: incidence, risk factors, and outcome analysis. *Spine.* 2005;30(4):468–474.
9. Ilharreborde B, et al. Bioactive glass as a bone substitute for spinal fusion in adolescent idiopathic scoliosis: a comparative study with iliac crest autograft. *J Pediatr Orthop.* 2008;28(3):347–351.
10. Sengupta DK, et al. Outcome of local bone versus autogenous iliac crest bone graft in the instrumented posterolateral fusion of the lumbar spine. *Spine (Phila Pa 1976).* 2006;31(9):985–991.
11. Khan SN, et al. The biology of bone grafting. *J Am Acad Orthop Surg.* 2005;13(1):77–86.
12. Steffen T, et al. Minimally invasive bone harvesting tools. *Eur Spine J.* 2000;9(suppl 1):S114–S118.
13. Ito Z, et al. Bone union rate with autologous iliac bone versus local bone graft in posterior lumbar interbody fusion (PLIF): a multicenter study. *Eur Spine J.* 2013;22(5):1158–1163.
14. Enneking WF, et al. Physical and biological aspects of repair in dog cortical-bone transplants. *J Bone Joint Surg Am.* 1975;57(2):237–252.

15. Enneking WF, Eady JL, Burchardt H. Autogenous cortical bone grafts in the reconstruction of segmental skeletal defects. *J Bone Joint Surg Am.* 1980;62(7):1039–1058.
16. Gitelis S, Cole BJ. The use of allografts in orthopaedic surgery. *Instr Course Lect.* 2002;51:507–520.
17. Morone MA, Boden SD. Experimental posterolateral lumbar spinal fusion with a demineralized bone matrix gel. *Spine.* 1998;23(2):159–167.
18. Martin Jr GJ, et al. New formulations of demineralized bone matrix as a more effective graft alternative in experimental posterolateral lumbar spine arthrodesis. *Spine (Phila Pa 1976).* 1999;24(7):637–645.
19. Oikarinen J. Experimental spinal fusion with decalcified bone matrix and deep-frozen allogeneic bone in rabbits. *Clin Orthop Relat Res.* 1982;162:210–218.
20. Ammerman JM, Libricz J, Ammerman MD. The role of Osteocel Plus as a fusion substrate in minimally invasive instrumented transforaminal lumbar interbody fusion. *Clin Neurol Neurosurg.* 2013;115(7):991–994.
21. Tohmeh AG, et al. Allograft cellular bone matrix in extreme lateral interbody fusion: preliminary radiographic and clinical outcomes. *Sci World J.* 2012;2012:263637.
22. Neman J, et al. Lineage mapping and characterization of the native progenitor population in cellular allograft. *Spine J.* 2013;13(2):162–174.
23. Rush SM. Trinity evolution. *Foot Ankle Spec.* 2010;3(3):140–143.
24. Temple HT, Malinin TI. Orthobiologics in the foot and ankle. *Foot Ankle Clin.* 2016;21(4):809–823.
25. Yuan H, et al. Osteoinductive ceramics as a synthetic alternative to autologous bone grafting. *Proc Natl Acad Sci U S A.* 2010;107(31):13614–13619.
26. Bucholz RW, Carlton A, Holmes R. Interporous hydroxyapatite as a bone graft substitute in tibial plateau fractures. *Clin Orthop Relat Res.* 1989;(240):53–62.
27. Hench LL, et al. Bonding mechanisms at the interface of ceramic prosthetic materials. *J Biomed Mater Res.* 1971;5(6):117–141.
28. Jones JR. Reprint of: review of bioactive glass: from Hench to hybrids. *Acta Biomater.* 2015;23:S53–S82.
29. Lieberman JR, Daluiski A, Einhorn TA. The role of growth factors in the repair of bone: biology and clinical applications. *JBJS.* 2002;84(6):1032–1044.
30. Heldin C-H, Miyazono K, ten Dijke P. TGF-[beta] signalling from cell membrane to nucleus through SMAD proteins. *Nature.* 1997;390(6659):465–471.
31. Nakase T, et al. Transient and localized expression of bone morphogenetic protein 4 messenger RNA during fracture healing. *J Bone Miner Res.* 1994;9(5):651–659.
32. Ishidou Y, et al. Enhanced expression of type I receptors for bone morphogenetic proteins during bone formation. *J Bone Miner Res.* 1995;10(11):1651–1659.
33. Onishi T, et al. Distinct and overlapping patterns of localization of bone morphogenetic protein (BMP) family members and a BMP type II receptor during fracture healing in rats. *Bone.* 1998;22(6):605–612.
34. Yazaki Y, et al. Immunohistochemical localization of bone morphogenetic proteins and the receptors in epiphyseal growth plate. *Anticancer Res.* 1998;18(4a):2339–2344.
35. Carlisle E, Fischgrund JS. Bone morphogenetic proteins for spinal fusion. *Spine J.* 2005;5(6):S240–S249.
36. Vaidya R. Transforaminal interbody fusion and the "off label" use of recombinant human bone morphogenetic protein-2. *Spine J.* 2009;9(8):667–669.
37. Carragee EJ, Hurwitz EL, Weiner BK. A critical review of recombinant human bone morphogenetic protein-2 trials in spinal surgery: emerging safety concerns and lessons learned. *Spine J.* 2011;11(6):471–491.
38. Cahill KS, et al. Prevalence, complications, and hospital charges associated with use of bone-morphogenetic proteins in spinal fusion procedures. *JAMA.* 2009;302(1):58–66.
39. Williams BJ, et al. Complications associated with BMP use in 11,933 cases of spinal fusion. *Spine J.* 2010;10(9):S98–S99.
40. Vaidya R, et al. Interbody fusion with allograft and rh-BMP-2 leads to consistent fusion but early subsidence. *J Bone Joint Surg Br.* 2007;89(3):342–345.
41. Carragee E, Wildstein M. 17. A controlled trial of BMP and unilateral transpedicular instrumentation in circumferential single or double level lumbar fusion. *Spine J.* 2007;7(5):8S–9S.
42. Smoljanovic T, Siric F, Bojanic I. Six-year outcomes of anterior lumbar interbody arthrodesis with use of interbody fusion cages and recombinant human bone morphogenetic protein-2. *JBJS.* 2010;92(15):2614–2615.
43. Kang BU, et al. An analysis of general surgery-related complications in a series of 412 minilaparotomic anterior lumbosacral procedures. *J Neurosurg Spine.* 2009;10(1):60–65.
44. Carragee EJ, et al. Retrograde ejaculation after anterior lumbar interbody fusion using rhBMP-2: a cohort controlled study. *Spine J.* 2011;11(6):511–516.
45. Helgeson MD, et al. Adjacent vertebral body osteolysis with bone morphogenetic protein use in transforaminal lumbar interbody fusion. *Spine J.* 2011;11(6):507–510.
46. Knox JB, Dai 3rd JM, Orchowski J. Osteolysis in transforaminal lumbar interbody fusion with bone morphogenetic protein-2. *Spine (Phila Pa 1976).* 2011;36(8):672–676.
47. Thawani JP, et al. Bone morphogenetic proteins and cancer review of the literature. *Neurosurgery.* 2010;66(2):233–246.
48. Arnold PM, et al. Efficacy of i-factor bone graft versus autograft in anterior cervical discectomy and fusion: results of the prospective, randomized, single-blinded food and drug administration investigational device exemption study. *Spine.* 2016;41(13):1075–1083.
49. Olivares-Navarrete R, et al. Rough titanium alloys regulate osteoblast production of angiogenic factors. *Spine J.* 2013;13(11):1563–1570.

50. Vlacic-Zischke J, et al. The influence of surface microroughness and hydrophilicity of titanium on the up-regulation of TGFbeta/BMP signalling in osteoblasts. *Biomaterials.* 2011;32(3):665–671.

51. Kieswetter K, et al. Surface roughness modulates the local production of growth factors and cytokines by osteoblast-like MG-63 cells. *J Biomed Mater Res.* 1996;32(1):55–63.

52. Gafni Y, et al. Stem cells as vehicles for orthopedic gene therapy. *Gene Ther.* 2004;11(4):417–426.

53. Peterson B, et al. Healing of critically sized femoral defects, using genetically modified mesenchymal stem cells from human adipose tissue. *Tissue Eng.* 2005;11(1–2):120–129.

54. Lo KW, et al. The role of small molecules in musculoskeletal regeneration. *Regen Med.* 2012;7(4):535–549.

55. Montgomery SR, et al. A novel osteogenic oxysterol compound for therapeutic development to promote bone growth: activation of hedgehog signaling and osteogenesis through smoothened binding. *J Bone Miner Res.* 2014;29(8):1872–1885.

56. Sintuu C, et al. Full-length bovine spp24 [spp24 (24-203)] inhibits BMP-2 induced bone formation. *J Orthop Res.* 2008;26(6):753–758.

57. Alanay A, et al. The adjunctive effect of a binding peptide on bone morphogenetic protein enhanced bone healing in a rodent model of spinal fusion. *Spine (Phila Pa 1976).* 2008;33(16):1709–1713.

58. Laurencin CT, et al. Delivery of small molecules for bone regenerative engineering: preclinical studies and potential clinical applications. *Drug Discov Today.* 2014;19(6):794–800.

59. Ding M, et al. Efficacy of a small cell-binding peptide coated hydroxyapatite substitute on bone formation and implant fixation in sheep. *J Biomed Mater Res Part A.* 2015;103(4):1357–1365.

60. Paesold G, Nerlich AG, Boos N. Biological treatment strategies for disc degeneration: potentials and shortcomings. *Eur Spine J.* 2007;16(4):447–468.

61. Vadalà G, et al. Intervertebral disc regeneration: from the degenerative cascade to molecular therapy and tissue engineering. *J Tissue Eng Regen Med.* 2015;9(6):679–690.

62. Masuda K, Oegema Jr TR, An HS. Growth factors and treatment of intervertebral disc degeneration. *Spine (Phila Pa 1976).* 2004;29(23):2757–2769.

63. Yoon ST, Patel NM. Molecular therapy of the intervertebral disc. *Eur Spine J.* 2006;15(suppl 3):379–388.

64. Thompson JP, Oegema Jr TR, Bradford DS. Stimulation of mature canine intervertebral disc by growth factors. *Spine (Phila Pa 1976).* 1991;16(3):253–260.

65. Richardson SM, et al. Mesenchymal stem cells in regenerative medicine: opportunities and challenges for articular cartilage and intervertebral disc tissue engineering. *J Cell Physiol.* 2010;222(1):23–32.

66. Henriksson HB, et al. Transplantation of human mesenchymal stems cells into intervertebral discs in a xenogeneic porcine model. *Spine.* 2009;34(2):141–148.

67. Orozco L, et al. Intervertebral disc repair by autologous mesenchymal bone marrow cells: a pilot study. *Transplantation.* 2011;92(7):822–828.

68. An HS, et al. Intradiscal administration of osteogenic protein-1 increases intervertebral disc height and proteoglycan content in the nucleus pulposus in normal adolescent rabbits. *Spine (Phila Pa 1976).* 2005;30(1):25–31; discussion 31-2.

69. Presciutti SM, Paglia DN, Karukonda T, et al. PDGF-BB inhibits intervertebral disc cell apoptosis in vitro. *J Orthop Res.* 2014;32(9):1181–1188.

70. Paglia DN, Singh H, Karukonda T, Drissi H, Moss IL. PDGF-BB delays degeneration of the intervertebral discs in a rabbit preclinical model. *Spine.* 2016;41(8):E449–E458.

71. Nishida K, et al. 1999 Volvo award winner in basic science studies: modulation of the biologic activity of the rabbit intervertebral disc by gene therapy: an in vivo study of adenovirus-mediated transfer of the human transforming growth factor β1 encoding gene. *Spine.* 1999;24(23):2419.

CHAPTER 16

Biologics in Foot and Ankle Surgery

ADAM D. LINDSAY, MD • VINAYAK SATHE, MD, MS, FRCS • JOHN PLAYFAIR
ROSS, BS, MD

ROLE OF BIOLOGICS IN ACHILLES TENDINOPATHY

Despite the Achilles tendon being one of the strongest tendons in the human body, it is one of the most frequently ruptured lower limb tendons and comprises roughly 20% of all large tendon injuries.[1] Unfortunately, healing of Achilles tendon has had unpredictable outcomes due to its limited bloody supply that diminishes usually after the third decade.[2] Tendon healing often results in a fibrovascular scar and tendon that is weaker than the previously uninjured healthy tendon.[3] This obviously leaves the tendon at increased risk of rerupture and stiffness. This has led to the investigation of biologics for Achilles tendinopathy. Although the role of biologics in Achilles tendinopathy is still under study, we will explore current findings of tendon healing with platelet-rich plasma (PRP) and bone marrow aspirate concentrate (BMAC). We will also discuss the use of acellular dermal matrices and their use in strengthening Achilles tendon rupture.

PRP and BMAC: Is There a Role?

PRP has received much more attention recently in its role to stimulate healing and even revascularization with in vitro studies with growing evidence in its use in the setting of foot and ankle pathology.[4] PRP is defined as plasma with a twofold or more platelet concentration above baseline level.[5] In vitro studies have shown PRP to release platelet-derived growth factors (PDGFs), multiple transforming growth factors including TGF-B1/B2, and growth factors used in healing and stimulating the inflammatory response.[4,6] The platelets also contain cytokines and chemical mediators such as histamine, fibrinogen, fibronectin, and serotonin to help induce the inflammatory response. Biologic studies have also shown that PRP can enhance type I and type III collagen synthesis by tendons.[7,8] The use of PRP has been investigated in mice with positive results.[9] Kaux et al. examined the use of PRP injection in mice after Achilles tendon rupture and found

that those with PRP injections had earlier tendon healing and stronger mechanical resistance at 30 days.[9]

PRP has been used in humans as well for chronic Achilles tendinopathy with mixed results.[10–12] de Jong et al. found that patients with chronic Achilles tendinopathy had no significant clinical or ultrasonographic tendon differences with PRP versus placebo at 1 year.[13] PRP may have more of a role in assisting in the healing of partial or full-thickness tendon tears. Several mice studies have demonstrated increased neovascularization and accelerated healing with Achilles tendon tears.[14,15] Filardo et al. presented a case report of a competitive athlete with partial Achilles tendon rupture who was treated nonoperatively with PRP injections. Their study found that with three injections within 3 weeks, the patient was able to go back to baseline sports performance within 75 days of the initial injury.[16] Plasma rich in growth factors has also been examined and has demonstrated superior tendon healing compared to control. Despite the more promising results of PRP in animal studies, its effect on human studies have been mixed. The literature has shown that PRP may be more useful with healing of the acute tendon rupture rather than chronic tendinopathies.

Along with PRP, bone marrow aspirate has also been used for possible treatment of Achilles tendinopathy. Bone marrow aspirate differs from PRP in that it contains mesenchymal and hematopoietic stems cells along with PDGFs.[17,18] The bone marrow concentrate is done via aspiration usually from the iliac crest and produced by centrifugation, isolating stem cells to be reinjected into the Achilles tendon. Stein et al. examined the use of bone marrow aspirate in a small cohort of patients who underwent open Achilles tendon repair with BMAC injections and found no rerupture, with 92% of patients returning to their sport at a mean of 5.9 months.[19] The use of bone marrow cell injection has also been supported in animal studies. Okamoto et al. compared the use of bone marrow cell transplantation versus mesenchymal stem cells in mice after Achilles tendon rupture.[20]

Biologics in Orthopaedic Surgery. https://doi.org/10.1016/B978-0-323-55140-3.00016-3

They found significantly increased type III collage at 1 week and type I collagen at 1 month with bone marrow cell transplantation.[20] Despite the early benefits seen in both the clinical and animal studies, long-term data in its use in Achilles tendon are not yet available.[21,22] This will help assess the risk of these stems developing into tumor lineages which is a potential concern of BMAC.[23]

Acellular Dermal Matrices for Strengthening Repairs

More recently, acellular dermal matrices (ADMs) have been examined for their use in Achilles tendon repair. ADM is derived from cadaveric skin with techniques that allow preservation of the extracellular matrix.[24] The matrix is used to act as scaffold for reepithialization, neovascularization, and fibroblast proliferation without theoretically inducing an inflammatory response.[25] The acellular matrix contains collagen, elastin, and proteoglycans along basement membrane connective tissues which allow for integration and support into the host tissue.[25] ADMs allow for mechanical support while enhancing healing through host cell infiltration.[26] Lee et al. examined the effectiveness of acellular dermal tissue matrix as an augment to Achilles tendon repair which was sutured circumferentially around the tendon.[27] They saw no cases of rerupture or recurrent pain at 20 months, with an average time to baseline activity by 11 weeks.[27]

Rerupture of an Achilles tendon repair after use of ADM augment has been reported.[51] Bertasi removed part of the ADM after rerupture for histological examination, which showed excellent attachment of the ADM to the paratenon at 8 weeks postoperatively.[51] They also identified vast vascularization in the graft paratenon interface. Their study showed excellent integration of the matrix with remodeling of the ADM into the tendon. The use of ADM augments in Achilles tendon ruptures is still in its infancy with limited available long-term data; however, the available studies have demonstrated good results with little complications with in vitro use.

ROLE OF ORTHOBIOLOGICS IN PLANTAR FASCIITIS

Plantar fasciitis is among the most common causes of plantar hindfoot pain among sedentary and active individuals in the United States and accounts for nearly 600,000 to 1 million physician visits annually, although this number may be greater.[28,29] The plantar "fascia" is a thick connective aponeurosis that originates proximally on the medial tubercle of the calcaneus and inserts distally in the form of five distinct bands onto the metatarsal heads and bases of the proximal phalanges.[30] The mechanical function of the plantar fascia is to maintain the integrity of the longitudinal arch of the foot and promote efficient gait via the windlass mechanism.[2,3] The pathophysiology of plantar fasciitis is likely multifactorial and not currently well understood, although repetitive microtrauma yielding an inflammatory cascade with failed healing likely plays a significant role. The diagnosis is primarily made through a thorough history and physical examination, with advanced imaging used primarily to exclude other likely manifestations from the differential. The symptomatology of plantar fasciitis can be variable but typically involves throbbing heel pain with weight-bearing activities. Therapies such as rest, activity modification, heel-stretching exercises, corticosteroid injections, and nonsteroidal antiinflammatory medications are the mainstay of conservative treatment and function beneficially in the majority patients.[3,31] Extracorporeal shock wave therapy also may provide benefits in certain patients, but recent randomized control trials (RCTs) showed no significant differences in pain alleviation between treatment and placebo groups.[32,33] Newer therapeutic strategies have focused on PRP injections with hopes of directly treating the aberrant manifestation of collagen matrix degradation and disordered vascularity in plantar fasciitis by restarting the inflammatory cascade and augmenting the healing response. PRP is the superficial portion of centrifuged blood and is relatively easy to obtain in a clinic setting.[34] A recent systematic review of 12 studies in which PRP was compared to controls of both placebo and corticosteroid preparations showed uniform improvement in symptoms without any complications other than temporary localized pain.[35] Sample sizes within these studies were small and had variable treatment protocols; however, although the data had limitations, the trend toward a beneficial response is promising, especially in the setting of trivial complications. Additional randomized trials also share similar findings.[36,37] PRP injections may also show measurable symptomatic benefit in patients with recalcitrant plantar fasciitis that is unresponsive to aggressive conservative measures.[38]

OPTIONS FOR TREATING THE ARTICULAR SURFACES

Articular cartilage is a complex tissue isolated from synovial joints and is coated by hyaline cartilage.[39] It is a highly organized substance divided into four unique zones, each with its own unique extracellular matrix (ECM), chondrocyte subtypes, cellular architecture, and varying proportions of proteoglycan and cartilage.[12,40]

The complexity of the cellular subtypes and their unique arrangement coupled with its relatively avascular structure makes articular cartilage defects notoriously difficult to heal. Primary reasons include poor ability of progenitor cells to migrate to the source of injury because of minimal clot formation as well as limited ability for sufficient ECM production by mature chondrocytes.[12] Furthermore, articular cartilage properties vary greatly among the load-bearing synovial joints in the body. Within the ankle, the articular cartilage appears to be thinner than its knee counterpart, and the chondrocytes themselves appear more spaced apart.[41] The ankle joint cartilage also appears more resistant to compressive loads due to a relatively greater proteoglycan concentration within its ECM.[42] Treatment strategies must consider the variability in articular cartilage structure, etiology, time course of presentation, and dimensions of the chondral lesion in question. Options include but are not limited to marrow stimulation via microfracture or direct drilling, auto/allograft osteochondral transplantation, chondrocyte implantation, concentrated bone marrow aspirate, and PRP injection.

Marrow Stimulation and Osteochondral Allografts in the Talar Dome

Following a trial of conservative therapy aimed at reducing symptoms rather than direct repair of the lesion, several treatment modalities exist. Microfracture involves penetrating subchondral bone in multiple areas causing stimulation of mesenchymal stem cells and a local inflammatory cascade that eventually produces fibrocartilagenous ingrowth into the defect.[43] This new tissue is predominantly type-1 collagen that has different mechanical and physiologic properties from the type-2 dominant articular cartilage.[44] In a prospective cohort study of 105 patients with osteochondral defects of varying size, 100% of patients with lesions <15 mm (n = 73) met the authors' criteria for successful outcome after microfracture.[45] In those remaining patients with lesions >15 mm, only one patient obtained a successful outcome.[18] These results were corroborated by a later study of 120 patients showing that lesions 12.3 mm and greater had an 80% rate of failure.[46] It should be noted that clinical improvement does not necessarily correlate with the quality of repair tissue or extent of consolidation within the chondral defect.[16,47]

For larger lesions, osteochondral grafting may be used. This approach attempts to replenish a localized defect with articular cartilage and subchondral bone of similar structural properties.[16] Autologous grafts, most commonly taken from the ipsilateral knee margin, have the benefit of a native immunologic profile that comes with the cost of donor site morbidity, whereas allografts taken from cadavers avoid this problem while increasing risks of systemic rejection and being constrained by limited availability.[16] Furthermore, allograft procurement falls in a narrow window of less than 1 week for fresh samples to maximize active chondrocyte availability, although frozen specimens can offer up to 4 weeks of viable tissue.[16,48] Results of these treatments are generally positive. At an average of 7 years follow-up, Imhoff et al. retrospectively reported excellent clinical results in 25 patients who underwent autograft implantation for symptomatic talar defects less than 3 cm².[49] 80% of patients reported return to their preoperative exercise capacity.[22] Relatively fewer studies exist evaluating allograft implantation outcomes; however, at an average of 37.7 months, El-Rashidy and colleagues reported good, very good, or excellent outcomes in 73% of their 38 patients treated with fresh allograft.[50]

BONE GRAFTING IN FOOT AND ANKLE SURGERY

Broadly, bone graft materials can be classified as either autograft, allograft, or synthetics. There has been considerable growth in both the development and use of nonautograft materials; however, iliac crest bone graft (ICBG) remains as the gold standard. Here we review the latest evidence comparing various graft options.

GRAFTING FOR MECHANICAL STABILITY

Graft material can be used to promote fracture healing, fill bony defects, and aid in arthrodesis. The ideal graft material is osteoconductive, osteoinductive, and osteogenic. Osteoconductive materials can be thought of as a scaffold for which bone formation can take place. These materials do not have any ability to simulate bone growth, but, instead, act as a framework into which ingrowth can occur. Osteoinductive materials have the ability to stimulate bone growth by inducing stem cells to mature down a bone-forming lineage via growth factors. Osteogenic materials have the greatest potential to promote bone formation as they contain mesenchymal stem cells, osteoblasts, and osteocytes.[52,53]

Although several studies have shown autograft to be the gold standard for bone grafting in foot and ankle surgery,[54–58] its use does have consequences. Donor site complications including pain, hematoma, infection, nerve injury, and muscle herniation have all been reported.[59–61] Quantity of graft can also be a problem. In an effort to avoid these issues, the use of allograft, growth factors, and various synthetics including hydroxyapatite, calcium sulfates, and calcium phosphates has become increasingly popular.[62–64]

Much of the literature regarding bone graft materials in foot and ankle surgery focuses on their biologic rather than mechanical utility, that is, using nonstructural graft materials to augment fusion or promote fracture union. For example, cancellous bone graft lacks the structural advantages of cortical graft but is more easily vascularized and incorporated into host bone. It is more suitable for use in arthrodesis as it can be manipulated to fill voids while providing osteoinductive potential.[59] However, when mechanical stability is paramount, structural bone graft in the form of corticocancellous autografts, allografts, or synthetics is required. Few studies specific to foot and ankle surgery have attempted to compare autograft to allograft in this setting; however, some evidence does exist in select procedures.[59,62,65]

Lateral Column Lengthening

In 2007 Dolan et al. performed a randomized prospective study comparing tricortical iliac crest autograft to allograft for lateral column lengthening as part of surgical correction for posterior tibial tendon dysfunction (PTTD). They followed up 33 patients (18 allograft group, 15 autograft) to 1 year and demonstrated union in both the groups at 12 weeks.[66] They concluded that allograft was a viable alternative to autograft while avoiding donor site morbidity.

Subtalar Bone Block Arthrodesis

In 1988 Carr et al. described incorporating a subtalar bone block into arthrodesis to restore calcaneal height and width lost in trauma.[67] In this setting the use of a structural graft during fusion is required as unrestored calcaneal height can lead to fibular abutment, peroneal impingement, and tibiotalar impingement.[67,68] Schepers, in a 2013 systematic review of level 4 retrospective case series reviewed 456 patients treated with subtalar distraction bone block arthrodesis for late complications of calcaneal fractures.[69] In most cases, authors preferred the use of tricortical iliac crest bone (ICB), and they achieved good results: an average-modified american orthopedic foot and ankle society (AOFAS) score of 73 points (range 64–83) at final follow-up, with an average union rate of 96%.[69] In three studies included in this review, allograft consisting of fresh frozen femoral head was used. One of these studies was performed by Trnka et al., in which a surprisingly high 80% nonunion rate was noted.[70]

This complication rate was inconsistent with that of the other studies in which allograft or iliac crest (IC) autograft was used.

GRAFTING TO PROMOTE OSSEOUS HEALING (PDGF, BMAC, AND BMP)

An extensive review of the published foot and ankle literature suggests that although limited, there is growing evidence to support the use of materials other than autograft in the appropriate clinical setting. Several adjuncts and/or alternatives to autologous graft are being used and investigated. Here we will review the most up-to-date highest level evidence for PDGF, BMAC, and BMP.

Recombinant Human PDGF

During the inflammatory response, PDGF is released from platelets and macrophages in response to tissue injury.[71] PDGF and other growth factors act by recruiting inflammatory cells, increasing collagen deposition, and promoting angiogenesis. Recombinant human PDGF-BB (rhPDGF-BB) is an isoform of PDGF, which, when combined with beta-tricalcim phosphate (B-TCP) as an osteoconductive scaffold, has been shown to promote healing in foot and ankle arthrodesis. To date, several high-quality studies exist.[72–78] In a 2013 prospective, randomized, noninferiority trial, DiGiovanni et al. demonstrated that patients undergoing ankle or hindfoot fusions using rhPDGF-BB/B-TCP (n = 285) had statistically similar fusion rates to those treated with autograft (n = 149), with less complications while avoiding donor site morbidity.[78] These findings were further supported by Daniels et al. in 2015 in another RCT in which 75 patients were randomized at a 5:1 ratio for treatment with rhPDGF-BB/B-TCP versus autograft and compared to 142 historical autograft controls. The mean time to fusion was not statistically different. Complete fusion at 24 weeks was present on CT in 84% of the rhPDGF-BB/B-TCP group and 65% of the controls. Ninety-one percent of fusions in the experimental and 78% of fusions in the control group were deemed a success at 1 year with no difference in complications. Younger et al. note that these findings have virtually eliminated the need for autograft harvest in high-risk patients and drastically lowered this need in patients for whom larger amounts of graft material are required.[76] Sun et al., in 2017, performed a systematic review and metaanalysis of these studies and found rhPDGF to be no different from autograft in terms of fusion potential or safety.[77] Clinical outcomes were identical with the exception of the autograft groups having better long-term Short Form-12 physical component scores. Additional clinical trials have suggested that sufficient graft quantity, rather than the type of graft material, is the essential variable for a successful fusion.[75] The support for rhPDGF-BB/b-tcp is strong and generated from high-level studies, making it the best evidence-based alternative to autograft to date. Further study is warranted to address its potential to replace autograft as the standard of care.

Bone Marrow Aspirate Concentrate

BMAC has the osteogenic properties of ICBG while having the benefit of being less invasive. It is typically harvested from the ipsilateral iliac crest under local anesthesia and concentrated via centrifuge. Lee et al. in a randomized trial of 20 patients (10 each arm) looked at the effect of using BMAC plus PRP injection at the osteotomy site versus no injection for patients undergoing distraction osteogenesis for bilateral tibial lengthening.[79] They noted no difference in mean external fixator index between the groups with improved mean cortical healing indexes in the experimental group. Average time to full weight-bearing, determined by the presence of healing at two cortices, was lower in the experimental group (avg. of 0.99 mos vs. 1.38 mos, $P < .001$).[79]

BMAC has also shown utility in the setting of non-union and nonunion prevention. Braly et al. in an 11-patient case series injected BMA under fluoroscopic guidance around distal tibial metaphyseal nonunion sites that were previously plated and went onto nonunion at an average of 8 months postoperatively.[80] Nine of the 11 patients had united by 6 months after the injection. Six of the nine with successful union were followed up for an average of 4.4 years and were noted to have significant improvements in validated pain and function metrics. Murawski et al. in a 26-patient case series used BMAC and a "Charlotte Carolina" screw to percutaneously fix zone II and III fifth metatarsal Jones fractures in athletes.[81] The authors note improvement at final follow-up in several metrics from preoperative values including foot and ankle orthopedic (FAO) score and short form - 12 (SF-12) score; however, this does not prove that BMAC was the reason for this finding. A total of 24 of 26 patients returned to their previous level of sport, and one patient had a delayed union. The authors concluded that BMAC use yielded more predictable results and allowed return to sport; however, with no control group, this claim is unsubstantiated. Overall, the support for BMAC in the foot and ankle literature is relatively weak and requires further investigation.

Bone Morphogenetic Proteins

Bone morphogenetic proteins are a group of proteins that belong to the TGF-B superfamily and found to influence a wide range of growth factor functions.[82]

Recombinant human BMP-2 (rhBMP-2) is one type, approved by the FDA for use in lumbar fusions and open tibial shaft fractures, often used off-label with good success. In 2009 Bibbo et al. evaluated 69 high-risk patients (64% smokers, 19% diabetic, 68% with history of high energy trauma, 32% with talar avascular necrosis (AVN)) undergoing ankle and hindfoot fusions at a total of 112 fusion sites.[83] All patients received rhBMP-2 in addition to no graft, autograft, or allograft with graft only used when necessary for defects or malalignment. They achieved a 96% union rate at 11 weeks and no significant difference in union or time to union between subgroups. They concluded that rhBMP-2 appears to be an effective and safe adjunct to bone healing in this setting.

In 2014 Rearick et al. retrospectively reviewed 51 cases of high-risk patients augmented with rhBMP-2 during foot and ankle fusions and revisions for fracture nonunions.[84] A proportion of 92.2% cases united with a per-site union rate of 95%. They found no significant difference in time to union (mean 111 days) or complication rates among patients for whom allograft, autograft, or differently sized rhBMP-2 kits were used. They concluded that rhBMP-2 is a safe and effective adjunct to these procedures and warrants further investigation.

SUMMARY

At present time, the foot and ankle literature has demonstrated, at best, noninferiority of allograft and synthetics in select procedures. In well-vascularized bone similar to the calcaneus, autograft may not be necessary; however, in less vascularized areas, incorporation of allograft and synthetics is problematic.[65,66,85–88] Autograft remains the gold standard as it is osteogenic, nonimmunogenic, and structurally superior. Allografts and synthetics are not ideal as they have immunogenic potential necessitating they undergo sterilization and preservation, a process that is nonuniform and structurally detrimental. Most authors continue to recommend using autograft tissue whenever possible, while supplementing with allograft and synthetics as needed.

The use of amniotic membrane in the setting of foot and ankle surgery has become increasingly popular in recent years. Surprisingly, this is not a new concept as publications describing its use in humans as a living surgical dressing date back to 1973.[1] Several recent high-quality studies have shown it to be effective in the management of chronic diabetic foot ulcers.[2-11] Most notably, Snyder et al. in a 2016 prospective, randomized control trial demonstrated its superiority over the standard of care in the healing of chronic diabetic foot ulcers with no reported adverse events.[2] The trial was conducted at 8 sites and only included 14 experimental and 15 control patients; nevertheless, the emerging data show promise. Additionally, amniotic membrane has shown utility in the treatment of plantar fasciitis as well as during tarsal coalition resection.[12-15]

REFERENCES

1. Haines JF. Bilateral rupture of the Achilles tendon in patients on steroid therapy. *Ann Rheum Dis.* 1983;(42): 652–654.
2. Lagergre C, Lindholm A. Vascular distribution in the Achilles tendon: an angiographic and microangiographic study. *Acta Chir Scand.* 1958/1959;116:491–495.
3. Gott M, et al. Tendon phenotype should dictate tissue engineering modality in tendon repair: a review. *Discov Med.* 2011;12(62):75–84.
4. Soomekh DJ. Current concepts for the use of platelet-rich plasma in the foot and ankle. *Clin Podiatr Med Surg.* 2011;28(1):155–170.
5. Fortier LA, et al. The role of growth factors in cartilage repair. *Clin Orthop Relat Res.* 2011;469(10):2706–2715.
6. Dhillon MS, et al. Orthobiologics and platelet rich plasma. *Indian J Orthop.* 2014;48(1):1–9.
7. De Mos M, van der Windt AE, Johr H, et al. Can platelet-rich plasma enhace tendon repair? A cell culture study. *Am J Sports Med.* 2008;36:1171–1178.
8. Visser LC, Arnoczky SP, Caballero O, Kern A, Ratcliffe A, Gardner KL. Growth factor-rich palsma increases tendon cell proliferation and matrix synthesis on a synthetic scaffold: an in vitro study. *Tissue Eng Part A.* 2010;16:1021–1029.
9. Kaux JF, et al. Effects of platelet-rich plasma (PRP) on the healing of Achilles tendons of rats. *Wound Repair Regen.* 2012;20(5):748–756.
10. Sadoghi P, et al. The role of platelets in the treatment of Achillestendon injuries. *J Orthop Res.* 2013;31(1):111–118.
11. Owens Jr RF, et al. Clinical and magnetic resonance imaging outcomes following platelet rich plasma injection for chronic mid substance Achilles tendinopathy. *Foot Ankle Int.* 2011;32(11):1032–1039.
12. de Jonge S, de Vos RJ, Weir A, et al. One-year follow-up of platelet-rich plasma treatment in chronic achilles tendinopathy: a double-blind randomized placebo-controlled trial. *Am J Sports Med.* 2011;39:1623–1629.
13. Schepull T, et al. Autologous platelets have no effect on the healing of human Achilles tendon ruptures: a randomized single-blind study. *Am J Sports Med.* 2011;39(1): 38–47.
14. Lyras DN, et al. The influence of platelet-rich plasma on angiogenesis during the early phase of tendon healing. *Foot Ankle Int.* 2009;30(11):1101–1106.
15. Aspenberg P, Virchenko O. Platelet concentrate injection improves Achilles tendon repair in rats. *Acta Orthop Scand.* 2004;75(1):93–99.
16. Filardo G, et al. Nonoperative biological treatment approach for partial Achilles tendon lesion. *Orthopedics.* 2010;33(2):120–123.
17. Tohidnezhad M, et al. Platelet-released growth factors can accelerate tenocyte proliferation and activate the anti-oxidant response element. *Histochem Cell Biol.* 2011;135(5):453–460.
18. Broese M, et al. Seeding a human tendon matrix with bone marrow aspirates compared to previously isolated hBMSCs—an in vitro study. *Technol Health Care.* 2011;19(6):469–479.
19. Stein BE, Stroh DA, Schon LC. *Int Orthop (SICOT).* 2015;39:901. https://doi.org/10.1007/s00264-015-2725-7.
20. Okamoto N, Kushida T, Oe K, Umeda M, Ikehara S, Iida H. Treating achilles tendon rupture in rats with bone-marrow-cell transplantation. *Ther Bone Joint Surg Am.* 2010;92(17):2776–2784.
21. Jia X, Peters PG, Schon L. The use of platelet-rich plasma in the management of foot and ankle conditions. *Oper Tech Sports Med.* 2011;19:177–184.
22. Yao J, Woon CY, Behn A, et al. The effect of suture coated with mesenchymal stem cells and bioactive substrate on tendon repair strength in a rat model. *J Hand Surg Am.* 2012;37:1639–1645.
23. Breitbach M, Bostani T, Roell W, et al. Potential risks of bone marrow cell transplantation into infarcted hearts. *Blood.* 2007;110:1362–1369.
24. Lee JH, Kim HG, Lee WJ. Characterization and tissue incorporation of cross-linked human acellular dermal matrix. *Biomaterials.* 2015:195–205.
25. Carlson TL, Lee KW, Pierce LM. Effect of cross-linked and non-cross-linked acellular dermal matrices on the expression of mediators involved in wound healing and matrix remodeling. *Plast Reconstr Surg.* 2013;131:697–705.
26. Aurora A, McCarron J, Iannotti JP, Derwin K. Commercially available extracellular matrix materials for rotator cuff repairs: state of the art and future trends. *J Shoulder Elbow Surg.* 2007;16:S171–S178.
27. Lee DK. A preliminary study on the effects of acellular tissue graft augmentation in acute Achilles tendon ruptures. *J Foot Ankle Surg.* 2008;47(1):8–12.
28. Cole C, Seto C, Gazewood J. Plantar fasciitis: evidence-based review of diagnosis and therapy. *Am Fam Phys.* 2005;72:2237–2242,2247-8.
29. Monto R. Plasma-rich plasma and plantar fasciitis. *Sports Med Arthrosc Rev.* 2013;21:220–224.
30. Cutts S, Obi N, Pasapula C, et al. Plantar fasciitis. *Ann R Coll Surg Engl.* 2012;94:539–542.
31. DiGiovanni BF, Nawoczenski DA, Lintal ME, et al. Tissue-specific plantar fasciastretching exercise enhances outcomes in patients with chronic heel pain. A prospective, randomized study. *J Bone Joint Surg Am.* 2003;85(1): 270–277.
32. Speed CA, Nichols D, Wies J, Humphreys H, et al. Extracorporeal shock wave therapy for plantar fasciitis. A double blind randomised controlled trial. *J Orthop Res.* 2003;21:937–940.
33. Haake M, Buch M, Schoellner C, et al. Extracorporeal shock wave therapy for plantar fasciitis: randomised controlled multicentre trial. *Br Med J.* 2003;327:75.

34. Soomekh D. Current concepts for the use of platelet-rich plasma in the foot and ankle. *Clin Podiatr Med Surg.* 2011;28:155–170.
35. Chiew SK, Ramasamy TS, Amini F. Effectiveness and relevant factors of platelet-rich plasma treatment in managing plantar fasciitis: a systematic review. *J Res Med Sci.* 2016;21:38.
36. Gogna P, Gaba S, Mukhopadhyay R, et al. Plantar fasciitis: a randomized comparative study of platelet rich plasma and low dose radiation in sportspersons. *Foot (Edinb).* 2016;28:16–19.
37. Vahdatpour B, Kianimehr L, Moradi A, et al. Beneficial effects of platelet-rich plasma on improvement of pain severity and physical disability in patients with plantar fasciitis: a randomized trial. *Adv Biomed Res.* 2016;5:179.
38. Shetty VD, Dhillon M, Hegde C, et al. A study to compare the efficacy of corticosteroid therapy with platelet-rich plasma therapy in recalcitrant plantar fasciitis: a preliminary report. *Foot Ankle Surg.* 2014;20:10–13.
39. Carballo C, Nakagawa Y, Sekiya I, et al. Basic science of articular cartilage. *Clin Sports Med.* 2017;36:413–425.
40. Johnstone B, Alini M, Cucchiarini M, et al. Tissue engineering for articular cartilage repair—the state of the art. *Eur Cell Mater.* 2013;25:248–267.
41. Kraeutler MJ, Kaenkumchorn T, Pascual-Garrido C, et al. Peculiarities in ankle cartilage. *Cartilage.* 2017;8:12–18.
42. Kuettner KE, Cole AA. Cartilage degeneration in different human joints. *Osteoarthr Cartil.* 2005;13:93–103.
43. Hannon CP, Smyth NA, Murawski CD, et al. Osteochondral lesions of the talus. *Bone Joint J.* 2014;96-B:164–171.
44. Furukawa T, Eyre DR, Koide S, Glimcher MJ. Biochemical studies on repair cartilage resurfacing experimental defects in the rabbit knee. *J Bone Joint Surg.* 1980;62-A:79–89.
45. Chuckpaiwong B, Berkson EM, Theodore GH. Microfracture for osteochondral lesions of the ankle: outcome analysis and outcome predictors of 105 cases. *Arthroscopy.* 2008;24:106–112.
46. Choi WJ, Park KK, Kim BS, Lee JW. Osteochondral lesion of the talus: is there a critical defect size for poor outcome? *Am J Sports Med.* 2009;37(10):1974–1980.
47. Looze C, Capo J, Ryan M, et al. Evaluation and management of osteochondral lesions of the talus. *Cartilage.* 2017;8:19–30.
48. Pearsall 4th AW, Tucker JA, Hester RB, Heitman RJ. Chondrocyte viability in refrigerated osteochondral allografts used for transplantation within the knee. *Am J Sports Med.* 2004;32:125–131.
49. Imhoff AB, Paul J, Ottinger B, et al. Osteochondral transplantation of the talus long-term clinical and magnetic resonance imaging evaluation. *Am J Sports Med.* 2011;39:1487–1493.
50. El-Rashidy H, Villacis D, Omar I, et al. Fresh osteochondral allograft for the treatment of cartilage defects of the talus: a retrospective review. *J Bone Joint Surg Am.* 2011;93:1634–1640.
51. Bertasi G, Cole W, Samsell B, Qin X, Moore M. Biological incorporation of human acellular dermal matrix used in Achilles tendon repair. *Cell Tissue Bank.* 2017;4:28–33.
52. Arner JW, Santrock RD. A historical review of common bone graft materials in foot and ankle surgery. *Foot Ankle Spec.* 2014;7(2):143–151.
53. DiDomenico LA, Thomas ZM. Osteobiologics in foot and ankle surgery. *Clin Podiatr Med Surg.* 2015;32(1):1–19.
54. Kopp FJ, Banks MA, Marcus RE. Clinical outcome of tibiotalar arthrodesis utilizing the chevron technique. *Foot Ankle Int.* 2004;25(4):225–230.
55. Davies MB, Rosenfeld PF, Stavrou P, Saxby TS. A comprehensive review of subtalar arthrodesis. *Foot Ankle Int.* 2007;28(3):295–297.
56. Danziger MB, Abdo RV, Decker JE. Distal tibia bone graft for arthrodesis of the foot and ankle. *Foot Ankle Int.* 1995;16(4):187–190.
57. Thompson IM, Bohay DR, Anderson JG. Fusion rate of first tarsometatarsal arthrodesis in the modified Lapidus procedure and flatfoot reconstruction. *Foot Ankle Int.* 2005;26(9):698–703.
58. Soohoo NF, Cracchiolo 3rd A. The results of utilizing proximal tibial bone graft in reconstructive procedures of the foot and ankle. *Foot Ankle Surg.* 2008;14(2):62–66.
59. Fitzgibbons TC, Hawks MA, McMullen ST, Inda DJ. Bone grafting in surgery about the foot and ankle: indications and techniques. *J Am Acad Orthop Surg.* 2011;19(2):112–120.
60. DeOrio JK, Farber DC. Morbidity associated with anterior iliac crest bone grafting in foot and ankle surgery. *Foot Ankle Int.* 2005;26(2):147–151.
61. Younger EM, Chapman MW. Morbidity at bone graft donor sites. *J Orthop Trauma.* 1989;3(3):192–195.
62. Yeoh JC, Taylor BA. Osseous healing in foot and ankle surgery with autograft, allograft, and other orthobiologics. *Orthop Clin North Am.* 2017;48(3):359–369.
63. Beuerlein MJ, McKee MD. Calcium sulfates: what is the evidence? *J Orthop Trauma.* 2010;24(suppl 1):S46–S51.
64. Larsson S. Calcium phosphates: what is the evidence? *J Orthop Trauma.* 2010;24(suppl 1):S41–S45.
65. Shibuya N, Jupiter DC. Bone graft substitute: allograft and xenograft. *Clin Podiatr Med Surg.* 2015;32(1):21–34.
66. Dolan CM, Henning JA, Anderson JG, Bohay DR, Kornmesser MJ, Endres TJ. Randomized prospective study comparing tri-cortical iliac crest autograft to allograft in the lateral column lengthening component for operative correction of adult acquired flatfoot deformity. *Foot Ankle Int.* 2007;28(1):8–12.
67. Carr JB, Hansen ST, Benirschke SK. Subtalar distraction bone block fusion for late complications of os calcis fractures. *Foot Ankle.* 1988;9(2):81–86.
68. Bednarz PA, Beals TC, Manoli 2nd A. Subtalar distraction bone block fusion: an assessment of outcome. *Foot Ankle Int.* 1997;18(12):785–791.

69. Schepers T. The subtalar distraction bone block arthrodesis following the late complications of calcaneal fractures: a systematic review. *Foot (Edinb)*. 2013;23(1):39–44.

70. Trnka HJ, Easley ME, Lam PW, Anderson CD, Schon LC, Myerson MS. Subtalar distraction bone block arthrodesis. *J Bone Joint Surg Br*. 2001;83(6):849–854.

71. Lin SS, Montemurro NJ, Krell ES. Orthobiologics in foot and ankle surgery. *J Am Acad Orthop Surg*. 2016;24(2):113–122.

72. Daniels T, DiGiovanni C, Lau JT, Wing K, Younger A. Prospective clinical pilot trial in a single cohort group of rhPDGF in foot arthrodeses. *Foot Ankle Int*. 2010;31(6):473–479.

73. Daniels TR, Younger AS, Penner MJ, et al. Prospective randomized controlled trial of hindfoot and ankle fusions treated with rhPDGF-BB in combination with a beta-TCP-collagen matrix. *Foot Ankle Int*. 2015;36(7):739–748.

74. Digiovanni CW, Baumhauer J, Lin SS, et al. Prospective, randomized, multi-center feasibility trial of rhPDGF-BB versus autologous bone graft in a foot and ankle fusion model. *Foot Ankle Int*. 2011;32(4):344–354.

75. DiGiovanni CW, Lin SS, Daniels TR, et al. The importance of sufficient graft material in achieving foot or ankle fusion. *J Bone Joint Surg Am*. 2016;98(15):1260–1267.

76. Younger A, Penner M, Montijo HE. Vancouver experience of recombinant human platelet-derived growth factor. *Foot Ankle Clin*. 2016;21(4):771–776.

77. Sun H, Lu PP, Zhou PH, et al. Recombinant human platelet-derived growth factor-BB versus autologous bone graft in foot and ankle fusion: a systematic review and meta-analysis. *Foot Ankle Surg*. 2017;23(1):32–39.

78. DiGiovanni CW, Lin SS, Baumhauer JF, et al. Recombinant human platelet-derived growth factor-BB and beta-tricalcium phosphate (rhPDGF-BB/beta-TCP): an alternative to autogenous bone graft. *J Bone Joint Surg Am*. 2013;95(13):1184–1192.

79. Lee DH, Ryu KJ, Kim JW, Kang KC, Choi YR. Bone marrow aspirate concentrate and platelet-rich plasma enhanced bone healing in distraction osteogenesis of the tibia. *Clin Orthop Relat Res*. 2014;472(12):3789–3797.

80. Braly HL, O'Connor DP, Brinker MR. Percutaneous autologous bone marrow injection in the treatment of distal meta-diaphyseal tibial nonunions and delayed unions. *J Orthop Trauma*. 2013;27(9):527–533.

81. Murawski CD, Kennedy JG. Percutaneous internal fixation of proximal fifth metatarsal jones fractures (Zones II and III) with Charlotte Carolina screw and bone marrow aspirate concentrate: an outcome study in athletes. *Am J Sports Med*. 2011;39(6):1295–1301.

82. Bibbo C, Nelson J, Ehrlich D, Rougeux B. Bone morphogenetic proteins: indications and uses. *Clin Podiatr Med Surg*. 2015;32(1):35–43.

83. Bibbo C, Patel DV, Haskell MD. Recombinant bone morphogenetic protein-2 (rhBMP-2) in high-risk ankle and hindfoot fusions. *Foot Ankle Int*. 2009;30(7):597–603.

84. Rearick T, Charlton TP, Thordarson D. Effectiveness and complications associated with recombinant human bone morphogenetic Protein-2 augmentation of foot and ankle fusions and fracture nonunions. *Foot Ankle Int*. 2014;35(8):783–788.

85. Mahan KT, Hillstrom HJ. Bone grafting in foot and ankle surgery. A review of 300 cases. *J Am Podiatr Med Assoc*. 1998;88(3):109–118.

86. McCormack AP, Niki H, Kiser P, Tencer AF, Sangeorzan BJ. Two reconstructive techniques for flatfoot deformity comparing contact characteristics of the hindfoot joints. *Foot Ankle Int*. 1998;19(7):452–461.

87. Danko AM, Allen Jr B, Pugh L, Stasikelis P. Early graft failure in lateral column lengthening. *J Pediatr Orthop*. 2004;24(6):716–720.

88. Cook EA, Cook JJ. Bone graft substitutes and allografts for reconstruction of the foot and ankle. *Clin Podiatr Med Surg*. 2009;26(4):589–605.

89. Trelford JD, Hanson FW, Anderson DG. Amniotic membrane as a living surgical dressing in human patients. *Oncology*. 1973;28(4):358–364.

90. Snyder RJ, Shimozaki K, Tallis A, et al. A prospective, randomized, multicenter, controlled evaluation of the use of dehydrated amniotic membrane allograft compared to standard of care for the closure of chronic diabetic foot ulcer. *Wounds*. 2016;28(3):70–77.

91. Rosenblum BI. A retrospective case series of a dehydrated amniotic membrane allograft for treatment of unresolved diabetic foot ulcers. *J Am Podiatr Med Assoc*. 2016;106(5):328–337.

92. Raphael AA. single-centre, retrospective study of cryopreserved umbilical cord/amniotic membrane tissue for the treatment of diabetic foot ulcers. *J Wound Care*. 2016;25(suppl 7):S10–S17.

93. Single-center Couture MA. Retrospective study of cryopreserved umbilical cord for wound healing in patients suffering from chronic wounds of the foot and ankle. *Wounds*. 2016;28(7):217–225.

94. Abdo RJ. Treatment of diabetic foot ulcers with dehydrated amniotic membrane allograft: a prospective case series. *J Wound Care*. 2016;25(suppl 7):S4–S9.

95. Kirsner RS, Sabolinski ML, Parsons NB, Skornicki M, Marston WA. Comparative effectiveness of a bioengineered living cellular construct vs. a dehydrated human amniotic membrane allograft for the treatment of diabetic foot ulcers in a real world setting. *Wound Repair Regen*. 2015;23(5):737–744.

96. Warner M, Lasyone L. An open-label, single-center, retrospective study of cryopreserved amniotic membrane and umbilical cord tissue as an adjunct for foot and ankle surgery. *Surg Technol Int*. 2014;25:251–255.

97. Shah AP. Using amniotic membrane allografts in the treatment of neuropathic foot ulcers. *J Am Podiatr Med Assoc*. 2014;104(2):198–202.

98. Zelen CM, Serena TE, Denoziere G, Fetterolf DE. A prospective randomised comparative parallel study of amniotic membrane wound graft in the management of diabetic foot ulcers. *Int Wound J.* 2013;10(5): 502–507.

99. Werber B, Martin E. A prospective study of 20 foot and ankle wounds treated with cryopreserved amniotic membrane and fluid allograft. *J Foot Ankle Surg.* 2013;52(5):615–621.

100. Garras DN, Scott RT. Plantar fasciitis treatment with particulated human amniotic memebrane. *Foot & Ankle Orthopaedics.* 2016;1(1):2473011416S2473000245.

101. Covell DJ, Cohen B, Ellington JK, Jones CP, Davis WH, Anderson RB. The use of cryo-preserved umbilical cord plus amniotic membrane tissues in the resection of tarsal coalition. *Foot & Ankle Orthopaedics.* 2016;1(1): 2473011416S2473000311.

101. Hanselman AE, Tidwell JE, Santrock RD. Cryopreserved human amniotic membrane injection for plantar fasciitis: a randomized, controlled, double-blind pilot study. *Foot Ankle Int.* 2015;36(2):151–158.

103. Zelen CM, Poka A, Andrews J. Prospective, randomized, blinded, comparative study of injectable micronized dehydrated amniotic/chorionic membrane allograft for plantar fasciitis—a feasibility study. *Foot & Ankle International.* 2013;34(10):1332–1339.

CHAPTER 17

Biologics in Fracture Care

STEPHEN L. DAVIS, MD

INTRODUCTION

Fractures are a common cause of morbidity, lost productivity in the work force, and a significant driver of costs in the medical economy.[1] Although exact numbers are difficult to identify, one Finnish registry study reported 53.4 fractures per 1000 person-years in women and 24.9 per 1000 person-years in men.[2] Delayed healing and nonunion remain as significant complications in the treatment of fractures. Reported rates of delayed healing and nonunion approach 600,000 and 100,000 per year, respectively, in the United States alone.[3]

Considerable research has been dedicated to improving the ultimate healing rate of fractures and preventing complications. Biologic augmentation and supplementation in the treatment of fractures is a pivotal area of development. The U.S. Food and Drug Administration definition of biologic treatment for fractures covers a wide range of therapies, including blood and blood components, stem cells, tissue grafts, recombinant proteins, and gene therapies.[4] Biologic treatments in general are aimed at enhancing one or more aspects of the natural process of fracture healing. This includes stimulating cells with the capacity to form bone to actually do so (osteoinduction), augmenting the number or availability of cells capable of producing bone (osteogenesis), enhancing vascular growth and proliferation, and providing a scaffold conducive for cellular attachment and bone construction (osteoconductive).[5] Although a comprehensive review of the available literature on biologic treatment of fractures is well beyond the scope of this textbook, this chapter seeks to provide an overview of currently available biologic treatments for fracture care.

WHEN TO CONSIDER BIOLOGIC AUGMENTATION

The majority of fractures (90%–95%) do not require biological enhancement and will heal uneventfully on their own with simple immobilization or standard internal fixation techniques.[6] No definitive indications for biologic augmentation of fracture treatments exist. However, common indications cited in the literature include fracture

nonunion and bony defects.[7,8] Critical sized bone defects, commonly defined as greater than 50% circumferential bone loss or a 2 cm defect, may result from bone loss in open fractures or secondary to resection of infected bone at a fracture site.[9] In either case, the healing potential of the fracture environment is not robust enough to result in bony union, whether the healing response is compromised or the size of the defect exceeds the body's natural capability for fracture healing.

The selection of a particular biological adjuvant will depend on the specific clinical scenario. For instance, bone marrow aspirate (BMA) injection may be useful in the setting of stably fixed, aseptic nonunions of the tibia.[10,11] Segmental defects may require more comprehensive treatment, such as autogenous bone graft, which contains vascular proliferative qualities and includes osteogenic, osteoinductive, and osteoconductive components.[12] Patient factors such as the presence of infection, soft tissue coverage, or other medical problems may influence the decision as well. The remainder of this chapter will discuss the various biologic materials available to solve the clinical problems of nonunion and bone defects.

Autograft

Autograft is currently regarded as the gold standard for treatment of nonunions and bone defects and is the standard against which all other treatments are compared. It has multiple advantages. It is easy to obtain; is cheaper than most commercially available substitutes; is osteogenic, osteoinductive, and osteoconductive; and has a long track record of success in the literature. It can be obtained from a variety of anatomic sites, and there is no risk of disease transmission with its use. Disadvantages include donor site morbidity and limitations on available graft volume for large defects.[13] The anterior and posterior iliac crests have historically been the most popular locations for graft harvesting. Chronic pain may be a complication at these sites, although there is evidence to show that the complication rate may be lower than previously reported.[14] The reamer irrigator aspirator (RIA, Synthes, West Chester, PA) is an aspirating reamer that can be used to harvest bone from

Biologics in Orthopaedic Surgery. https://doi.org/10.1016/B978-0-323-55140-3.00017-5

the intramedullary canal of the femur. There is evidence that bone harvested from the femur using the RIA has a higher concentration of growth factors than does iliac crest autograft.[15] Higher volumes may be harvested using the RIA, as well.[16] Studies have shown that the stem cells obtained from these reamings display similar osteogenic potential when compared with more conventionally harvested bone marrow stem cells.[17] It has also been shown that the waste fluid from the RIA has elevated levels of osteoprotegerin, osteocalcin, and osteopontin, which are all known stimulators of bone formation.[18] There is also level 1 evidence showing equivalent union rates and increased graft volume using the RIA compared with anterior iliac crest graft.[19] Unique complications are possible, however, including iatrogenic femur fracture and exsanguination if appropriate technique is not used.[20]

BONE VOID FILLERS

Synthetic bone void fillers, for the purposes of this chapter, are considered as biologic adjuvants because they provide an osteoconductive matrix to facilitate proliferation of bone.[21] Some help to provide mechanical support, whereas others are meant to act as carriers for autogenous grafts, such as BMA.[22] Bone void fillers, for example calcium phosphate and calcium sulfate, have no osteoinductive or osteogenic properties and may pose a challenge in the treatment of infections, as they can be difficult to completely remove without destroying normal bone.

Calcium phosphate is an injectable paste that hardens in the warm environment in the body, forming a mineral similar to, but with a higher compressive strength than, the mineral phase of bone.[22] It is commonly used to augment fixation and stabilize metaphyseal defects, especially in the setting of periarticular fractures such as in the tibial plateau or distal radius.[23] It is especially useful to support depressed articular fragments after reduction.[24] There is level 1 evidence supporting the use of calcium phosphate over autogenous graft for preventing subsidence in depressed tibial plateau fractures[25] (Fig. 17.1).

Calcium phosphate is slowly resorbed by osteoclasts and replaced by lamellar bone over a period of usually a year or more.[26] (Fig. 17.2)

Calcium sulfate is another option that typically comes in pellets or a powder that can be mixed with autogenous graft sources or powdered antibiotics and then molded into specific shapes. Calcium sulfate differs from calcium phosphate in that it has a lower compressive strength and is resorbed much more

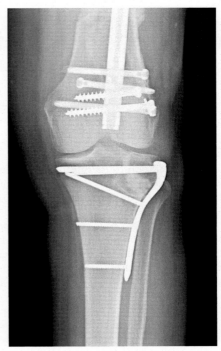

FIG. 17.1 Calcium phosphate cement is visible as radiodense material supporting a large, depressed articular segment in this radiograph of a tibia plateau fracture. The injectable quality of calcium phosphate allows it fill the entirety of a defect and then harden for optimal support of the cavity. (Stephen L. Davis, MD.)

quickly.[27] Because of this rapid resorption and weaker mechanical properties, it is more useful for increasing graft volume and for managing dead space while delivering antibiotics for the treatment of infection.[28] An advantage over the use of poly-methyl methacrylate, which is nonresorbable, for making antibiotic beads is that a second surgery is not required for removal of the beads (Fig. 17.3). However, wound drainage is a reported complication in the use of calcium sulfate.[29]

BONE MORPHOGENIC PROTEIN IN FRACTURE HEALING

Bone morphogenic proteins (BMPs) are a group of signaling molecules that are part of the transforming growth factor beta (TGF-β) family and are known to be strong osteoinductive agents.[30] For this reason there has been a great deal of interest to harness them for clinical use. There are currently two FDA-approved BMP products on the market: recombinant human BMP-2 (rhBMP-2) and recombinant human BMP-7 (rhBMP-7).

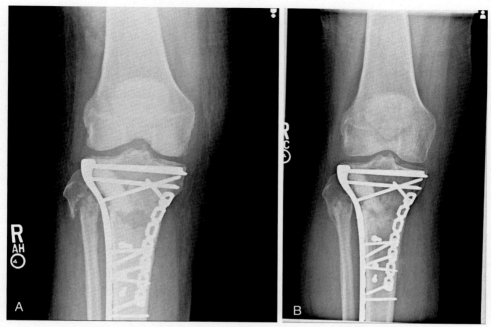

FIG. 17.2 Calcium phosphate is slowly resorbed from bone, as seen in radiographs of this tibia plateau fracture at 2 weeks postoperative **(A)** and at 8 months postoperative **(B)** (Stephen L. Davis, MD.)

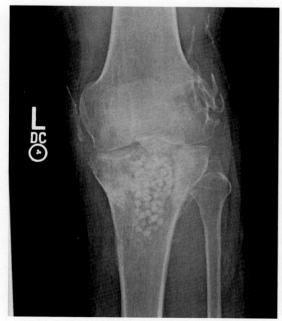

FIG. 17.3 Calcium sulfate beads mixed with antibiotics for the treatment of osteomyelitis of the proximal tibia. (Stephen L. Davis, MD)

Two of the most notable randomized clinical trials investigating the use of rhBMP-2 are the BESTT trial[31] and the BESTT-ALL[32] trial. The BESTT trial reported on the effect of three treatment groups for open tibial shaft fracture: standard intramedullary nailing, intramedullary nailing plus rhBMP-2 in an absorbable collagen sponge at a concentration of 0.75 mg/mL, and intramedullary nailing plus rhBMP-2 in an absorbable collagen sponge at a concentration of 1.50 mg/mL. A total of 450 patients were randomized to these three groups, and a dose-dependent decrease in secondary intervention was observed. Additionally, a 21% increase in union rate at 6 months was found in the 1.50 mg/mL group when compared with control. Finally, there was a significant decrease in infection rate for Gustilo-Anderson type IIIA and IIIB fractures when the 1.50 mg/mL group was compared with control. It is difficult to determine at this time if a true relationship exists between BMP and infection prevention.

In the BEST-ALL trial, 30 patients with an average 4 cm residual cortical defect following intramedullary nailing for tibial shaft fractures were treated with either ICBG or a combination of allografts chips with an overlay of rhBMP-2 on an absorbable collagen sponge at a mean of 11 weeks after original nailing. The results were statistically equivalent between the two groups with union observed in 10/15 in the ICBG group and 13/15 in the rhBMP-2 group. No difference was found in functional outcomes.

Studies regarding rhBMP-7 have primarily focused on aseptic nonunion of the tibia. A randomized controlled trial comparing application of rhBMP-7 versus standard autograft (ICBG) found similar rates of union (81% and 84%) when used in conjunction with intramedullary nailing of tibial shaft nonunions.[33] These results have been replicated in some case series, with a union rate of 89%[34] seen for rhBMP-7 application with revision internal fixation of tibial shaft nonunion and a union rate of 87%[35] seen for rhBMP-7 with revision fixation of long bone nonunion.

In summary, the literature supports the use of rhBMP-7 as a viable alternative to autogenous bone graft in long bone nonunion, although there should certainly be consideration for the increased price. The use of rhBMP-2 should likely be restricted to use in Gustilo-Anderson type III open fractures of the tibia.

CELL-BASED THERAPY

One of the more researched and promising biologics to aid fracture healing is cell-based therapy, commonly referred to as "stem cell" therapy. In this treatment, progenitor cells consisting of either mesenchymal stem cells (MSCs) and/or connective tissue progenitor cells (CTPs) are delivered to a site of fracture or nonunion to aid in healing. MSCs are multipotent cells that have the capability of dividing into osteoblasts, tenocytes, myoblasts, chondrocytes, fibroblasts, and adipocytes.[36] MSCs are truly "stem cells" in that they can self-replicate. CTPs, on the other hand, are multipotent and capable of differentiating into all the above-listed cell lineages but have lost the ability to self-replicate. The rationale behind cell-based therapy is that delivery of a healthy population of cells that are capable of differentiation into mature osteoblasts can help to form bone at an atrophic nonunion site that is lacking in biology.

These cells can be obtained and delivered different ways. The first, and more common, method is BMA. BMA contains both MSCs and CTPs in varying concentrations. BMA is typically harvested via a minimally invasive technique using a cannula directed into the iliac crest and has the advantage of less donor site morbidity than traditional iliac crest bone graft harvesting. It then can be either delivered to the operative site directly (BMA) or after concentration via centrifuge (concentrated bone marrow aspirate [cBMA]). The optimal amount of progenitor cells is unknown, but there is evidence to suggest that a minimum concentration of 1500 progenitors per cm^3 may be needed to adequately stimulate bony healing, which is a concentration that could only be reached with centrifugation.[37] A recent systematic review found support for the use of cBMA in a range of clinical applications including nonunion. This study also importantly noted that the exact concentrations and centrifugation settings remain highly variable across studies.[38] Much of the literature for this reason has focused on cBMA.

Another therapy involves isolation of MSCs from BMA. There are various ways to isolate MSCs from BMA; however, the details of this process are out of the scope of this chapter. Growth factors can be added to the MSCs in vitro to help steer differentiation into an osteocyte lineage. A recent study using a murine nonunion model demonstrated improved bone formation and torsional stiffness after delivering cultured MSCs to the nonunion in a fibrin glue matrix.[39] This type of therapy, while exciting, is mostly experimental at this point given the increased complexity and processing involved in the use of isolated and cultured MSCs. For this reason, most human cell-based therapy is limited to BMA.

There are three general clinical scenarios in which cell-based therapy can be used to aid fracture healing. One is at the time of fixation for an acute fracture. A second is percutaneous injection into a site of nonunion. A third is augmentation of graft products during revision open reduction internal fixation for a nonunion.

There is limited evidence to support BMA in the treatment of acute fractures without critical sized defects. A randomized controlled trial of patients with extra-articular distal tibia fractures investigated the difference between treatment with surgery alone or surgery plus injection of a mixture of Platelet rich plasma (PRP), MSCs, and demineralized bone matrix (DBM) at 3–6 weeks after the index procedure.[40] Treatment with cell-based therapy showed a statistically significant decrease in time to clinical and radiographic union. There were no nonunions in either group, raising questions as to the cost-effectiveness of the treatment.

Percutaneous injection of BMA for treatment of aseptic, atrophic nonunions has more literature support. A retrospective study demonstrated a 79.6% rate of union after percutaneous injection of cBMA into the site of long bone nonunion.[41] Similar studies have shown union rates of 82%,[42] 60%,[43] 95%,[44] 50%,[45] 67%,[10] and 75%[46] following percutaneous injection of BMA. Most of these studies are retrospective with small sample sizes. However, there is a trend showing improved clinical and radiographic union rates for aseptic long bone nonunions.

BMA can also be used with bone void fillers or other graft carriers in the setting of revision open reduction and internal fixation for nonunions. Autograft, usually from the iliac crest, is still the accepted gold standard in this situation. However, there has been interest in using cBMA in place of standard ICBG. One study compared a series of 10 patients with atrophic nonunions treated with open reduction internal fixation (ORIF) augmented with either cBMA mixed with hydroxyapatite crystals or standard ICBG. Both groups showed equivalent results in radiographic union, pain scores, and functional outcomes at 12 months.[47]

SUMMARY

There is good support in the literature for the use of biologic adjuvants to promote healing in the setting of fracture care. The ideal type, timing, and method of application all remain unclear but likely depend on the specific clinical scenario.

Autogenous bone graft remains the gold standard for treatment of a variety of conditions, including nonunion and small critical sized defects. Iliac crest bone graft has a long track record of success, but intramedullary reamings show good promise for the future.

Bone void fillers are useful for filling bony defects, providing an osteoconductive matrix, and augmenting the stability of internal fixation. They also are helpful for augmenting the volume of graft for filling bony defects and delivering antibiotics to the site of deep infection while managing dead space.

BMA can be used either as percutaneous injection into a nonunion site or mixed with bone void fillers at the time of revision ORIF as an alternative to open autograft bone grafting. There is growing support in the literature for its use. BMP use in the treatment of fractures is currently indicated only for high-grade open tibia fractures or tibial shaft nonunion, although careful consideration of cost may limit its use. The evidence to use biologics in the setting of acute fracture without critical-sized defects is less compelling, and certainly cost and donor site morbidity are both a consideration.

Although not discussed in this chapter, the induced membrane technique shows great promise for reconstruction of critical-sized defects and can be utilized with autograft, BMP, cell-based therapies, and bone void fillers. A full discussion of the induced membrane technique is beyond the scope of this chapter, as there is extensive literature supporting its use and largely replacing bone transport and other techniques for treatment of large bone defects.

Future directions for biologic treatment of fractures include investigations into systemic administration of antisclerostin antibody, anti-Dkk-1 antibody, recombinant parathyroid hormone (PTH), and gene therapy, to name a few. At this point, these types of treatments remain highly experimental but are exciting and may play a substantial role in human fracture care of the future.

REFERENCES

1. Heckman JD, Sarasohn-kahn J. The economics of treating tibia fractures. The cost of delayed unions. *Bull Hosp Jt Dis.* 1997;56(1):63–72.
2. Piirtola M, Vahlberg T, Isoaho R, Aarnio P, Kivelä SL. Incidence of fractures and changes over time among the aged in a Finnish municipality: a population-based 12-year follow-up. *Aging Clin Exp Res.* 2007;19(4):269–276.
3. Miranda MA, Moon MS. Treatment strategy for nonunions and malunions. In: Stannard JP, Schmidt AH, Kregor PJ, eds. *Surgical Treatment of Orthopaedic Trauma.* Vol. 1. New York, NY: Thieme; 2007:77–100.
4. Virk MS, Lieberman JR. Biologic adjuvants for fracture healing. *Arthritis Res Ther.* 2012;14(6):225.
5. Lieberman JR. Orthopaedic gene therapy. Fracture healing and other nongenetic problems of bone. *Clin Orthop Relat Res.* 2000;(suppl 379):S156–S158.
6. Axelrad TW, Kakar S, Einhorn TA. New technologies for the enhancement of skeletal repair. *Injury.* 2007;38(suppl 1):S49–S62.
7. Emara KM, Diab RA, Emara AK. Recent biological trends in management of fracture non-union. *World J Orthop.* 2015;6(8):623–628.
8. Bostrom MP, Saleh KJ, Einhorn TA. Osteoinductive growth factors in preclinical fracture and long bone defects models. *Orthop Clin North Am.* 1999;30(4):647–658.
9. Mackenzie EJ, Jones AS, Bosse MJ, et al. Health-care costs associated with amputation or reconstruction of a limb-threatening injury. *J Bone Joint Surg Am.* 2007;89(8):1685–1692.
10. Braly HL, O'connor DP, Brinker MR. Percutaneous autologous bone marrow injection in the treatment of distal meta-diaphyseal tibial nonunions and delayed unions. *J Orthop Trauma.* 2013;27(9):527–533.
11. Hernigou P, Mathieu G, Poignard A, Manicom O, Beaujean F, Rouard H. Percutaneous autologous bone-marrow grafting for nonunions. Surgical technique. *J Bone Joint Surg Am.* 2006;88(suppl 1 Pt 2):322–327.
12. Schwartz AM, Schenker ML, Ahn J, Willett NJ. Building better bone: the weaving of biologic and engineering strategies for managing bone loss. *J Orthop Res.* 2017.
13. Cyril M, Barlow BT, Smith W. Management of segmental bone defects. *JAAOS.* 2015;(23):143–153.
14. Loeffler BJ, Kellam JF, Sims SH, Bosse MJ. Prospective observational study of donor-site morbidity following anterior iliac crest bone-grafting in orthopaedic trauma reconstruction patients. *J Bone Joint Surg Am.* 2012;94(18):1649–1654.

15. Sagi HC, Young ML, Gerstenfeld L, Einhorn TA, Tornetta P. Qualitative and quantitative differences between bone graft obtained from the medullary canal (with a Reamer/Irrigator/Aspirator) and the iliac crest of the same patient. *J Bone Joint Surg Am.* 2012;94(23):2128–2135.
16. Belthur MV, Conway JD, Jindal G, Ranade A, Herzenberg JE. Bone graft harvest using a new intramedullary system. *Clin Orthop Relat Res.* 2008;466(12):2973–2980.
17. Kuehlfluck P, Moghaddam A, Helbig L, et al. RIA fractions contain mesenchymal stroma cells with high osteogenic potency. *Injury.* 2015;46(suppl 8):S23–S32.
18. Crist BD, Stoker AM, Stannard JP, Cook JL. Analysis of relevant proteins from bone graft harvested using the reamer irrigator and aspirator system (RIA) versus iliac crest (IC) bone graft and RIA waste water. *Injury.* 2016;47(8):1661–1668.
19. Dawson J, Kiner D, Gardner W, Swafford R, Nowotarski PJ. The reamer-irrigator-aspirator as a device for harvesting bone graft compared with iliac crest bone graft: union rates and complications. *J Orthop Trauma.* 2014;28(10):584–590.
20. Dimitriou R, Mataliotakis GI, Angoules AG, Kanakaris NK, Giannoudis PV. Complications following autologous bone graft harvesting from the iliac crest and using the RIA: a systematic review. *Injury.* 2011;42(suppl 2):S3–S15.
21. Bajada S, Harrison PE, Ashton BA, Cassar-pullicino VN, Ashammakhi N, Richardson JB. Successful treatment of refractory tibial nonunion using calcium sulphate and bone marrow stromal cell implantation. *J Bone Joint Surg Br.* 2007;89(10):1382–1386.
22. Hak DJ. The use of osteoconductive bone graft substitutes in orthopaedic trauma. *J Am Acad Orthop Surg.* 2007;15(9):525–536.
23. Dickson KF, Friedman J, Buchholz JG, Flandry FD. The use of bone source hydroxyapatite cement for traumatic metaphyseal bone void filling. *J Trauma.* 2002;53(6):1103–1108.
24. Lobenhoffer P, Gerich T, Witte F, Tscherne H. Use of an injectable calcium phosphate bone cement in the treatment of tibial plateau fractures: a prospective study of twenty-six cases with twenty-month mean follow-up. *J Orthop Trauma.* 2002;16(3):143–149.
25. Russell TA, Leighton RK. Comparison of autogenous bone graft and endothermic calcium phosphate cement for defect augmentation in tibial plateau fractures. A multicenter, prospective, randomized study. *J Bone Joint Surg Am.* 2008;90(10):2057–2061.
26. Frankenburg EP, Goldstein SA, Bauer TW, Harris SA, Poser RD. Biomechanical and histological evaluation of a calcium phosphate cement. *J Bone Joint Surg Am.* 1998;80(8):1112–1124.
27. Walsh WR, Morberg P, Yu Y, et al. Response of a calcium sulfate bone graft substitute in a confined cancellous defect. *Clin Orthop Relat Res.* 2003;406:228–236.
28. Turner TM, Urban RM, Gitelis S, Kuo KN, Andersson GB. Radiographic and histologic assessment of calcium sulfate in experimental animal models and clinical use as a resorbable bone-graft substitute, a bone-graft expander, and a method for local antibiotic delivery. One institution's experience. *J Bone Joint Surg Am.* 2001;83-A(suppl 2(Pt 1)):8–18.
29. Kelly CM, Wilkins RM, Gitelis S, Hartjen C, Watson JT, Kim PT. The use of a surgical grade calcium sulfate as a bone graft substitute: results of a multicenter trial. *Clin Orthop Relat Res.* 2001;382:42–50.
30. Wang EA, Rosen V, D'alessandro JS, et al. Recombinant human bone morphogenetic protein induces bone formation. *Proc Natl Acad Sci USA.* 1990;87(6):2220–2224.
31. Govender S, Csimma C, Genant HK, et al. Recombinant human bone morphogenetic protein-2 for treatment of open tibial fractures: a prospective, controlled, randomized study of four hundred and fifty patients. *J Bone Joint Surg Am.* 2002;84-A(12):2123–2134.
32. Jones AL, Bucholz RW, Bosse MJ, et al. Recombinant human BMP-2 and allograft compared with autogenous bone graft for reconstruction of diaphyseal tibial fractures with cortical defects. A randomized, controlled trial. *J Bone Joint Surg Am.* 2006;88(7):1431–1441.
33. Friedlaender GE, Perry CR, Cole JD, et al. Osteogenic protein-1 (bone morphogenetic protein-7) in the treatment of tibial nonunions. *J Bone Joint Surg Am.* 2001;83-A(suppl 1(Pt 2)):S151–S158.
34. Kanakaris NK, Calori GM, Verdonk R, et al. Application of BMP-7 to tibial non-unions: a 3-year multicenter experience. *Injury.* 2008;39(suppl 2):S83–S90.
35. Calori GM, Tagliabue L, Gala L, D'imporzano M, Peretti G, Albisetti W. Application of rhBMP-7 and platelet-rich plasma in the treatment of long bone non-unions: a prospective randomised clinical study on 120 patients. *Injury.* 2008;39(12):1391–1402.
36. Pittenger MF, Mackay AM, Beck SC, et al. Multilineage potential of adult human mesenchymal stem cells. *Science.* 1999;284(5411):143–147.
37. Hernigou P, Poignard A, Beaujean F, Rouard H. Percutaneous autologous bone-marrow grafting for nonunions. Influence of the number and concentration of progenitor cells. *J Bone Joint Surg Am.* 2005;87(7):1430–1437.
38. Gianakos AL, Sun L, Patel JN, Adams DM, Liporace FA. Clinical application of concentrated bone marrow aspirate in orthopaedics: a systematic review. *World J Orthop.* 2017;8(6):491–506.
39. Hao C, Wang Y, Shao L, Liu J, Chen L, Zhao Z. Local injection of bone mesenchymal stem cells and fibrin glue promotes the repair of bone atrophic nonunion in vivo. *Adv Ther.* 2016;33(5):824–833.
40. Liebergall M, Schroeder J, Mosheiff R, et al. Stem cell-based therapy for prevention of delayed fracture union: a randomized and prospective preliminary study. *Mol Ther.* 2013;21(8):1631–1638.
41. Desai P, Hasan SM, Zambrana L, et al. Bone mesenchymal stem cells with growth factors successfully treat nonunions and delayed unions. *HSS J.* 2015;11(2):104–111.

42. Hernigou P, Guissou I, Homma Y, et al. Percutaneous injection of bone marrow mesenchymal stem cells for ankle non-unions decreases complications in patients with diabetes. *Int Orthop.* 2015;39(8):1639–1643.

43. Emadedin M, Labibzadeh N, Fazeli R, et al. Percutaneous autologous bone marrow-derived mesenchymal stromal cell implantation is safe for reconstruction of human lower limb long bone atrophic nonunion. *Cell J.* 2017;19(1):159–165.

44. Kassem MS. Percutaneous autogenous bone marrow injection for delayed union or non union of fractures after internal fixation. *Acta Orthop Belg.* 2013;79(6):711–717.

45. Guimarães JA, Duarte ME, Fernandes MB, et al. The effect of autologous concentrated bone-marrow grafting on the healing of femoral shaft non-unions after locked intramedullary nailing. *Injury.* 2014;45(suppl 5): S7–S13.

46. Goel A, Sangwan SS, Siwach RC, Ali AM. Percutaneous bone marrow grafting for the treatment of tibial nonunion. *Injury.* 2005;36(1):203–206.

47. Ismail HD, Phedy P, Kholinne E, et al. Mesenchymal stem cell implantation in atrophic nonunion of the long bones: a translational study. *Bone Joint Res.* 2016;5(7):287–293.

CHAPTER 18

Biologics in Musculoskeletal Oncology

ZACHARY CAVENAUGH, MD • ADAM D. LINDSAY, MD

TARGETED THERAPIES IN ORTHOPEDIC ONCOLOGY

As we continue to learn more about the pathophysiology of bone and soft tissue neoplasms, we are presented with new molecular targets for treatment. No chapter on the use of biologics in musculoskeletal oncology would be complete without a discussion of the use of biologics to treat these tumors. Targeted therapies, which use normal biology to manipulate pathologic genes and proteins, are evolving as an alternative to traditional cytotoxic chemotherapy.

Denosumab Treatment of Giant Cell Tumor of Bone

Giant cell tumor of bone (GCTB) is characterized as a benign, yet locally aggressive, tumor that can result in significant osteolysis and destruction of bone. Previous research has demonstrated that the neoplastic cells responsible for GCTB have roots drawing from aberrant and incomplete differentiation of mesenchymal stem cells along the osteoblast lineage. The histology is characterized by layers of mononuclear cells with high Receptor activator of nuclear factor k-beta (RANK) ligand (RANKL) expression, RANK-positive mononuclear cells of myeloid lineage, and large osteoclast-like giant cells which also express RANK. Each of these histologic features of GCTB makes denosumab an ideal treatment strategy. Denosumab is a human monoclonal antibody that specifically binds to RANK ligand. This provides therapeutic benefit by targeting the two physiologic pathways responsible for the aggressive osteolytic process: (1) reducing the number of RANK-positive giant cells and (2) reducing the number of mononuclear stromal cells that overexpress RANKL, which some authors believe is the true neoplastic cell in GCTB.

Early clinically trials, although small in size, show promising results. One previous cohort study evaluating denosumab treatment for GCTB found no disease progression in 96% (163/169) patients with surgically unsalvageable disease treated only with denosumab.[1] The same study also found that of 100 eligible patients planned for surgical intervention, 74% did not need to undergo surgery after treatment, and of those remaining, 62% underwent a significantly less morbid procedure.

Tyrosine Kinase Inhibitors for Sarcoma

Recent advances in oncologic research have identified angiogenesis as a common pathway, critical in the growth, invasion, and subsequent metastases of multiple tumor types. Multiple growth factors are implicated in both the normal physiologic as well as pathologic processes. The importance of Vascular endothelial growth factor (VEGF) and platelet derived growth factor (PDGF) has been identified as these growth factors initiate a cascade of intracellular signaling that culminates in the stimulation of endothelial cell proliferation, migration, and inhibition of apoptosis. This signaling process occurs through binding the external component of a transmembrane receptor linked to an intercellular tyrosine kinase, which initiates the aforementioned cascade of cellular events.[2]

In sarcomas the interaction between VEGF and its tyrosine kinase receptor has recently been shown to be critical in tumor progression. These growth factors have also demonstrated their utility as prognostic indicators, with higher serum levels of VEGF strongly correlated with the poorest differentiated soft tissue sarcomas,[3,4] and specifically in leiomyosarcoma, higher levels are associated with worse prognosis and shorter survival.[5,6] As a result of these findings, the VEGF tyrosine kinase receptors have emerged as a key target in the development of new anticancer agents within the "cancer cell"–specific therapies. Initial clinical studies evaluating the efficacy of pazopanib in the treatment of soft tissue sarcomas have encouraging early results. A recent phase III trial demonstrated a significant improvement in progression-free survival in patients receiving pazopanib compared with placebo, yet no difference in overall survival was detected in the study.[7] In light of these findings, the FDA approved the use of pazopanib for treatment of patients with advanced soft tissue sarcomas who have previously received chemotherapy. Although these early medications are still in

Biologics in Orthopaedic Surgery. https://doi.org/10.1016/B978-0-323-55140-3.00018-7

the infancy of their development, they serve to high-light the critical clinical significance of these proangio-genic tyrosine kinase receptors and their potential as therapeutic targets to impair and inhibit progression of tumor grown.

VOID FILLERS FOR BENIGN BONE TUMORS: WHAT ARE THE CLINICAL RESULTS?

Management of symptomatic benign bone tumors and tumor-like lesions typically requires excision and curet-tage of the entire lesion. This leaves behind an often-sizable defect in the bone, which must be filled to restore mechanical integrity and structural support of the affected bone. The gold standard has long been autologous bone grafting, often from the iliac crest. However, this pro-vides additional morbidity away from the primary surgi-cal site, with complication rates reported from 8% up to 13% from graft harvest alone,[8,9] and offers a finite, and at times, insufficient amount of graft to fill the defect.[10]

Alternative methods to fill these defects have been developed, which include allograft bone chips, poly-methylmethacrylate (PMMA) bone cement, and syn-thetic bone substitutes. Allograft avoids the problems associated with donor site morbidity but provides no immediate mechanical stability. Additionally, resorp-tion of allograft bone chips can be difficult to discern from tumor recurrence. Filling defects with PMMA bone cement has the advantage of providing immediate mechanical stability while also serving as an adjuvant treatment through thermo-necrosis of remaining super-ficial tumor cells. However, PMMA does not preserve bone stock and does not allow for any bony ingrowth. To help overcome the shortcomings of each of these methods, the use of synthetic bone graft substitutes for defects after tumor excision has been proposed.

Multiple variations of calcium products are cur-rently commercially available to fill bone defects after tumor surgery, including calcium hydroxyapatite (HA), calcium phosphate, and calcium sulfate. A series of 60 patients with benign bone tumors treated with curettage and grafting using calcium HA ceramic chips identified good outcomes with no local recurrences, yet three patients sustained a major complication in the form of a pathological fracture.[11] More recently, Yamamoto et al. evaluated a series of 75 patients using calcium HA with tricalcium phosphate. The group found that HA was incorporated into the healing bone at a mean of 4.2 months. However, despite excellent incorporation, there was never resorption of the synthetic graft, and a 9% complication rate was still encountered.[12]

In contrast to calcium HA or calcium phosphate, calcium sulfate resorbs at a rate that keeps pace with the rate of new bone formation through the process of creeping substitution.[13] In addition, the subsequent trabecular bone that grows into the prior defect has been shown to be histologically equivalent to the tra-becular bone formed from the current gold standard, autogenous bone graft.[13–15] A prospective multicenter trial assessing use of calcium sulfate as a bone graft sub-stitute found 99% resorption at 6 months, and 88% of the defect filled with trabecular bone.[16] While this trial included patients with defects attributable to trauma, revision arthroplasty, and fusion supplementation, a subset of 46 benign bone tumors showed identical results.[16]

For treatment of enchondromas of the hand, clinical studies have demonstrated good functional outcomes and minimal recurrence with calcium phosphate,[17] HA,[18] and sterile plaster of Paris.[19] Pianta et al. evaluated the mechanical strength of different void filler substi-tutes using a biomechanical model for enchondromas in the hand. The study found that two separate calcium phosphate bone cements provided excellent structural support and immediate restoration of mechanical sta-bility almost comparable to that of an intact metacar-pal bone.[20] In contrast, the demineralized bone matrix added no additional stability to an empty bone cavity, which weakened the bone to 70% of its initial strength. The authors concluded that use of calcium phosphate bone cements may allow early range of motion in the hand and prevent potential complications due to stiff-ness and postoperative immobilization.[20]

Overall, although autogenous bone graft remains the gold standard, the advances in recent void filler substitutes has provided an alternative method that avoids potential donor site morbidity and complica-tions while also bypassing difficulties encountered due to the limited quantity of available autograft. However, these potential benefits must be weighed against the disadvantages. The current synthetic fillers are osteo-conductive only without the osteoinductive properties seen with autogenous bone graft and provide an added financial cost that would otherwise be spared.

OSTEOARTICULAR ALLOGRAFTS: STILL AN OPTION?

Osteoarticular allografts have been used since the 1970s for limb-sparing reconstructions when the tumor resec-tion requires complete resection of the native articular surface. This technique allows for the preservation of a biologic articular surface without necessitating an endoprosthesis. Osteoarticular allografts have provided overall acceptable functional outcomes in the literature, with reported Musculoskeletal Tumor Society (MSTS) scores ranging from 70% to 91%.[21] Advantages of this technique include the ability to directly reattach a patient's preserved native tendons and ligaments, which may increase strength and overall stability of the joint. Furthermore, the use of osteoarticular allografts allows for bone preservation that becomes increasingly more important in younger patients, who likely require at least one to two revisions during their lifetime.[21]

In addition, the advantages of an osteoarticular allograft are also largely impacted by the anatomic site that is reconstructed. Joints with extensive soft tissue, tendon, and ligament attachments can take advantage of the retained soft tissue attachments on the allograft for added stability and function. In particular, osteoarticular allografts of the proximal tibia allow for reconstruction of the extensor mechanism.[22–24] In contrast, a location such as the distal femur with few soft tissue attachments does not derive the same benefit.

However, the risk of failure and overall complications with the use of these grafts remains high, with overall complication rates ranging from 40% to 70%.[21] A long-term study by Toy et al. found complications in 19 of 26 patients undergoing distal femoral osteoarticular allografts, which required 30 additional surgical procedures. Of note, 73% of these secondary surgeries occurred in the first 5 years after surgery.[25] Mankin et al. reviewed their use of osteoarticular allografts in 386 patients over 24 years, finding good-to-excellent results in 73% of patients. The study also brought out the critical period in the lifespan of an allograft replacement. If an allograft survives past the increased risk of infection in the first year after implantation of 10% and 19% risk of fracture in first 3 years, they became stable with 75% retained for more than 20 years.[26] Stability with 5- and 10-year survival has also been reported for distal femoral,[27] unicondylar[28] (femur & tibia), and proximal tibial[29] allografts as 78%, 85%, and 65%, respectively.

Unfortunately, complications are not an infrequent occurrence in allograft reconstruction, with overall complication rates in up to 52% of patients.[26] While the risk of fracture is the most common complication, infection can be far more devastating. In one series, despite infection in only 11% of patients, graft infection accounted for 43% of overall graft failures.[26] As the most common complication, fracture risk is highest when intramedullary nail fixation is used, and this risk may be mitigated by instead providing stability with plate fixation. Fracture risk may be further reduced with a dual plating technique to provide greater stability at the allograft-host bone interface. However, this often requires greater soft tissue dissection and may increase the risk of graft or hardware infection.

There are also concerns over the potential viability of cryopreserved articular cartilage. Enneking and Campanacci performed a histological examination of the articular cartilage in their allografts, finding that 86% had no viable chondrocytes within 5 years.[30] A series by Toy et al. evaluating distal femoral osteoarticular allografts found that 31% of patients required further surgery as a result of joint deterioration at a mean of 7.2 years. While this is a relatively large proportion of patients requiring secondary surgery before 10 years, it is a known and expected late complication of this procedure. Similarly, Mankin et al. found that 16%–20% of the surviving osteoarticular allografts required total joint arthroplasty,[26] and Ogilvie found 25% conversion to arthroplasty at a mean of 6.6 years.[31]

Alternative Techniques
Articular sparing resections & implants
Recent advances in computer navigation–assisted surgical procedures have allowed surgeons to push the envelope with resection margins in ways that were previously not possible. There is little room for error with respect to surgical margins as recurrence rates are directly related to the adequacy of resection.[32] In addition, as tumor proximity approaches even closer to the physis and articular margin, navigation can help allow for retention of maximal bone stock to allow for preservation of the native joint and even maintain ability for growth. Initial reports demonstrate excellent accuracy of the navigated resection and no major complications.[33] However, more long-term studies are needed to further evaluate these techniques before their widespread use.

INTERCALARY ALLOGRAFTS IN LIMB SALVAGE SURGERY

Intercalary allografts have a proven track record in terms of longevity and durability, with 10-year survival rates up to 80%.[34] There are many advantages to support the use of intercalary allografts. First, it allows for the preservation of host bone stock. This allows more surgical options when additional revision procedures are needed, which become critically important in the younger population (Fig. 18.1). In certain areas of the body, they also allow for anatomic restoration of tendon and ligamentous attachments.

However, there are also disadvantages and complications with the use of these grafts. Up to 70% of patients

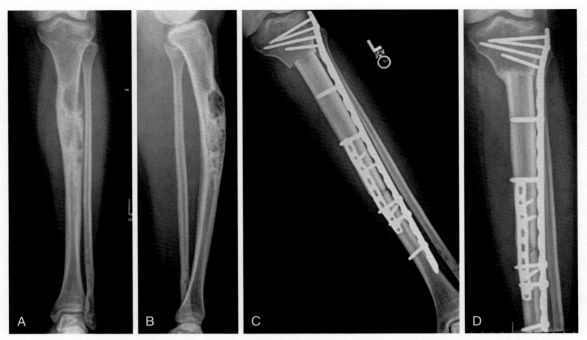

FIG. 18.1 Preoperative Anteroposterior (AP) **(A)** and lateral **(B)** radiographs of a patient with an adamanti-noma arising in the setting or previously diagnosed osteofibrous dysplasia of the left tibia. This was treated with wide resection and intercalary reconstruction **(C)**. Radiographs 6 months postoperatively show healing of the proximal junction and incomplete healing of the distal junction **(D)**.

who receive an intercalary allograft will require a return to the operating room for at least one additional surgical procedure.[35] Reasons for additional surgical procedures are most often due to the "triad" of complications, comprised of infection, nonunion, and graft fracture. Overall failure rates have been reported to range from 10% up to 39%, and similar to osteoarticular allografts, the vast majority of these complications occur within the first 3–4 years from the initial surgical procedure.[36] Prior studies have suggested that if an intercalary allograft is able to survive this initial time period, then the risk of late failure is negligible. Mankin et al. demonstrated good-to-excellent results in 84% of their intercalary allografts and failure in only 13%.[26]

Controversy exists over the best method of host-allograft fixation to optimize union rates and reduce risk of fracture. Fixation techniques include intramedullary nailing, plate fixation, or a combination of both (Fig. 18.2). Plate fixation provides better compression at the host-allograft interface to maximize the rate of union. However, to obtain this compression, screws must be placed into the allograft bone, which can increase the subsequent risk of late graft fracture. This

risk may be mitigated with the use of a long plate to span the entire allograft or with the use of 90–90 plating techniques.[34]

In contrast, an intramedullary nail allows the surgeon to span the entire bone, offering support and stability across the host-allograft interface without requiring screw placement into the allograft bone. This technique has been shown to reduce the risk of allograft fracture, but in turn, it becomes more difficult to obtain compression, thereby increasing the risk of nonunion.[34]

Alternative Techniques

Beginning in the late 1970s, the free vascularized fibular graft (FVFG) has served as an alternative to the intercalary allograft for limb reconstruction. The primary advantage with this technique lies in the ability to maintain normal bone healing and biology through preservation of the periosteal cuff and nutrient vessels of the fibula. This becomes increasingly more crucial to graft healing and incorporation in patients with prior surgery or radiation therapy, in which case the harvested blood supply can allow for immediate viability even in those areas of soft tissue compromise.

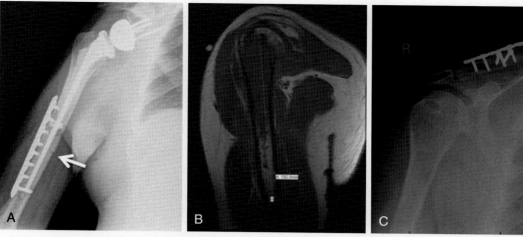

FIG.18.2 Preoperative radiograph **(A)** and preoperative MRI **(B)** in a patient with an intermediate-grade chondrosarcoma of the right proximal humerus. Postoperative radiograph **(C)** shows reconstruction after wide resection of the proximal humerus. An allograft prosthetic composite was used for reconstruction. Both intramedullary (humeral stem) and extramedullary fixation are used to bridge the graft-host junction (*arrow*).

Free vascularized fibular autografts are typically used in one of two forms: (1) intercalary graft supplied by the peroneal vessels or (2) proximal grafts supplied by the anterior tibial vessels. In children the use of a vascularized proximal fibular graft can serve to preserve the epiphysis of the fibula and subsequently allow for some longitudinal growth of the reconstructed bone. However, the postoperative protocol for FVFG requires at least 3 months of strict immobilization of the affected extremity, followed by passive range of motion exercises. Initiation of protected weight-bearing begins only when bony union is visualized on radiographs, which typically occurs 5–7 months from the time of surgery. Zaretski et al. reviewed a cohort of 30 patients with malignant or aggressive bone tumors treated with free fibular vascularized graft. All patients were immobilized in a plaster cast for at least 3 months, and there was a 100% union rate with average time to union 4.8 months in lower extremity and 3.8 months in the upper extremity. Despite appearance of radiographic union, full weight-bearing was not achieved until an average of 9.2 months from surgery.[36]

Extracorporeal devitalized autograft reconstructions

Tumor resections that result in either very large defects or those with irregular anatomic contours create a unique surgical challenge. Initially described in 1968 by Spira and Lubin, the use of extracorporeal devitalized autografts has helped provide a possible solution to this unique surgical dilemma. By using the patient's own bone stock after tumor eradication, it essentially provides a massive allograft, which is perfectly contoured to fit the specific anatomy of that patient.[37] This technique becomes particularly advantageous with tumors arising from the pelvis. However, this technique is not without its own risks and complications. Prior studies have demonstrated an association between complications and the dose of radiation used to sterilize the autograft. Using a dose of 50 Gy, both deep infection and stress fracture occurred at a rate of 7.7%, with no local recurrences reported.[38] In contrast, Sys et al. reported 13 complications in 16 patients treated with extracorporeally irradiated autografts that received 300 Gy for intraoperative sterilization and 46.7% mortality after local recurrence of the tumor.[39]

Ultimately, each technique has its own pros and cons. The decision to proceed with any procedure should be made according to each patient's prognosis as well as his/her own goals and expectations of life after surgery.

REFERENCES

1. Thomas D, Henshaw R, Skubitz K, et al. Denosumab in patients with giant-cell tumour of bone: an open-label, phase 2 study. *Lancet Oncol.* 2010;11(3):275–280. https://doi.org/10.1016/S1470-2045(10)70010-3.

2. Ranieri G, Mammì M, Donato Di Paola E, et al. Pazopanib a tyrosine kinase inhibitor with strong anti-angiogenetic activity: a new treatment for metastatic soft tissue sarcoma. *Crit Rev Oncol Hematol*. 2014;89(2):322–329. https://doi.org/10.1016/j.critrevonc.2013.08.012.

3. Graeven U, Andre N, Achilles E, Zornig C, Schmiegel W. Serum levels of vascular endothelial growth factor and basic fibroblast growth factor in patients with soft-tissue sarcoma. *J Cancer Res Clin Oncol*. 1999;125(10):577–581. http://www.ncbi.nlm.nih.gov/pubmed/10473871.

4. Chao C, Al-Saleem T, Brooks JJ, Rogatko A, Kraybill WG, Eisenberg B. Vascular endothelial growth factor and soft tissue sarcomas: tumor expression correlates with grade. *Ann Surg Oncol*. 2001;8(3):260–267. http://www.ncbi.nlm.nih.gov/pubmed/11314944.

5. Potti A, Ganti AK, Foster H, et al. Immunohistochemical detection of HER-2/neu, c-kit (CD117) and vascular endothelial growth factor (VEGF) overexpression in soft tissue sarcomas. *Anticancer Res*. 2004;24(1):333–337. http://www.ncbi.nlm.nih.gov/pubmed/15015617.

6. Potti A, Ganti AK, Tendulkar K, et al. Determination of vascular endothelial growth factor (VEGF) overexpression in soft tissue sarcomas and the role of overexpression in leiomyosarcoma. *J Cancer Res Clin Oncol*. 2004;130(1):52–56. https://doi.org/10.1007/s00432-003-0504-0.

7. van der Graaf WT, Blay J-Y, Chawla SP, et al. Pazopanib for metastatic soft-tissue sarcoma (PALETTE): a randomised, double-blind, placebo-controlled phase 3 trial. *Lancet*. 2012;379(9829):1879–1886. https://doi.org/10.1016/S0140-6736(12)60651-5.

8. Jäger M, Westhoff B, Wild A, Krauspe R. Bone Harvesting from the iliac crest. *Orthopäde*. 2005;34(10):976–994. https://doi.org/10.1007/s00132-005-0839-0.

9. Younger EM, Chapman MW. Morbidity at bone graft donor sites. *J Orthop Trauma*. 1989;3(3):192–195. http://www.ncbi.nlm.nih.gov/pubmed/2809818.

10. Le Guéhennec L, Layrolle P, Daculsi G. A review of bioceramics and fibrin sealant. *Eur Cell Mater*. 2004;8:1–10-1 http://www.ncbi.nlm.nih.gov/pubmed/15494929.

11. Uchida A, Araki N, Shinto Y, Yoshikawa H, Kurisaki E, Ono K. The use of calcium hydroxyapatite ceramic in bone tumour surgery. *J Bone Joint Surg Br*. 1990;72(2):298–302. https://doi.org/10.1302/0301-620X.72B2.2155908.

12. Yamamoto T, Onga T, Marui T, Mizuno K. Use of hydroxyapatite to fill cavities after excision of benign bone tumours. Clinical results. *J Bone Joint Surg Br*. 2000;82(8):1117–1120. http://www.ncbi.nlm.nih.gov/pubmed/11132269.

13. Turner TM, Urban RM, Gitelis S, Kuo KN, Andersson GB. Radiographic and histologic assessment of calcium sulfate in experimental animal models and clinical use as a resorbable bone-graft substitute, a bone-graft expander, and a method for local antibiotic delivery. One institution's experience. *J Bone Joint Surg Am*. 2001;83-A(suppl 2(Pt 1):8–18. http://www.ncbi.nlm.nih.gov/pubmed/11685848.

14. Turner TM, Urban RM, Hall DJ, Cheema N, Lim TH. Restoration of large bone defects using a hard-setting, injectable putty containing demineralized bone particles compared to cancellous autograft bone. *Orthopedics*. 2003;26(suppl 5):s561–s565. http://www.ncbi.nlm.nih.gov/pubmed/12755226.

15. Kelly CM, Wilkins RM. Treatment of benign bone lesions with an injectable calcium sulfate-based bone graft substitute. *Orthopedics*. 2004;27(suppl 1):s131–s135. http://www.ncbi.nlm.nih.gov/pubmed/14763545.

16. Kelly CM, Wilkins RM, Gitelis S, Hartjen C, Watson JT, Kim PT. The use of a surgical grade calcium sulfate as a bone graft substitute: results of a multicenter trial. *Clin Orthop Relat Res*. 2001;382:42–50. http://www.ncbi.nlm.nih.gov/pubmed/11154003.

17. Yasuda M, Masada K, Takeuchi E. Treatment of enchondroma of the hand with injectable calcium phosphate bone cement. *J Hand Surg Am*. 2006;31(1):98–102. https://doi.org/10.1016/j.jhsa.2005.08.017.

18. Joosten U, Joist A, Frebel T, Walter M, Langer M. The use of an in situ curing hydroxyapatite cement as an alternative to bone graft following removal of enchondroma of the hand. *J Hand Surg Am*. 2000;25(3):288–291. https://doi.org/10.1054/jhsb.2000.0383.

19. Gaasbeek RDA, Rijnberg WJ, van Loon CJM, Meyers H, Feith R. No local recurrence of enchondroma after curettage and plaster filling. *Arch Orthop Trauma Surg*. 2005;125(1):42–45. https://doi.org/10.1007/s00402-004-0747-5.

20. Pianta TJ, Baldwin PS, Obopilwe E, Mazzocca AD, Rodner CM, Silverstein EA. A biomechanical analysis of treatment options for enchondromas of the hand. *HAND*. 2013;8(1):86–91. https://doi.org/10.1007/s11552-012-9476-3.

21. Bus MPA, van de Sande MAJ, Taminiau AHM, Dijkstra PDS. Is there still a role for osteoarticular allograft reconstruction in musculoskeletal tumour surgery? *Bone Joint J*. 2017;99-B(4):522–530. https://doi.org/10.1302/0301-620X.99B4.BJJ-2016-0443.R2.

22. Abed YY, Beltrami G, Campanacci DA, Innocenti M, Scoccianti G, Capanna R. Biological reconstruction after resection of bone tumours around the knee. *J Bone Joint Surg Br*. 2009;91-B(10):1366–1372. https://doi.org/10.1302/0301-620X.91B10.22212.

23. Ayerza MA, Aponte-Tinao LA, Abalo E, Muscolo DL. Continuity and function of patellar tendon host-donor suture in tibial allograft. *Clin Orthop Relat Res*. 2006;450:33–38. https://doi.org/10.1097/01.blo.0000229291.21722.b5.

24. Brien EW, Terek RM, Healey JH, Lane JM. Allograft reconstruction after proximal tibial resection for bone tumors. An analysis of function and outcome comparing allograft and prosthetic reconstructions. *Clin Orthop Relat Res*. 1994;(303):116–127. http://www.ncbi.nlm.nih.gov/pubmed/8194221.

25. Toy PC, White JR, Scarborough MT, Enneking WF, Gibbs CP. Distal femoral osteoarticular allografts: long-term survival, but frequent complications. *Clin Orthop Relat Res*. 2010;468(11):2914–2923. https://doi.org/10.1007/s11999-010-1470-x.

26. Mankin HJ, Gebhardt MC, Jennings LC, Springfield DS, Tomford WW. Long-term results of allograft replacement in the management of bone tumors. *Clin Orthop Relat Res.* 1996;(324):86–97. http://www.ncbi.nlm.nih.gov/pubmed/8595781.

27. Muscolo DL, Ayerza MA, Aponte-Tinao LA, Ranalletta M. Use of distal femoral osteoarticular allografts in limb salvage surgery. *J Bone Jt Surg.* 2005;87(11):2449. https://doi.org/10.2106/JBJS.D.02170.

28. Muscolo DL, Ayerza MA, Aponte-Tinao LA, Abalo E, Farfalli G. Unicondylar osteoarticular allografts of the knee. *J Bone Jt Surg.* 2007;89(10):2137. https://doi.org/10.2106/JBJS.F.01277.

29. Muscolo DL, Ayerza MA, Farfalli G, Aponte-Tinao LA. Proximal tibia osteoarticular allografts in tumor limb salvage surgery. *Clin Orthop Relat Res.* 2010;468(5):1396–1404. https://doi.org/10.1007/s11999-009-1186-y.

30. Enneking WF, Campanacci DA. Retrieved human allografts: a clinicopathological study. *J Bone Joint Surg Am.* 2001;83-A(7):971–986. http://www.ncbi.nlm.nih.gov/pubmed/11451965.

31. Ogilvie CM, Crawford EA, Hosalkar HS, King JJ, Lackman RD. Long-term results for limb salvage with osteoarticular allograft reconstruction. *Clin Orthop Relat Res.* 2009;467(10):2685–2690. https://doi.org/10.1007/s11999-009-0726-9.

32. Picci P, Sangiorgi L, Rougraff BT, Neff JR, Casadei R, Campanacci M. Relationship of chemotherapy-induced necrosis and surgical margins to local recurrence in osteosarcoma. *J Clin Oncol.* 1994;12(12):2699–2705. https://doi.org/10.1200/JCO.1994.12.12.2699.

33. Wong KC, Kumta SM. Joint-preserving tumor resection and reconstruction using image-guided computer navigation. *Clin Orthop Relat Res.* 2013;471(3):762–773. https://doi.org/10.1007/s11999-012-2536-8.

34. Panagopoulos GN, Mavrogenis AF, Mauffrey C, et al. Intercalary reconstructions after bone tumor resections: a review of treatments. *Eur J Orthop Surg Traumatol.* 2017;27(6):737–746. https://doi.org/10.1007/s00590-017-1985-x.

35. Bus MPA, Dijkstra PDS, van de Sande MAJ, et al. Intercalary allograft reconstructions following resection of primary bone tumors. *J Bone Jt Surg.* 2014;96(4):e26. https://doi.org/10.2106/JBJS.M.00655.

36. Zaretski A, Amir A, Meller I, et al. Free fibula long bone reconstruction in orthopedic oncology: a surgical algorithm for reconstructive options. *Plast Reconstr Surg.* 2004;113(7):1989–2000. http://www.ncbi.nlm.nih.gov/pubmed/15253188.

37. Spira E, Lubin E. Extracorporeal irradiation of bone tumors. A preliminary report. *Isr J Med Sci.* 2018;4(5):1015–1019. http://www.ncbi.nlm.nih.gov/pubmed/5251288.

38. Krieg AH, Mani M, Speth BM, Stalley PD. Extracorporeal irradiation for pelvic reconstruction in Ewing's sarcoma. *J Bone Joint Surg Br.* 2009;91-B(3):395–400. https://doi.org/10.1302/0301-620X.91B3.21164.

39. Sys G, Uyttendaele D, Poffyn B, Verdonk R, Verstraete K. Extracorporeally irradiated autografts in pelvic reconstruction after malignant tumour resection. *Int Orthop.* 2002;26(3):174–178. https://doi.org/10.1007/s00264-002-0352-6.

CHAPTER 19

Regenerative Engineering in the Field of Orthopedic Surgery

CATO T. LAURENCIN, MD, PHD • MARY A. BADON, MD, MBA

The field of regenerative engineering seeks to address the most complex and relevant questions in the realm of future of regeneration, namely, how to regenerate complex structures comprised of multiple types of tissues to improve the quality of life and the scope of structural and biological ailments that can be treated by modern biomedical science. To accomplish this task, the regenerative engineer must use tools from many traditional fields of study including tissue engineering, materials science, bioengineering, and developmental biology, as well as observations and applications from medicine and surgery. Regenerative engineering focuses on a number of areas, but the development of novel materials, in addition to redeveloping existing materials, which are then used to facilitate biological processes and the growth and development of tissues directly into functional and complete structures that are identical to their native tissues has taken center stage.

This chapter will provide some background into both the materials that have been developed as scaffolds for facilitating tissue growth as wells as insights into the biological processes that must be harnessed or modified for the cells within those regenerated tissues to reenter the cell cycle and redifferentiate into functional adult cells. In addition, we will describe the importance of innovation in this field and how regenerative engineering groups bring together scientists, engineers, and clinicians to facilitate not only sustaining or incremental improvements but also innovations that can be truly disruptive and change the way health care is delivered in the field orthopedic surgery.

Although applications should not dictate the scope or direction of basic science, it is important to highlight some of the most challenging conditions that face the modern orthopedic surgeon. This includes bone and tissue loss due to trauma, infection, cancer, and inflammation. Surgeons are skilled at rearranging and reconstructing tissues to create functional structures and are at the same time limited by the tissues present at the time of surgery. Herein lie the potential contributions of the field of regenerative engineering, to create the building blocks with which the orthopedic surgeon can reconstruct and recreate a functional musculoskeletal system, where one was missing or has been lost.

TISSUE REGENERATION AND THE ROLE OF REGENERATIVE ENGINEERING

Regeneration mimics the natural processes of tissue formation that occurs during several stages of an organism's development. Tissues normally form during fetal phase of life termed embryonic tissue formation, tissue growth and development (fetal and postnatal), remodeling (degradation-formation), and healing (repair vs. regeneration). It is important to distinguish the difference in functionality that exists in repaired tissue that forms during the normal healing process, and that tissue would be created through regenerative engineering methods.

One aspect of regenerative engineering focuses on using cues from earlier tissue-formation periods and applies them to situations and injuries that occur later. This is performed in the hopes of directing adult tissue away from simple repair, where a defect in the tissue fills with relatively biologically inactive, nonfunctional tissues such as scar. Wound healing is a conserved evolutionary process among species and encompasses processes including inflammation, blood clotting, and cellular proliferation and extracellular matrix (ECM) remodeling[1] which leads to distinct scar formation. Regeneration on the other hand would result in tissues where the defect or injury fills with a regenerate that is indistinguishable from the original surrounding native tissues.

Tissue gaps or large scars present biological challenges that have significant clinical consequences. For example, infarcts secondary to pulmonary emboli or myocardial infarctions result in relatively noncompliant scars taking the place of biologically active tissues that reduce the overall function of the organ as the scar cannot carry out the roll of the organ. The inferior scar tissue fails to emulate the tissue's original structure and composition. In addition to the scar replacing the native, functional tissue, the scar also impedes the function of the rest of the organ due to physical forces restricting the dynamic movement of the tissue. These gaps or scars can be focused in a single area as in the case of infarction but can also be diffusely distributed in the native, normal tissue as in the case of infection. Even focal injuries can result in congestive heart failure in the case of myocardial infarction and restrictive lunch disease in the case of pulmonary embolism. Disease processes can also result in more diffuse changes in the affected tissue. Classically in the case of hand cellulitis, the compliance of the soft tissues is reduced after the infection has cleared, resulting in joint capsule contracture as well as generation restriction throughout the skin and muscle resulting in reduced range of motion, discomfort, and difficulty with fine motor movements.[2] Similarly, diffuse changes that affect the compliance of tissues can be seen in certain autoimmune disorders such as systemic sclerosis, a chronic multisystem autoimmune disease characterized by a vasculopathy, diffuse fibrosis of skin and various internal organs, and immune abnormalities.[3]

Regenerative engineering seeks to create physical and biological solutions for biological deficiencies. Ideally, when materials are used, engineered matrices are involved so that they can create appropriate and appropriately timed biological and physical signals to pluripotent cells within the surrounding tissues to stimulate the formation of bioidentical tissues that are contiguous with the surrounding biological environment. The implants simultaneously act as templates and guides for tissue ingrowth and incorporation. The choice of materials used for these scaffolds, any biologics that are incorporated into their physical arrangement and structure, and the nature in which they are assembled can have dramatic impacts on the ability of the stem cells to differentiate into tissues and ultimately function in the context of the musculoskeletal system.

When a regenerative engineering problem is approached, the engineer must decide on what strategy they would like to use for multitissue structure regeneration. In nature, most tissue development occurs during embryonic development, remodeling of existing tissues, or injury healing. Each regeneration strategy may include completely differing signaling cues as to stimulate growth. For example, the engineer needs to recapitulate embryonic/developmental conditions with appropriate precursor cells and/or extracellular matrices or, if appropriate, instead provide conditions (cells and matrix) that favor tissue formation of regenerated tissue from surrounding adult tissue.

The most common approach is to establish the growth of tissues within scaffolds in vitro. This traditional approach is an important testing ground to establish proof of concept experiments that determine which developmental biochemical cues induce the desired tissue proliferation. The developmental signals used during in vitro tissue engineering and propagation can include signal transduction molecules, cofactors, and growth factors. The in vitro approach can be controlled but is limited and does not fully recapitulate the in vivo environment.

The in vivo environment may have many other, complex, structural, physical, or systemic cues that contribute to tissue development and function. For example, one must consider gradient signals associated with tissues, such as hypoxia to stimulate angiogenesis,[4] interactions with the endocrine system or hormones, or physical load to stimulate bone growth and remodeling.[5] However, there are other challenges associated with the in vivo environment which make experiments in live animals challenging to control and interpret.

To take advantage of the in vivo setting and thus the biological environment surrounding the injured area and mechanical stimuli, the regenerative engineer will lose some of the overall control of the experimental settings. An in vivo approach, in combination with implants that use advanced technology in materials engineering, signal transduction, and surgical techniques to facilitate the growth of complex tissues and structures, increases the scope of medical problems that can be addressed and also minimizes the duration of time tissue regeneration takes by simultaneously growing multiple types of tissue rather than needing sequential reconstructive procedures. Through the formation of implants using advanced biomaterials and techniques, the regenerative engineer is setting the stage for tissue growth and development to happen in vivo rather than solely in a petri dish.

THE CLINICAL RELEVANCE AND IMPORTANCE OF REGENERATIVE ENGINEERING

The evolution of regenerative engineering can be marked by similar breakthroughs in biomedical history. The field of regenerative engineering can trace its origins to the 1970s and 1980s when IntegraTM

(Integra Life Sciences Corporation Plainsboro, New Jersey), a collagen-glycosaminoglycan (GAG) matrix that is used to help complex wounds and burns heal, first emerged.[6] Similar to bone, skin is another tissue that is capable of and can be steered toward regeneration rather than healing under certain conditions. IntegraTM is manufactured in the form of a wound dressing that is placed over a debrided wound. The scaffold, made up of collagen-GAG provides the needed structure that angiogenesis and ingrowth of dermal skin cells need to remodel the damaged site. Reliably, over the course of 14–21 days after placement of this dressing, fibroblasts and mesenchymal stem cells migrate into the scaffold. After migration of the precursor cells, the collagen scaffold is resorbed and replaced with the patient's own tissue, and the wound gradually healed. This breakthrough resulted in a user friendly product that was rapidly integrated into clinical practice and is still routinely used today.

Scaffolds have found other uses in medicine and surgery including aiding in bone regeneration. Bone, when fractured, crushed, or otherwise damaged, is unique in its ability to heal without the formation of scar tissue. The stages of fracture healing includes coordinated responses of the bone marrow, bone cortex, periosteum, the surrounding soft tissues, the immune system, including regulation of cellular proliferation, and migration and differentiation of mesenchymal stem cells.[7] However, because bone has the innate ability to regenerate, the primary use of the scaffolds was to overcome physical gaps that precluded normal healing. This is different from the goal of the development of new tissues that do not possess some regeneration capacity on their own. Examples of other tissues that spontaneously regenerate include bone, epithelia (including stomach lining, intestinal lining, and skin) and smooth muscle. Areas of active research for the development of scaffold for regeneration of tissues that do not spontaneously regenerate include articular cartilage,[8] ligaments (predominantly collagen type I),[9] both the nucleus pulposus,[10] and annulus fibrosis[11] of intervertebral discs of the spine, cardiac muscle,[12] skeletal muscle,[13] and nerves.[14]

Bone is an interesting example as there are several options for scaffolds to aid in bone-defect healing. Bone is a highly structured and dynamic tissue made up of both organic and inorganic matrices. Primarily made of collage type I and hydroxyapatite (HA), it is also both innervated and vascularized as it regenerates. However, factors such as the size of defects (defects or gaps greater than 2 mm are at risk of not healing), unfavorable environments such as the collapse of tissues

into defects preventing opposing ends of the bone from opposing in the case of fractures or occupying space in the case of periodontal defects, and inappropriate physical forces across the injured area in the case of unstable or over-stabilized fracture resulting in hypertrophic or atrophic nonunions (ideal strain is thought to be 2% for bone healing to occur). Options for scaffolds for bone defects include autograft, allograft, and bone substitute or synthetic materials. The tissue regeneration capacity of these bone grafts is measured in terms of their osteogenic, osteoconductive, and osteoinductive potentials. As described in a review by Liliana Polo-Corrales et al. in the Journal of Nanoscience and Nanotechnology,[15] the table below demonstrates that many materials can be made into scaffolds conducive to bone regeneration.

Category	Material
Natural polymer	Collagen hydrogel
	Chitosan
	Silk fibroin
	Alginate
	Hyaluronic acid
	Peptide hydrogels
Synthetic polymers	Polyesters (polyglycolic acid, poly-lactic acid, and polycaprolactone)
	Poly(diisopropyl fumarate) (PDIPF)
	Poly(L-lactide-co-ε-caprolactone (poly(LLA-co-CL)) and poly(L-lactide-co-1,5-dioxepan-2-one), (poly(LLA-co-DXO))
Ceramic scaffolds	Bioglass
	Calcium phosphate
	Coral
Metal scaffolds	Titanium/titanium oxide
	Aluminate/melatonin
Composites	Polymer/ceramics
	Metal/ceramic
	Metal/polymer

Collagen type I is also the predominant type of collagen in ligaments. The intraarticular environment of the knee is not conducive to ligament healing due to the presence of synovial fluid. Attempts at supportive care to promote anterior cruciate ligament (ACL) healing have a substantially high rate of failure (40% -100%), even after surgical repair using suture.[16] Synovial fluid provides necessary nutrition and lubrication to articular cartilage and also presents an obstacle to ligament healing. Polymer fibers made of poly(lactic acid) (PLLA), polyglycolic acid, and polylactic-co-glycolic acid can be wound into scaffolds and implanted surgically using the same techniques as an allograft or autograft.[17–19] These polymer scaffolds, especially when combined with biologics such as bone morphogenetic protein and other growth factors, provide soft tissue reconstruction solutions for both articular cartilage and ligaments in the presence of synovial fluid.

The potential market for application of synthetic ACL grafts is growing. Current trends in the United States suggest that regenerative engineering advances in ACL reconstruction would be timely as between 1994 and 2006, the population-adjusted estimate of the rate of ACL reconstructions increased by 37% (33.0/100,000 capita or 86,837 total procedures to 45.1/100,000 capita or 134,421 total procedures). Synthetic ACL grafts would provide a real option for patients who prefer to not undergo tissue harvest and avoid the associated donor site morbidity associated with hamstring or patellar tendon harvest; who wish to avoid the small, but real, risk of disease transmission and higher graft failure rates associated with donor grafts (allograft); and those patients who require revision surgery due to previous ACL graft reconstruction failures in the setting of autografts or allografts.

While primary repair of torn anterior cruciate ligaments fell out of favor, the advent of scaffold has brought about a renewed interest in the ability to suture repair cruciate ligaments in the intraarticular milieu.[20,21] Bridge-enhanced ACL repair (BEAR), involves suture repair of the ligament in the presence of a bioactive scaffold to bridge the gap between the torn ligament ends and facilitate healing. In a cohort study with 20 patients, 10 patients underwent BEAR and were compared with 10 patients who underwent reconstruction with hamstring autograft. There were no differences between groups in effusion or pain and no failures by Lachman examination criteria. Magnetic resonance images from all the BEAR and ACL-reconstructed patients demonstrated a continuous ACL or intact graft. Patients who underwent BEAR had significantly greater hamstrings strength at 3 months postoperatively than the autograft control group. The authors concluded that these promising results should lead to future studies with larger groups so more conclusive results can be obtained.[21]

THE EVOLUTION OF MATERIALS AND THEIR APPLICATION IN REGENERATIVE ENGINEERING

The variety of materials that can be used to develop biologically compatible scaffolds capable of supporting bone growth provides a stage for what engineers can use to address tissue engineering challenges. Implant development no longer centers on how to create implants that are biologically inert but rather on how the implant can impart the desired biological effect on the body.

When implants and scaffolds are placed in an organism, they must survive a highly corrosive environment for sufficient time for tissue ingrowth and maturation. As a simplification, scaffolds generally are broken into categories of synthetic polymers, natural polymers, metals, ceramics, and composites. Each material has its benefits and challenges. Metals in the corrosive environment can react and corrode, creating inflammation and ultimately destroying surrounding tissues. Polymers can fatigue and fail as they do not undergo remodeling as natural tissues in the body. Ceramics can be brittle and fracture. The use of composite materials and the introduction of three-dimensional printing provide new methods to overcome the shortcomings of earlier scaffold materials and designs.

A good example of the evolution of a material is the use of ceramics. Used first in implants due to their biologic inertness, first-generation ceramics included alumina, zirconia, as well as porous ceramics whose physical structure facilitates bone ingrowth. Alumina, in the form of alpha-Al_2O_3, was first reported as a component of a femoral head in a joint arthroplasty in 1972.[22,23] Ceramic materials were later used for acetabular cups. Ceramics make good implant materials as they have low wear rates, resistance to corrosion, high strength, and good biocompatibility when compared with previous acetabular cups made of polyethylene. Despite all these favorable characteristics and improved biocompatibility when compared to polyethylene which shed particles, which would result in osteolysis, ceramic acetabular cups had low fracture toughness resulting in catastrophic failures. Currently, ceramics such as alumina and zirconia are used for total joint arthroplasty in conjunction with other types of materials such as ceramic femoral heads with polyethylene liners.

None of those early designs really took advantage of ceramics as a scaffold until the modification of surface characteristics on the implant to improve bone ingrowth. In addition, porous ceramics intuitively would provide an opportunity for native tissues to integrate into the structure of the scaffold. Alumina and zirconia can be made into porous forms with foaming agents that produce gases while the ceramic is setting, resulting in relatively diffuse and random distribution of pores.[24] These porous ceramics could then be implanted in the hopes that surrounding osteocytes and fibroblasts would occupy those gas-created spaces and whiten the ceramic, integrating the ceramic into the surrounding bone. These experiments, however, led to disappointing results as the risk of mechanical collapse. One of the problems with porous ceramics is that they were too brittle and would fail catastrophically in a predictable fashion under stress.[25] This does not happen in normal bone because the combination of inorganic HA (approximately 70%) and organic components such as collagen (approximately 30%) adds elasticity and flexibility.[26]

Scientists also looked at nature for inspiration, where hierarchal patterns are common. Bone has two characteristic patterns, dense cortical bone as well as trabecular (also referred to as cancellous or spongy bone). The relatively heavy cortical bone provides strength and is load bearing. Human mandibular cortical bone has a porosity of approximately 3.5%.[27] Its thickness and density varies with the amount of force that is imparted on it, referred to as Wolff's law with higher load–bearing bones such as the femur having thicker and denser cortical bone than the upper extremities. In addition to being responsive to mechanical forces, the cortical bone also has a complex microstructure including canals and conduits for blood supply, innervation, and cell-to-cell communication between osteocytes, as well as providing specialized pores for cells involved in bone turnover such as osteoblasts and osteoclasts.

Trabecular bone with its honeycomb-like structure is contained within the cortical bone shell. Trabecula (plural trabeculae, from Latin for "small beam") is a small, often microscopic, tissue element in the form of a small beam, strut, or rod. The rod and beam structure of trabecular bone, in contrast to the denser cortical bone, creates a lightweight network of cavities within the bone. Human mandibular trabecular bone is less dense with porosity of about 79.3%.[27] This reflects its function in the body. The trabecular bone does contribute to the overall strength of the bone, and it also provides space for both fatty and red bone marrow as well as blood cell production.

Looking elsewhere in nature for hierarchal structures that could dissipate forces, scientists noticed that the calcium carbonate structure of certain corals mimic trabecular bone. Beginning in the 1970s scientists began exploring the use of natural coral graft substitutes derived from the exoskeleton of marine madreporic corals as ostoconductive bone xenograph.[28] The porite, which is the structural unit of coral, is similar to that of cancellous bone, both in their scaffold-like network of channels and cavities as well as some of their mechanical properties. Made up of primarily calcium carbonate, treated coral proved to be biocompatible being relatively inert like many other ceramics, osteoconductive providing channels for blood vessel ingrowth similar to trabecular bone, and bioresorbable

over time. To minimize and prevent bioresorbability for creating a longer lasting implant, coral can be treated using a hydrothermal process to convert it to a nonresorbable HA material.[29] However, the hierarchal structure of corals, while mimicking native trabecular bone, did not have osteoinductive or osteogenic properties unless combined with other biologics.[30] Coraline matrix is currently sold as calcified matrix for use in orthopedic surgery.

Another source of calcium minerals from nature for bone scaffold is avian eggshell.[31-33] Similar to both bone and coral, eggshell is composed primarily of calcium and phosphate. Although eggshell as a natural biomaterial is biodegradable, readily available, and inexpensive, it requires surface modification to improve cell interactions. These modifications include hydrothermal treatment of eggshell to calcium-deficient HA with surface microstructure. This resulted in higher osteoblast viability on surface-modified ES than a commercially available bone substitute, bovine bone (Bio-Oss, BO).[31] In in vivo studies, there was significantly greater new bone formation and mineralized bone-to-graft contact of surface-modified ES, especially with hydrothermally treated ES, compared with BO in 5-mm diameter calvarial defects in rats at 4 and 8 weeks of healing on both histological and histomorphometric analysis.[31] In 2011, scientists synthesize 3D calcium carbonate interwoven nanofibrous platforms from eggshells using high-repetition femtosecond laser irradiation.[32] This was the first study looking at synthesizing 3D nanofibrous structures from eggshell. Three-dimensional (3D) nanostructures are preferred to act as growth-support platforms for bone and stem cells.

While coral and eggshell, both calcium-based natural bioceramics, seem intuitively modifiable to form bone scaffolds, another source of natural xenograft is, surprisingly, trees. In 2009 Italian scientists announced a breakthrough in the use of wood as a bone substitute.[26] Trees and other vascularized plants contain as hierarchal microstructure consisting of channels which bring water and sap up and down the organism through canals called xylem and phloem. Similar to bone, these channels are organized in a hierarchal fashion. A HA scaffold can be made from native wood through a sequence of thermal and hydrothermal chemical processes. These reactions, though highly caustic, ultimately yield calcium carbonate (the same component in untreated coraline xenografts) and then undergo phosphatization through hydrothermal treatment to achieve HA. This yields an inorganic biomorphic scaffold providing a biomimetic nanostructure surface for orthopedic and engineering applications.

The inventors of this wood-derived, HA scaffold claim that their material will permit better penetration during bone growth and allow more flexion than metal or hard ceramic grafts. This demonstrates that scientists can look to nature for inspiration and ways to repurpose materials that evolved to serve other purposes.

Scientists no longer have to be limited to random pattern ceramics through chemical reactions or rely on nature to repurpose other hierarchal patterns into scaffolds. Three-dimensional printing (3DP) can overcome the limitations of using natural tissues and open up the possibility of high-precision microstructural engineering of materials to take advantage of the physical characteristics of novel hierarchal designs and patterns. Take for example, our discussion of avian eggshell nature-derived scaffolds. The eggshells could be crushed into a powder and then pressed into blocks to be used in their native form as bone scaffolds, or 3DP could be used to construct the biomaterial into a new structure altogether. Eggshell was explored as a precursor for the biologically active bone implant. Park et al. fabricated 3D-lattice-patterned scaffolds from slurry created from crushed *Gallus gallus* eggshells via coagulation-assisted extrusion-based printing.[33] Notably, compared to contemporary methods, a multiphasic CaP-based 3D scaffold with hierarchical porosity was prepared using a simple slurry processing, followed by a single heat-treatment cycle. When compared to a similar scaffold fabricated from a chemically synthesized calcium phosphate powder, the naturally sourced eggshell scaffold had improved biological activity in comparison with the synthetic one. Enhanced cell activity promoted significant ECM deposition during in vitro biological assessment as well as higher cell adhesion and rapid differentiation into osteogenic lineage. In sense, the use of 3DP enhanced and modified the biologic activity that the original material imparts on the surrounding host cells.

This theme of remanufacturing and redesigning existing materials has been the focus of Markus Buehler's group of the Department of Civil and Environmental Engineering at the Massachusetts Institute of Technology. "Metamaterials" is the term coined by this group for creating new composites with novel, emergent properties not found in their component materials. This group integrates advanced design, computational modeling, and 3-D assembly with chemistry, materials engineering, and tissue engineering to generate entirely new "metamaterials" that are then printed into novel structures using a 3D printer. In other words, materials can be arranged into new structures to generate scaffolds that today do not exist in either engineered or biological forms. These metamaterials can be chemically or physically resurfaced to interact and direct the growth of surrounding tissues, degrade at predetermined rates, have complex structures including channels and pores to direct the development of structures such as blood vessels and nerves, and have specific physical and mechanical behaviors.

In 2013 Mueller's group published a novel, 3DP composite material that consisted of two materials, one with high compliance, and the other highly brittle, printed into three distinct biologically inspired patterns. These patterns included a bone-like pattern, a biocalcite pattern, and a rotated bone pattern. From the base materials that are brittle and exhibit catastrophic failure, synthetic composites are created with superior fracture mechanical properties exhibiting deformation and fracture mechanisms reminiscent of mineralized biological composites. The fact that the experimental fracture behaviors resembled the computer models of failure also indicated that computer models to design composite materials to exhibit tailored fracture properties and then use 3D printing to synthesize materials with such mechanical performance.[34]

The scope of novel designs and composite materials becomes possible by combining computer design, microengineering, and 3DP may be essential for the fabrication of scaffolds capable of inducing complex tissue regeneration such as in organ or limb regeneration. This would include the growth of gradient tissues and structures such as joints which are made up of multiple types of tissue. Cell- and growth factor–based tissue engineering, especially if those signals can be geographically localized by binding signaling molecules to materials in predetermined specific locations yielding "intelligent" scaffolds that can direct the growth and behavior of the surrounding native tissue. This can include stimulating ingrowth of the surrounding native tissue and directing the development of local stem cells in the local native tissue to yield new tissue types distinct from the surrounding tissues.

Some of the ways scaffolds can be fabricated to direct the propagation, migration, and differentiation of surrounding cells by modifying their surface characteristics,[31] their ultrastructure in the case of nanofibers,[35–37] or by the inclusion of bound growth factors and biologics. Growth factors that have been surface adsorbed or encapsulated in scaffolds include vascular endothelial growth factor (VEGF),[38] platelet derived growth factor (PDGF),[39] epidermal growth factor (EGF),[40] and bone morphogenic protein (BMP).[41] These scaffolds can then trigger specific biological processes such as angiogenesis, bone formation, and fibroblast ingrowth. The method of cross-linking or embedding growth factors onto or into scaffolds can control the timing of their release and thus the biological signal into surrounding tissues.

Similar to biologics, physical factors such as the ultrastructure of a scaffold can influence cell behavior, just as dramatically as signal transduction and growth factors. Advances in textiles and materials science have given rise to electrospinning as a fiber and scaffold production method which uses electric force to draw charged threads of polymer solutions or polymer melts up to fiber diameters in the order of some 100 nanometers.[36,37] Working with polymers of this scale creates a very large surface area to volume ratio (this ratio for a nanofiber can be as large as 103 times of that of a microfiber), increase flexibility in surface functionalities, and superior mechanical performance (e.g., stiffness and tensile strength) compared with other materials and scaffolds even made with the same type of polymer.[35]

These fibers can then be further woven into scaffolds in the form of patches, meshes, tubes, or cords with precise and complicated microarchitecture structures that in themselves can influence cell behavior. These nanofiber scaffolds can be so finely engineered so that their morphological is similar to the native ECM.[42,43] Nanoscale alterations in scaffold topography elicit diverse cell behavior, ranging from changes in cell adhesion,[44] motility and migration,[45] activation of specific signal transduction cascades such as tyrosine kinases,[46] and even lead to upregulation or downregulation of gene expression.[46] For example, skeletal muscle can be cultured in vitro; however, if the fibers are not oriented in a systematic fashion, the resulting tissue will not be functional. A nanoscale polycaprolactone scaffold can be constructed and seeded with myoblasts which then orient themselves in a uniform pattern as well as change their morphology with a larger length to diameter ratio which is compatible with force production characteristic of skeletal muscle tissue.[47]

Nanofibers can also be conductive of physical forces and charges. Piezoelectric effect is the ability of certain materials to generate an electric charge in response to applied mechanical stress. The word Piezoelectric is derived from the Greek piezein, which means to squeeze or press, and piezo, which is Greek for "push." Bone tissues have the ability to generate electrical signals. This bioelectrical current is generated by the shear force of collagen and the deformation of fluid-filled channels within the bone. The stress-generated electrical stimuli might play a determining role in impacting osteogenic growth.[48]

In orthopedics, the use of electric and electromagnetic fields has focused primarily on promoting healing of bony nonunions.[49] There are multiple strategies for applying electrical forces across nonunions and bony

deficiencies. Direct current (DC) involves the surgical implantation of a cathode at the fracture site and an anode in the nearby subcutaneous tissue, with the production of an electric current between them.[50] Pulsed electromagnetic fields (PEMFs) therapy is a noninvasive mode of bone-growth stimulation involving placement of a wire coil over the fracture site.[50] Capacitive coupling (CC) is where the electrical field is created by an oscillating electric current produced between two capacitor plates placed on the skin on opposite sides of the fracture.[50] Finally, combined magnetic fields (CMFs) are produced through the combination of alternating and DC electric stimulation and are delivered by an external pair of coils applied over the fracture site which is worn by patients for 30 min a day.[50]

Similarly, certain nanofiber scaffolds, by their ability to conduct charges, can affect the bone marrow stroma, which consists of a heterogeneous population of cells that provide the structural and physiological support for hematopoietic cells.[51] The bone marrow stroma also contains precursor cells, with stem cell–like character, which can differentiate into bone, cartilage, adipocytes, and hematopoietic supporting tissues.[51] In addition to hypoxia and growth factors as development signals to differentiate cells within the bone marrow stroma, electrical stimulation (ES) is known to be able to promote osteogenic differentiation of bone marrow storm cells (BMSCs).[52]

External stimulation, in the form of magnetic fields, electrical currents, or electromagnetic forces, is known to play a role in articular cartilage maintenance and regeneration as well as in bone remodeling and enhances bone healing.[53–55] This effect can also be enhanced by nanofiber scaffolds, and this effect opens the door for bone healing strategies that take advantage of both external stimulation and smart scaffold design. In one study, to enhance the local electrical stimulation effect on surrounding BMSCs, parallel-aligned conductive nanofibers were electrospun from the mixtures of poly(L-lactide) (PLLA) and multi-walled carbon nanotubes (MWCNTs) and used for cell culture. Cultured BMSCs were exposed to ES (direct current, 1.5 V; 1.5 h/ day) applied perpendicular to the nanofiber scaffold fibers within the BMSC culture. They found that in comparison with ES-free groups, bone-related markers and genes were found significantly upregulated when ES was applied on BMSCs growing on nanofibers having higher conductivity, especially when the ES signal was applied earlier in the stem cell differentiation.[52] Similar results were observed in a rat calvarium model in which polarized nanocomposite membranes were applied to 5-mm calvarial defects in 8-week-old male rats. Each rat underwent the creation of two calvarial defects, with the right-sided defect implanted with electroconductive scaffold and the left undergoing implantation with nonconductive scaffold as a control. Micro-CT analysis showed that the polarized nanocomposite membranes lead to an increase in the amount of regenerated bone volume and bone mineral density, and the nascent bone was indistinguishable from the surrounding host bone after 12 weeks implantation of polarized nanocomposite membranes when imaged with X-rays.[56]

REGENERATIVE ENGINEERING, STEM CELL APPLICATIONS

One of the frontiers in orthopedic surgery lies in the ability to reconstruct badly traumatized tissue which has been removed for one reason or another. Many of the tissues most often treated by orthopedic surgeons do not undergo regeneration, including muscles, articular cartilage, ligaments, and nerves. Even bone, which in general can regenerate and change through remodeling, can be difficult to reconstruct in the presence of infection or cases of severe bone loss. Current reconstructive options include replacement of the diseased or absent tissue with implants or sequential and painful procedures using autograft or donor allografts to replace the diseased/missing tissue, or in severe cases, amputations to maximize function through prostheses.

The prospect of stem cell therapy, particularly mesenchymal stem cell (MSC) applications, may be the future treatment of many orthopedic ailments including osteoarthritis, osteochondral lesions, sprains/strains, and other trauma to muscles or ligaments, tendinoses, as well as meniscal and rotator cuff pathologies. The precursor, MSCs, can easily be isolated from the patient from many anatomic locations, including marrow aspirate, peripheral blood, muscle, and adipose[57] giving rise to personalized medicine and minimizing the effects of immune rejection or risk of disease transmission through the use of allografts.

Strategically, the regenerative orthopedic surgeon must carefully select the biopsy site from which they isolate the MSCs. In general, the closer the biopsy tissue is to the target tissue into which the isolated MSCs are to be differentiated into, the more successful they will be. For example, equine MSCs derived from bone marrow (bm-MSCs) had better chondrogenic potential and more readily produced hyaline-like matrix and GAGs than adipose tissue–derived MSCs (a-MSCs).[58] Similarly, in another study, synovial MSCs (closest to the target tissue of cartilage) had better chondrogenesis than bm-MSCs.[59]

Once MSCs have been harvested from the patient, which many times can be an office procedure, the cells must then be grown to sufficient number to be used for therapeutic applications. This is performed through cell culture where the harvested MSCs are grown in a monolayer in nutrient broth, and in doing so, their number amplified through cell division. However, in vitro expansion cannot be carried out indefinitely as the pluripotency of the MSCs decrease the "older" or more in vitro divisions they undergo,[60] and so the biopsies must be of sufficient quantity and quality to obtain an adequate number of progenitor cells.

Experiments using mesenchymal stem cells in animal and some human trials show enhancement in cartilage healing, meniscal repairs, tendon repair, and intervertebral disc treatment. MSC therapy appears to be promising for the treatment of early osteoarthritis, both through their regenerative capacity as well as through an anti-inflammatory effect.[61] For example, injections containing MSCs seem to be a potential treatment for early osteoarthritis. A study evaluating adipose-derived MSC injection into elderly patients (age >65 years) with knee osteoarthritis (OA) found that 88% demonstrated improved cartilage status at 2-year follow-up during second-look arthroscopy.[62] Another randomized trial of 30 patients with chronic knee pain unresponsive to conservative treatments and who also showed radiological evidence of osteoarthritis showed promising radiographic and clinical results in response to a single injection of allogenic bm-MSCs. When compared to the control group who received a single hyaluronic acid injection, the experimental group showed improved pain, disability, and quality-of-life ratings 1 year out, as well as articular cartilage as assessed by quantitative magnetic resonance imaging T2 mapping was also improved.[63] Larger scale studies are necessary to truly evaluate the potential regenerative potential of MSCs in chronic osteoarthritis. Potential frontiers could include the use of hydrogels or other scaffolds to stabilize mesenchymal stem cells, potentially directing them toward the articular cartilage surface to maximize any paracrine signal, anti-inflammatory, or direct regenerative effects on the target tissue.

Mesenchymal stem cell therapy has also been studied in acute articular cartilage injury. Current treatments include microfracture, microdrilling, osteochondral transplantation, and matrix autologous chondral implantation.[64] Autologous mesenchymal stem cell recruitment through microfracture or microdrilling creates a perforation through cortical bone into the bone marrow which subsequently induces a fibrin clot formation in the osteochondral defect containing platelets, growth factors, vascular elements, and MSCs.[65] Similarly, platelet-rich plasma (PRP) and bone marrow aspirate concentrate (BMAC) can be a source of isolated bm-MSCs that can be injected and contribute to the healing of osteochondral lesions either when used in isolation or in conjunction with microfracture.[66] Commercial kits for PRP and BMAC are now available. More sophisticated strategies for cartilage regeneration involve synovial stem cells as an additional source for MSCs, and their use has demonstrated chondrogenic potential. In one animal study, synovial MSCs were injected into acute cartilage defects created in porcine knees. The knees were immobilized for 10 min, which as demonstrated by fluorescent microscopy was sufficient time for stem cell adherence to take place. The animals were then followed up, and treated knees showed first a membrane formation and later cartilage formation which was native-appearing on histology.[67] There are also promising results for the treatment of osteochondral lesions with mesenchymal stem cells with or without scaffolds in humans. In humans, stem cell use for chondral repair has also proven promising.[68] For example, BMAC has been used in a prospective trial to treat focal chondral defects of an average size of 9.2 cm sq in 15 patients. The localization of the BMAC was aided by covering it with a collagen I/III matrix. This treatment produced significant improvements in patient-reported outcome scores, and magnetic resonance imaging demonstrated complete hyaline-like cartilage coverage in 80%. The improvement in cartilage quality was confirmed with second-look arthroscopy demonstrating normal to nearly normal tissue.[69] Similar results were found for superiority of chondral defects treated with BMAC compared with matrix-induced autologous chondrocyte implantation (MACI) for patellofemoral lesions in 37 patients. Posttreatment magnetic resonance imaging showed complete filling of defects in 81% of BMAC-treated patients when compared with 76% of MACI-treated patients.[70]

Upper extremity disorders have also been studied as potential targets for MSC treatment. Rotator cuff pathologies are difficult to treat because the rotator cuff tendons are relatively avascular, and the injuries tend to be chronic. There is a highly specialized fibrocartilaginous transition zone between the rotator cuff and the bone which does not regenerate after repair.[71–73] As described previously in this chapter, most surgical techniques simply reapproximate the torn end of the tendon to its insertion point on the humeral head, hoping for at best simple scar formation and healing which has inferior mechanical properties when compared with the native enthesis. Regenerative engineering and

medicine's efforts have been used to redirect the rotator cuff away from simple healing and to regenerate a functional bone-to-tendon interface.

The native enthesis is a sophisticated biological solution to a significant mechanical challenge. The stiffness difference between tendon and bone is responsible for significant mechanical stress in the regeneration zone.[74] The tissue that presents bone-to-tendon transition gradually changes its microstructure to accommodate the energy transmission from the bone and across to the tendon itself. The biomechanics of the four zones of the enthesis, namely the tendon area (zone 1) where there is a predominance of type I collagen fibers, the nonmineralized fibrocartilage area (zone 2), mineralized fibrocartilage (zone 3), and bone-alike composition in zone 4.[75] A fibrocartilage scar that would form in simple healing after reapproximation would have neither the functionality nor the durability that a regenerated enthesis might have.

Similar to MSC-based treatment approaches for articular cartilage injury, mesenchymal stem cells can be harvested from the patient from a variety of tissues and applied to the injured area either independently or in conjunction with reparative surgery depending on the stage and severity of the injury. These approaches can include platelet-rich plasma injections, bone marrow aspirate, growth factor supplements, and cell- and gene-modified cell therapy.[76] Scaffold-based strategy to enhance rotator cuff healing is based on two basic types of interactions. Scaffolds that act as vehicles that maintain the rounded shape of the cells and avoid contact in between them, promote the chondrogenic differentiation, and avoid expression of type I collagen. The other strategy involves porous gelatin scaffolds or those that use fibrin which favor a fibrocartilaginous phenotype due to the expression of collagen types I and II.[73,77] Both of these scaffold strategies are important for the complicated microstructure of the enthesis.

There are several commercially available ECM scaffolds being tested clinically to improve enthesis repair after rotator cuff (RC) repair. These extracellular matrices include GraftJacket, TissueMend, Restore, and CuffPatch.[78] However, these extracellular matrices fail to regenerate the fibrocartilage gradient at the enthuses because their structural properties degrade over time and do not match the rate of new ECM formation.[79] Synthetic matrices may lead to better regeneration of the bone-to-tendon junction. Combining an electrospun scaffold mimicking the tissue microenvironment with the structural signaling cues nanostructure can create as well as deliver MSC to take advantage of paracrine signaling and their regenerative potential in a rat rotator cuff repair model.[80] The combination of mesenchymal stem cells and physical signals from the scaffold, in a gradient fashion, is likely the strategy that will result in ethesis formation.

INNOVATION AND THE DELIVERY OF CARE

Current frontiers in regenerative engineering focus on not only tissue propagation but more sophisticated questions which involve function, development, and a focus on structure regeneration as opposed to individual tissues. The enthesis of the rotator cuff is a prime example where simple tissue engineering which could yield organized collagen in the form of a tendon would not be sufficient to recreate the sophisticated mechanics of the four zones of the bone-to-tendon transition zone in the rotator cuff. A well-designed material, phased scaffold, or implant has immediate applications in the clinical world as physicians and surgeon seek to improve patient outcomes as well as patient experience to reduce the duration and number of interventions necessary to restore structure and function.

In addition to increasing the scope and complexity of biological ailments that can be addressed by the modern orthopedic surgeon, regenerative engineering has the potential to change the manner and pace at which many orthopedic conditions are treated. This could be viewed as a disruptive innovation.

Sustaining innovations are common in medicine and surgery. They represent incremental and logical improvements in technologies, such as, a better implants, a wider lens in an arthroscope, and stronger anti-inflammatory medication. Disruptive innovations are unique in a way that they offer an often simpler solution or method to fulfill a need that is more convenient than sustaining innovation would be. An example of a disruptive innovation in consumer technology was the cellular phone that could take pictures. At the time, digital cameras were more common, and each year their charge coupled device sensor resolution would improve and price adjusts appropriately. Sales of digital cameras significantly decreased when cell phones with built in cameras that could connect to the internet were introduced because they fulfilled the social need of people to share their photos with families and friends. People were willing to sacrifice photo resolution for the convenience of one elegant device that could take (albeit lower resolution) photographs to share with their friends.

Regenerative engineering solutions in orthopedic surgery could decrease the overall costs and utilization of the health-care system through disease prevention or modification. Osteoarthritis no longer has to progress to the point that it causes disability, decreases productivity, and requires invasive joint replacement surgery when perhaps the cartilage degeneration process could be slowed, halted, or even reversed through a series of injections after office-based liposuction or a blood draw to obtain MSCs. Fracture surgery with implants might be replaced with a minimally invasive injection of "bone glue" scaffold where after a brief period of immobilization, people could mobilize without needing metallic implants. Similarly, for traumatic injuries, infections, and reconstruction after cancer, tissues could be regenerated in a single procedure through the implantation of sophisticated and personalized scaffolds that could be custom designed and printed on a three-dimensional printer with integrated signal transduction molecules to regenerate all tissues over the course of several weeks or months rather than months to years of sequential and painful procedures to reconstruct and rearrange what little injuries and scarred tissue might be left.

Regenerative engineering represents the next frontiers in orthopedic surgery, creating elegant and simple solutions to restoration of the structure and function of the musculoskeletal system.

DISCLOSURE STATEMENT

Dr. Laurencin is an owner of hot-bone, healing orthopedic technologies, natural polymer devices, and soft tissue regeneration. He receives royalties from Globus Inc. Dr Badon has no Disclosures.

REFERENCES

1. Seifert AW, et al. Skin regeneration in adult axolotls: a blueprint for scar-free healing in vertebrates. *PLoS One.* 2012;7(4):e32875.
2. Osterman M, Draeger R, Stern P. Acute hand infections. *J Hand Surg Am.* 2014;39(8):1628–1635; quiz 1635.
3. Liu H, et al. A preliminary study of skin ultrasound in diffuse cutaneous systemic sclerosis: does skin echogenicity matter? *PLoS One.* 2017;12(3):e0174481.
4. Nauta TD, van Hinsbergh VW, Koolwijk P. Hypoxic signaling during tissue repair and regenerative medicine. *Int J Mol Sci.* 2014;15(11):19791–19815.
5. Nagaraja MP, Jo H. The role of mechanical stimulation in recovery of bone loss-high versus low magnitude and frequency of force. *Life (Basel).* 2014;4(2):117–130.
6. Template for Skin Regeneration.pdf.
7. Dimitriou R, Tsiridis E, Giannoudis PV. Current concepts of molecular aspects of bone healing. *Injury.* 2005;36(12):1392–1404.
8. Han L, et al. Construction and biocompatibility of a thin type I/II collagen composite scaffold. *Cell Tissue Bank.* 2018;19(1):47–59.

9. Park SH, et al. Three-dimensional bio-printed scaffold sleeves with mesenchymal stem cells for enhancement of tendon-to-bone healing in anterior cruciate ligament reconstruction using soft-tissue tendon graft. *Arthrosc J Arthrosc Relat Surg.* 2018;34(1):166–179.

10. Gan Y, et al. An interpenetrating network-strengthened and toughened hydrogel that supports cell-based nucleus pulposus regeneration. *Biomaterials.* 2017;136:12–28.

11. Borem R, et al. Angle-ply biomaterial scaffold for annulus fibrosus repair replicates native tissue mechanical properties, restores spinal kinematics, and supports cell viability. *Acta Biomater.* 2017;58:254–268.

12. Wu Y, et al. Interwoven aligned conductive nanofiber yarn/hydrogel composite scaffolds for engineered 3D cardiac anisotropy. *ACS Nano.* 2017;11(6):5646–5659.

13. Eren Cimenci C, et al. Laminin mimetic peptide nanofibers regenerate acute muscle defect. *Acta Biomater.* 2017 15;60:190–200.

14. Zhang Z, et al. Electrically conductive biodegradable polymer composite for nerve regeneration: electricity-stimulated neurite outgrowth and axon regeneration. *Artif Organs.* 2007;31(1):13–22.

15. Pol0-Corrales L, Latorre-Esteves M, Ramirez-Vick J. Scaffold design for bone Regeneration. *J Nanosci Nanotechnol.* 2014;14(1):15–56.

16. Kiapour AM, Murray MM. Basic science of anterior cruciate ligament injury and repair. *Bone Joint Res.* 2014;3(2):20–31.

17. Lu HH, et al. Anterior cruciate ligament regeneration using braided biodegradable scaffolds: in vitro optimization studies. *Biomaterials.* 2005;26(23):4805–4816.

18. Ouyang HW, et al. Assembly of bone marrow stromal cell sheets with knitted poly (L-lactide) scaffold for engineering ligament analogs. *J Biomed Mater Res B Appl Biomater.* 2005;75(2):264–271.

19. Freeman J, Woods M, Laurencin C. Tissue engineering of the anterior cruciate ligament using a braid-twist scaffold design. *PMC.* 2007;40(9):2029–2036.

20. Kiapour AM, Fleming BC, Murray MM. Biomechanical outcomes of bridge-enhanced anterior cruciate ligament repair are influenced by sex in a preclinical model. *Clin Orthop Relat Res.* 2015;473(8):2599–2608.

21. Murray MM, et al. The bridge-enhanced anterior cruciate ligament repair (BEAR) procedure: an early feasibility cohort study. *Orthop J Sports Med.* 2016;4(11):2325967116672176.

22. P B. Arthroplastie totale de la hanche par prothèse en alumine frit,e: etude exp,rimentale et premères applications cliniques. *Rev Chir Orthop Reparatrice Appar Mot.* 1972;58:229–246.

23. Hamadouche M, et al. Alumina-on-Alumina articulation in total hip arthroplasty: from bench-side to bedside. *Semin Arthroplasty.* 2006;17(3–4):125–133.

24. Peroglio M, et al. Toughening of bio-ceramics scaffolds by polymer coating. *J Eur Ceram Soc.* 2007;27(7):2679–2685.

25. Ryshkewitch E. Compression strength of porous sintered alumina and zirconia. *J Am Ceram Soc.* 1953;34(10):322–326.

26. Tampieri A, et al. From wood to bone: multi-step process to convert wood hierarchical structures into biomimetic hydroxyapatite scaffolds for bone tissue engineering. *J Mater Chem.* 2009;19(28).

27. Renders GA, et al. Porosity of human mandibular condylar bone. *J Anat.* 2007;210(3):239–248.

28. C D, et al. Natural coral exoskeleton as a bone graft substitute: a review. *Biomed Mater Eng.* 2002;12(1):15–35.

29. Hu J, et al. Production and analysis of hydroxyapatite from Australian corals via hydrothermal process. *J Mater Sci Lett.* 2007;20(1):85–87.

30. Nandi SK, et al. Converted marine coral hydroxyapatite implants with growth factors: in vivo bone regeneration. *Mater Sci Eng C Mater Biol Appl.* 2015;49:816–823.

31. Park JW, et al. Evaluation of bone healing with eggshell-derived bone graft substitutes in rat calvaria: a pilot study. *J Biomed Mater Res A.* 2008;87(1):203–214.

32. Tavangar A, Tan B, Venkatakrishnan K. Synthesis of three-dimensional calcium carbonate nanofibrous structure from eggshell using femtosecond laser ablation. *J Nanobiotechnol.* 2011;9:1.

33. Dadhich P, et al. A simple approach for an eggshell-based 3D-printed osteoinductive multiphasic calcium phosphate scaffold. *ACS Appl Mater Interfaces.* 2016;8(19):11910–11924.

34. Dimas LS, et al. Tough composites inspired by mineralized natural materials: computation, 3D printing, and testing. *Adv Funct Mater.* 2013;23(36):4629–4638.

35. Huang Z-M, et al. A review on polymer nanofibers by electrospinning and their applications in nanocomposites. *Compos Sci Technol.* 2003;63(15):2223–2253.

36. Yang F, et al. Electrospinning of nano/micro scale poly (L-lactic acid) aligned fibers and their potential in neural tissue engineering. *Biomaterials.* 2005;26(15):2603–2610.

37. Li M, et al. Electrospinning polyaniline-contained gelatin nanofibers for tissue engineering applications. *Biomaterials.* 2006;27(13):2705–2715.

38. Henry JJD, et al. Engineering the mechanical and biological properties of nanofibrous vascular grafts for in situ vascular tissue engineering. *Biofabrication.* 2017;9(3):035007.

39. Lee J, et al. The effect of controlled release of PDGF-BB from heparin-conjugated electrospun PCL/gelatin scaffolds on cellular bioactivity and infiltration. *Biomaterials.* 2012;33(28):6709–6720.

40. Pulavendran S, Thiyagarajan G. Three-dimensional scaffold containing EGF incorporated biodegradable polymeric nanoparticles for stem cell based tissue engineering applications. *Biotechnol Bioproc Eng.* 2011;16(2):393–399.

41. Zhao X, et al. BMP-2 immobilized PLGA/hydroxyapatite fibrous scaffold via polydopamine stimulates osteoblast growth. *Mater Sci Eng C Mater Biol Appl.* 2017;78:658–666.

42. PX M, Ruiyun Z. Synthetic nano-scale fibrous extracellular matrix. *J Biomed Mater Res.* 1999;46(1):60–72.

43. Geckil H, et al. Engineering hydrogels as extracellular matrix mimics. *Nanomed (Lond).* 2010;5(3):469–484.

44. Jahan H, et al. The effect of aligned and random electrospun fibrous scaffolds on rat mesenchymal stem cell proliferation. *Cell J.* 2012;14(1):31–38.
45. Ottosson M, Jakobsson A, Johansson F. Accelerated wound closure - differently organized nanofibers affect cell migration and hence the closure of artificial wounds in a cell based in vitro model. *PLoS One.* 2017;12(1):e0169419.
46. Brown JL, et al. Composite scaffolds: bridging nanofiber and microsphere architectures to improve bioactivity of mechanically competent constructs. *J Biomed Mater Res A.* 2010;95A(4):1150–1158.
47. X T, Y K, C L. Electroconductive nanofiber scaffolds for muscle regenerative engineering. *Front Bioeng Biotechnol.* 2016.
48. Isaacson BM, Bloebaum RD. Bone bioelectricity: what have we learned in the past 160 years? *J Biomed Mater Res A.* 2010;95(4):1270–1279.
49. JT R. Clinical effects of electromagnetic and electric fields on fracture healing. *Clin Orthop Relat Res.* 1998;(suppl 355):S205–S215.
50. Goldstein C, Sprague S, Petrisor BA. Electrical stimulation for fracture healing: current evidence. *J Orthop Trauma.* 2010;24:S62–S65.
51. PH K, et al. Bone marrow stromal cells: characterization and clinical application. *Crit Rev Oral Biol Med.* 1999;10(2):165–181.
52. Zhu S, et al. Time-dependent effect of electrical stimulation on osteogenic differentiation of bone mesenchymal stromal cells cultured on conductive nanofibers. *J Biomed Mater Res Part A.* 2017;105(12):3369–3383.
53. Shao S, et al. Osteoblast function on electrically conductive electrospun PLA/MWCNTs nanofibers. *Biomaterials.* 2011;32(11):2821–2833.
54. Ribeiro C, et al. Dynamic piezoelectric stimulation enhances osteogenic differentiation of human adipose stem cells. *J Biomed Mater Res A.* 2015;103(6):2172–2175.
55. Yun HM, et al. Magnetic nanocomposite scaffolds combined with static magnetic field in the stimulation of osteoblastic differentiation and bone formation. *Biomaterials.* 2016;85:88–98.
56. Zhang X, et al. Nanocomposite membranes enhance bone regeneration through restoring physiological electric microenvironment. *ACS Nano.* 2016;10(8):7279–7286.
57. A A, JJ M. Mesenchymal stem cells: isolation and therapeutics. *Stem Cells Dev.* 2004;13(4):436–448.
58. Vidal MA, et al. Comparison of chondrogenic potential in equine mesenchymal stromal cells derived from adipose tissue and bone marrow. *Vet Surg.* 2008;37(8):713–724.
59. Yoshimura H, et al. Comparison of rat mesenchymal stem cells derived from bone marrow, synovium, periosteum, adipose tissue, and muscle. *Cell Tissue Res.* 2007;327(3):449–462.
60. A B, et al. Proliferation kinetics and differentiation potential of ex vivo expanded human bone marrow stromal cells- Implications for their use in cell therapy. *Exp Hematol.* 2000;28(6):707–715.
61. Pers YM, et al. Mesenchymal stem cells for the management of inflammation in osteoarthritis: state of the art and perspectives. *Osteoarthr Cartil.* 2015;23(11):2027–2035.
62. Koh YG, et al. Clinical results and second-look arthroscopic findings after treatment with adipose-derived stem cells for knee osteoarthritis. *Knee Surg Sports Traumatol Arthrosc.* 2015;23(5):1308–1316.
63. Vega A, et al. Treatment of knee osteoarthritis with allogeneic bone marrow mesenchymal stem cells: a randomized controlled trial. *Transplantation.* 2015;99(8):1681–1690.
64. Mirza Y, Oussedik S. Is there a role for stem cells in treating articular injury? *Br J Hosp Med (Lond).* 2017;78(7):372–377.
65. Nukavarapu S, et al. Regeneration of hyaline-like cartilage in situ with SOX9 stimulation of bone marrow-derived mesenchymal stem cells. *Plos One.* 2017;12(6).
66. Mosna F, Sensebé L, Krampera M. Human bone marrow and adipose tissue mesenchymal stem cells- a user's guide. *Stem Cells Dev.* 2010;19(10):1449–1470.
67. Nakamura T, et al. Arthroscopic, histological and MRI analyses of cartilage repair after a minimally invasive method of transplantation of allogeneic synovial mesenchymal stromal cells into cartilage defects in pigs. *Cytotherapy.* 2012;14(3):327–338.
68. Chahla J, et al. Concentrated bone marrow aspirate for the treatment of chondral injuries and osteoarthritis of the knee: a systematic review of outcomes. *Orthop J Sports Med.* 2016;4(1):2325967115625481.
69. Gobbi A, et al. One-step cartilage repair with bone marrow aspirate concentrated cells and collagen matrix in full-thickness knee cartilage lesions: results at 2-year follow-up. *Cartilage.* 2011;2(3):286–299.
70. Gobbi A, et al. Matrix-induced autologous chondrocyte implantation versus multipotent stem cells for the treatment of large patellofemoral chondral lesions: a nonrandomized prospective trial. *Cartilage.* 2015;6(2):82–97.
71. Galatz LM, et al. Characteristics of the rat supraspinatus tendon during tendon-to-bone healing after acute injury. *J Orthop Res.* 2006;24(3):541–550.
72. Kobayashi M, et al. Expression of growth factors in the early phase of supraspinatus tendon healing in rabbits. *J Shoulder Elbow Surg.* 2006;15(3):371–377.
73. Valencia Mora M, et al. Stem cell therapy in the management of shoulder rotator cuff disorders. *World J Stem Cells.* 2015;7(4):691–699.
74. Lui P, et al. Biology and augmentation of tendon-bone insertion repair. *J Orthop Surg Res.* 2010;5:59.
75. S T, GM G, LM G. The development and morphogenesis of the tendon-to-bone insertion - what development can teach us about healing. *J Musculoskelet Neuronal Interact.* 2010;10(1):35–45.
76. Nixon AJ, Watts AE, Schnabel LV. Cell- and gene-based approaches to tendon regeneration. *J Shoulder Elbow Surg.* 2012;21(2):278–294.

77. Gimble JM, Bunnell BA, Guilak F. Human adipose-derived cells: an update on the transition to clinical translation. *Regen Med.* 2012;7(2):225–235.

78. KA D, et al. Commercial extracellular matrix scaffolds for rotator cuff tendon repair. Biomechanical, biochemical, and cellular properties. *J Bone Joint Surg Am.* 2006;88(12):2665–2672.

79. Smietana MJ, et al. Tissue-engineered tendon for enthesis regeneration in a rat rotator cuff model. *BioResearch Open Access.* 2017;6(1):47–57.

80. Peach MS, et al. Engineered stem cell niche matrices for rotator cuff tendon regenerative engineering. *PLoS One.* 2017;12(4):e0174789.

Index

A

Abduction with external rotation (ABER) position, 77
Acellular dermal matrices (ADMs), 55, 66, 176
Achilles tendinopathy
  acellular dermal matrices (ADMs), 176
  bone marrow aspirate concentrate (BMAc), 175–176
  platelet-rich plasma (PRP), 175
  tendon healing, 175
Adipose-derived stem cells (ADSCs)
  cartilage restoration, 89
  orthopaedic surgery, 40–41
  osteoarthritis (OA), 89
  peripheral nerve repair, 152
Allogenic bone graft
  bone graft extenders, 167
  fresh allografts, 167
  immunogenicity, 167
  osteoinductivity, 167
  processed allografts, 167
Allografts, 4
  anterior cruciate ligament (ACL) reconstruction
    benefits, 108
    disadvantages, 108–109
    MOON cohort analyses, 109
    quality, 108–109
    soft tissue allografts, 109
  hand surgery, 135
  processing steps, 49
American Association of Tissue Banks (AATB), 50, 65–66
American Orthopaedic Society for Sports Medicine (AOSSM), 66
American Shoulder and Elbow Society score (ASES), 69–70
Amniotic fluid mesenchymal stem cells (AF-MSCs), 153
  orthopaedic surgery, 42–43
  peripheral nerve repair, 153
Amniotic membrane products, 66
Angel System, 2f
Anterior cruciate ligament (ACL) reconstruction
  allografts
    benefits, 108
    disadvantages, 108–109
    MOON cohort analyses, 109
    quality, 108–109
    soft tissue ACL allografts, 109

Anterior cruciate ligament (ACL) reconstruction (Continued)
  autografts
    bone patella tendon bone, 107–108
    hamstring, 107
    quadriceps, 108
  graft maturation, 113–114
  synthetic grafts, 106–107, 109
  tendon-to-bone healing
    ACL insertion, 110
    bone tunnel widening, 112
    "ligamentization", 111
    mechanical stability, 110–111
    "proliferative" phase, 110
    soft tissue integration, 110
    stem cells, 113
    vascularity, 112–113
  xenografts, 106–107, 109–110
Articular cartilage
  marrow stimulation, 177
  osteochondral allografts, 177
  zones, 31–32, 32f, 176–177
Articular hyaline cartilage, 101
Articular sparing resections & implants, 195
Autogenous biological conduits, 146
Autografts, 49
  anterior cruciate ligament (ACL) reconstruction
    bone patella tendon bone, 107–108
    hamstring, 107
    quadriceps, 108
  cancellous grafts, 167
  fracture, 185–186
  iliac crest, 166–167
Autologous blood injections (ABI), 2–3
Autologous bone grafting, 3–4
Autologous chondrocyte implantation (ACI), 65
  applications of, 36–37
  bone grafting, 33–34
  first generation, 34–35
  focal cartilage defects, 93–94
  graft bed preparation, 34–35
  inaugural techniques, 34–35
  matrix-induced ACI (MACI), 34f
  postprocedure healing and rehabilitation
    arthroscopy, 36
    continuous passive motion (CPM), 35
    transition phase, 35–36

Autologous chondrocyte implantation (ACI) (Continued)
  safety, 37
  second generation, 35
Autologous conditioned plasma (ACP). See Platelet-rich plasma (PRP)
Autologous matrix induced chondrogenesis (AMIC), 90–91
Axons, 141

B

BEAR scaffold, 115
Beta-tricalcim phosphate (B-TCP), 178–179
Bio4, 168
Bioactive glasses, 168
Bioburden reduction methods, 51
BioCartilage, 91
Biologic therapies
  bone graft, 63
  enhanced healing, 63
  restoration, 63
  sports medicine. See Sports medicine
  tissue grafting and banking, 63
Bisphosphonates, spontaneous osteonecrosis of the knee (SPONK), 128
Bone allografts
  bone formation and growth, 53
  cellular bone allografts, 54
  demineralization, 54
  filling bone voids, 53–54
  proteinaceous factors, 53
Bone graft extenders, 167
Bone grafting
  foot and ankle surgery
    mechanical stability, 177–178
    osseous healing, 178–179
  hand surgery, 135
Bone impaction grafting
  secondary osteonecrosis (SON), 130
  standard TKA, 130
Bone loss, upper extremity
  glenohumeral dislocation, 75
  glenoid bone loss. See Glenoid bone loss
  Hill–Sachs lesion. See Hill–Sachs lesion
  platelet-rich plasma (PRP), 80–82
  shoulder dislocations, 75

Note: Page numbers followed by "f" indicate figures, "t" indicate tables.

Bone marrow aspirate concentrate (BMAC)
  achilles tendinopathy, 175–176
  fracture, 188–189
  orthopaedic surgery
    application, 30–31
    bone healing, 27
    cellular composition, 27
    contents, 27, 28f
    growth factors and cytokines, 27–29
    mesenchymal stem cells (MSCs), 27
    safety, 31
    sources, 29
    technique, 29, 30t
  osseous healing, 179
  osteoarthritis (OA), 89
Bone marrow stem cells (BMSCs)
  orthopaedic surgery, 39–40
  osteoarthritis (OA), 89
  partial anterior cruciate ligament (ACL) reconstruction, 115–116
  peripheral nerve repair, 153
Bone morphogenic protein (BMP), 4, 168–169
  fracture
    BESTT trial, 187–188
    recombinant human BMP-2 (rhBMP-2), 187
    rhBMP-7, 188
  hand surgery, 135
  osseous healing, 179
  osteoarthritis (OA), 101
Bone patellar tendon bone (BPTB) autograft, 107–108
Bone tunnel widening, 112
Bone void fillers
  benign bone tumors, 194
  calcium phosphate, 186, 186f–187f
  calcium sulfate, 186, 187f
  synthetic, 186
Bridge-enhanced ACL repair (BEAR), 204

C

Calcium hydroxyapatite (HA), 194
Calcium phosphate, 186, 186f–187f
Calcium sulfate, 135–136, 186, 187f
Cancellous grafts, 167
Cartiform, 4f
Cartilage autograft implantation system (CAIS), 95
Cartilage structure
  collagen fibrils, 86
  focal chondral defect, 87
  glycosaminoglycans (GAGs), 86
  hyaline cartilage, 85
  structural zones, 86–87
  synovial fluid, 86
Cellular allograft, 167–168
Cellular augments, 71–72

Cements, hand surgery, 136
Ceramics, 168
  hand surgery, 135
  regenerative engineering, 204–205
Chondral/osteochondral defects, knee
  autologous chondrocyte implantation (ACI), 93–94
  microfracture (MFx), 89–91
  osteoarthritis (OA)
    adipose-derived mesenchymal stem cells, 89
    bone marrow–derived stem cells, 89
    hyaluronic acid (HA), 87–88
    platelet-rich plasma (PRP), 88–89, 88f
  osteoarticular transfer system (OATS), 91
  osteochondral allograft transplantation, 92–93
  particulated minced cartilage, 94–95
Ciliary neuronotrophic factor (CNTF), 142
Clostridium histolyticum collagenases (CHCs), 137–138
Code of Federal Regulations, 12
Collagen conduits, 149
Collagen-covered autologous chondrocyte implantation (CCACI), 65
Collateral ligament, 106
Connective tissue progenitor cells (CTPs)
  fracture, 188
Coralline hydroxyapatite, hand surgery, 135
Core decompression of osteonecrotic lesions, 128
Cortico-cancellous grafts, 167
Cruciate ligaments
  anterior cruciate ligament (ACL), 105
  posterior cruciate ligament (PCL), 105–106
Cryopreservation, human allografts, 56–57

D

Decellularized nerve allografts (DCAs), 147
Demineralized bone matrix (DBM), 4, 49, 135, 167
Denosumab, giant cell tumor of bone (GCTB), 193
Dense cortical bone, 205
Diffuse osteoarthritis (OA), 85
Distal tibial allograft (DTA), 77–78, 78f

E

Electrospinning, 154
Embryonic stem cells (ESCs), 4–5, 151–152
Enchondromas, 136, 194

End-organ atrophy, 145
Endothelial growth factor (EGF), 21t
Extracellular matrix patches, 71
Extracorporeal devitalized autograft reconstructions, 197
Extracorporeal shock wave therapy, 176

F

Fascial allograft, 71–72
Federal Food and Drug Association (FDA)
  chemical testing, 9–10
  Code of Federal Regulations, 12
  direct-to-consumer marketing, 10
  "Food, Drug, and Cosmetic Act", 10
  history, 9–10
  Human Cells, Tissues, and Cellular and Tissue-based Products (HCT/P), 12, 13f
  International Society for Stem Cell Research (ISSCR) guidelines, 16
  new approval system, 15
  "1976 Medical Device Amendments", 10
  organization, 10, 11f
  precedent
    guidance documents, 14
    Tissue Reference Group (TRG) recommendations, 14–15
    Untitled Letters and Warning Letters, 14
  Public Health Service Act (PHSA), 12
  "Pure Food and Drugs Act", 9–10
  REGROW Act, 15
  responsibilities, 10, 11f
  RMAT designation, 15
  safety and efficacy, 10
  21st Century Cures Act, 15–16
  351 product development pathway, 12, 13f
Fibrin, peripheral nerve injuries, 153–154
Fibroblast growth factors (FGFs), 27–29, 28t
"Food, Drug, and Cosmetic Act", 10
Foot and ankle surgery
  achilles tendinopathy
    acellular dermal matrices (ADMs), 176
    bone marrow aspirate concentrate (BMAc), 175–176
    platelet-rich plasma (PRP), 175
    tendon healing, 175
  articular cartilage, 176–177
  bone grafting
    mechanical stability, 177–178
    osseous healing, 178–179
  plantar fasciitis, 176
Fracture
  biologic augmentation
    autograft, 185–186
    bone marrow aspirate (BMA) injection, 185

Fracture *(Continued)*
    critical sized bone defects, 185
    indications, 185
    segmental defects, 185
    stimulating cells, 185
    bone morphogenic proteins (BMPs)
        BESTT trial, 187–188
        recombinant human BMP-2
            (rhBMP-2), 187
        rhBMP-7, 188
    bone void fillers
        calcium phosphate, 186,
            186f–187f
        calcium sulfate, 186, 187f
        synthetic, 186
    cell-based therapy, 188
    delayed healing and nonunion, 185
Free vascularized fibular graft (FVFG),
    196–197
Freeze-drying, human allografts, 57

G
Gamma-irradiated allografts
    chemical pretreatments, 52
    dose range, 52
    target dose, 52
    temperature, 52–53
    tissue recovery and processing
        methods, 53
Giant cell tumor of bone (GCTB), 193
Glenohumeral dislocation, 75
Glenoid bone loss
    accepted numerical value, 76
    arthroscopic Bankart repair, 76
    bony lesions, 75
    distal tibial allograft (DTA), 77–78, 78f
    failure rate, 75
    iliac crest bone graft (ICBG), 77
    Latarjet procedure
        arthroscopic Latarjet, 76–77
        coracoid postharvesting before
            fixation, 76
        limitation, 76
        subscapularis split and
            subscapularis tenotomy
            techniques, 77
    Pico method, 75–76
    3-dimensional (3-D) computed
        tomography, 75f
Growth factors
    bone marrow aspirate concentrate
        (BMAC), 27–29
    cellular effects, 21t
    hand surgery, 137
    platelet-derived growth factor
        (PDGF), 20
    platelet rich plasma (PRP)
        activation, 21
        commercial PRP systems, 21
        leukocyte-and platelet-rich fibrin
            (L-PRF), 22
        leukocyte-and platelet-rich plasma
            (L-PRP), 22

Growth factors *(Continued)*
        muscle injuries, 23
        osteoarthritis, 23–24
        platelet concentration, 20
        preparation, 20–21, 22t
        pure platelet-rich fibrin (P-PRF),
            22
        pure platelet-rich plasma (P-PRP),
            22
        randomized controlled trials
            (RCTs), 20
        rotator cuff, 23
        tendinopathy, 23
    spinal fusion, 168–169
    TGF-β1, 20
    vascular endothelial growth factor
        (VEGF), 20

H
Hamstring autografts, 107
Hand surgery
    bone grafts and substitutes, 135
    cements, 136
    collagenases, 137–138
    growth factor, 137
    mineral substitutes, 135–136
    platelet-rich plasma (PRP), 137
Hepatocyte growth factor (HGF), 21t
High tibial osteotomy (HTO), 128
Hill–Sachs lesion
    definition, 78
    engaging lesions, 78
    glenoid track concept, 78–79
    humeral head allograft, 79, 80f
    nonengaging lesions, 78
    osteochondral talus allograft, 79–80,
        81f
    primary anterior dislocation, 78
    recurrent dislocations, 78
Human allografts
    allogeneic cortical bone fragments,
        49
    bioburden reduction methods, 51
    bone allografts
        bone formation and growth, 53
        cellular bone allografts, 54
        demineralization, 54
        filling bone voids, 53–54
        proteinaceous factors, 53
    bone banks, 49–50
    decellularization
        chemical and mechanical
            extraction, 54
        DNA content, 55
        glutaraldehyde, 54
        immunogenicity issues, 54
        recellularization, 55
    disease transmission risk reduction,
        51
    gamma irradiation
        chemical pretreatments, 52
        dose range, 52
        target dose, 52

Human allografts *(Continued)*
        temperature, 52–53
        tissue recovery and processing
            methods, 53
    hepatitis C virus (HCV) infections,
        50–51
    HIV-infected donor, 50–51
    infection rate, 50–51
    limitations and considerations, 58
    preservation and storage methods,
        56t
        considerations, 55
        cryopreservation methods,
            56–57
        freeze-drying, 57
        media-derived preservation,
            57–58
        refrigeration, 55–56
    sterility test guidelines, 51–52
    tendon allografts, 49–50
    terminal sterilization, 52
    tissue bank standards and
        regulation, 50
Humeral head allograft, 80f
Hyaline cartilage, 85
Hyaluronic acid (HA)
    intraarticular hyaluronic acid
        (IAHA), 1–2
    osteoarthritis (OA), 87–88
    viscosupplementation, 1–2

I
i-FACTOR Bone Graft, 171
Iliac crest bone graft, 166–167
Iliac crest bone graft (ICBG), 77
Induced pluripotent stem cells (iPSCs),
    152
Inflammatory phase, wound healing,
    19–20
Insulin-like growth factor-1 (IGF-1),
    21t, 27–29, 28t
Intercalary allografts
    adamantinoma, 196f
    advantages, 195
    disadvantages and complications,
        195–196
    intermediate-grade chondrosarcoma,
        197f
    plate fixation, 196
"Interim Rule", 50
International Cartilage Repair Society
    (ICRS) grading system, 32–33
International Knee Documentation
    Committee (IKDC) score,
    36–37
International Society for Stem Cell
    Research (ISSCR) guidelines, 16
Intervertebral disc regeneration,
    171
Intraarticular hyaluronic acid (IAHA),
    1–2
Investigational New Drug Application
    (IND), 12

J

Joint arthroplasty, 1

K

Knee
  anatomy and biomechanics
    bony articulations, 105
    cruciate ligaments, 105–106
    ligaments, 105
    load-elongation curve, tensile
      failure, 105
  articular cartilage, 86f
  chondral lesions, 85
  diffuse osteoarthritis (OA), 85
  hyaline articular cartilage, 85
Knee Injury and Osteoarthritis
  Outcome Score (KOOS) subscales,
  40–41
Koshino staging system
  secondary osteonecrosis (SON), 130
  spontaneous osteonecrosis of the
    knee (SPONK), 126

L

Latarjet procedure
  arthroscopic Latarjet, 76–77
  coracoid postharvesting before
    fixation, 76
  limitation, 76
  subscapularis split and subscapularis
    tenotomy techniques, 77
Lateral collateral ligament (LCL), 106
Lateral column lengthening, 178
Lateral epicondylitis, 137
Leukocyte-and platelet-rich fibrin
  (L-PRF), 22
Leukocyte-and platelet-rich plasma
  (L-PRP), 22, 81f
Ligament Advanced Reinforcement
  System (LARS) ligament, 109

M

Magnetic resonanace imaging (MRI)
  postarthroscopic osteonecrosis, 131
  secondary osteonecrosis (SON), 130
  spontaneous osteonecrosis of the
    knee (SPONK), 126, 126f–127f
Matrix-associated autologous
  chondrocyte implantation (MACI),
  65, 89
Matrix metalloproteinase 3 (MMP3),
  145
Media-derived preservation, human
  allografts, 57–58
Medial collateral ligament (MCL), 106
Medial patellofemoral ligament
  (MPFL), 106
Mesenchymal stem cells (MSCs), 4–5,
  65
  fracture, 188
  orthopaedic surgery
    adipose-derived MSCs, 40–41
    allogenic adult derived, 43

Mesenchymal stem cells (MSCs)
  (Continued)
    amniotic-derived, 42–43
    bone marrow–derived MSCs
      (BMSCs), 39–40
    definition, 38
    derivation, 37–38, 38f
    differentiation, 38–39
    peripheral blood–derived stem
      cell (PBSC), 41–42
    qualities and functions, 37–38
    sources, 39
    synovium-derived, 41
  partial anterior cruciate ligament
    (ACL) reconstruction, 115–116
  regenerative engineering, 208–210
  spinal fusion, 170
Microfracture (MFx)
  augmentation, 90
  autologous matrix induced
    chondrogenesis (AMIC), 90–91
  exogenous scaffolds, 91
  long-term outcomes, 90
  technique, 89–90
Mineral substitutes, hand surgery,
  135–136
Multicenter Orthopaedic Outcome
  Network (MOON) data, 107
Muscle injuries, platelet rich plasma
  (PRP), 23
Musculoskeletal human allograft
  tissue, 65–66

N

Nanofiber scaffolds, 170–171
NeuraGen conduit, 149
Neural crest cells, 152–153
NeuroLac, 149–150
Neuron, 141
Nonautogenous biological conduits,
  146–148

O

Orthobiologics
  autologous bone grafting, 3–4
  autologous form, 1, 2f
  bone marrow aspirate concentrate
    (BMAC), 5
  bone repair and fracture healing, 3
  cell sheet technology, 5
  cell therapies, 1
  function, 1
  gene therapy, 5
  nerve regeneration, 5
  platelet-enriched plasma (PR)
    autologous blood injections
      (ABI), 2–3
    chronic lateral epicondylar
      tendinopathy, 3
    Ehrenfest classification, 3t
    fracture healing, 2
    growth factors, 2–3
    for knee osteoarthritis, 3

Orthobiologics (Continued)
    musculoskeletal conditions, 2
    platelet count, 2
    preparation, 2–3
    sports medicine classification, 3t
  stem cell–based therapy, 4–5
  synthetic bioactive growth factors, 4
  synthetic bone grafts, 4
  viscosupplementation, 1
Orthopaedic surgery
  articular cartilage injury
    autologous chondrocyte
      implantation. See Autologous
      chondrocyte implantation
      (ACI)
    biopsy sites, 34f
    chondral lesions, 33
    classifications systems, 33t
    bone marrow aspirate concentrate
      (BMAC)
      application, 30–31
      bone healing, 27
      cellular composition, 27
      contents, 27, 28f
      growth factors and cytokines,
        27–29
      mesenchymal stem cells (MSCs),
        27
      safety, 31
      sources, 29
      technique, 29, 30t
    mesenchymal stem cells (MSC)
      adipose-derived MSCs, 40–41
      allogenic adult derived, 43
      amniotic-derived, 42–43
      bone marrow–derived MSCs
        (BMSCs), 39–40
      definition, 38
      derivation, 37–38, 38f
      differentiation, 38–39
      peripheral blood–derived stem
        cell (PBSC), 41–42
      qualities and functions, 37–38
      sources, 39
      synovium-derived, 41
Orthopedic oncology
  articular sparing resections &
    implants, 195
  extracorporeal devitalized autograft
    reconstructions, 197
  free vascularized fibular graft
    (FVFG), 196–197
  giant cell tumor of bone (GCTB),
    193
  intercalary allografts, 195–197
  osteoarticular allografts, 194–195
  sarcoma, 193–194
  void fillers, 194
Osteoarthritis (OA)
  adipose-derived mesenchymal stem
    cells, 89
  articular hyaline cartilage, 101
  bone marrow–derived stem cells, 89

Osteoarthritis (OA) *(Continued)*
  bone morphogenic protein (BMP), 101
  burden of disease, 101
  hyaluronic acid (HA), 87–88
  nonsurgical treatments, 101
  pharmacologic treatments, 101
  platelet-rich plasma (PRP)
    cartilage regeneration, 101–102
    intraarticular injections, 102
    modulatory effect, 101
    procedure, 101
  stem cell–based treatment approaches
    intraarticular injection, 102–103
    mesenchymal stems cells (MSCs), 102
Osteoarticular allografts, orthopedic oncology, 194–195
Osteoarticular transfer system (OATS), 91
Osteocel Plus, 167–168
Osteochondral allograft transplantation, 92–93
Osteochondral grafting, 128, 177
Osteochondral talus allograft, 79–80, 81f
Osteoinductive agents, 165
Osteonecrosis
  postarthroscopic osteonecrosis, 131
  secondary osteonecrosis (SON). *See* Secondary osteonecrosis (SON)
  spontaneous osteonecrosis of the knee (SPONK). *See* Spontaneous osteonecrosis of the knee (SPONK)
Oxysterol, osteogenesis, 170

P
P-15, 171
Partial anterior cruciate ligament (ACL) reconstruction
  platelet-rich plasma, 114–115
  PRP plus collagen scaffold, 115
  stem cell therapy, 115–116
Particulated juvenile articular cartilage, 66
Particulated minced cartilage, 94–95
Patch augmentation
  cellular augments, 71–72
  extracellular matrix patches, 71
  xenograft and synthetic augment, 71
Patellar tendon autografts, 109
Peripheral blood–derived stem cell (PBSC), 41–42
Peripheral nerve regeneration, 5
  end-organ atrophy, 145
  nerve reconstruction outcomes, 142–143
  rate of, 144
  roadblocks to recovery, 142–143
  segmental nerve defects, 144–145
  specificity of, 144

Peripheral nerve repair
  autogenous biological conduits, 146
  biologic augments, 145
  exogenous agents
    BDNF and CTNF, 150
    betamethasone, 150
    GDNF, 150
    NGF, 150
    rapamycin and tacrolimus, 150–151
    thyroid hormone (T3), 150
    vitamin E and and pyrroloquinoline (PQQ), 150
  fibrin, 153–154
  nerve response, 142
  nerve tissue engineering and, 154–155
  nonautogenous biological conduits, 146–148
  physiological and histopathological changes, 141
  SC transplantation, 151
  sensory and motor deficits, 141
  stem cells transplantation
    adipose-derived stem cells (ADSCs), 152
    amniotic fluid mesenchymal stem cells (AF-MSCs), 153
    bone marrow stem cells (BMSCs), 153
    embryonic stem cells, 151–152
    induced pluripotent stem cells (iPSCs), 152
    neural crest cells, 152–153
  synthetic conduits
    collagen conduits, 149
    fibrin matrix, 148
    poly D, L lactide-co-epsilon-caprolactone conduits (PCL), 149–150
    polyglycolic acid (PGA), 148–149
Peripheral nerves, microanatomy, 141
Peyronie disease, 137–138
Photoacoustic shock, postarthroscopic osteonecrosis, 131
Pico method, 75–76
Piezoelectric effect, 207
Plantar fasciitis, 176
Platelet-derived angiogenic factor (PDAF), 21t
Platelet-derived endothelial growth factor (PDEGF), 21t
Platelet-derived growth factor (PDGF), 20, 21t, 27–29, 28t, 114
Platelet-derived growth factor-BB (PDGF-BB), 64
Platelet-rich plasma (PRP)
  achilles tendinopathy, 175–176
  activation, 21
  autologous blood injections (ABI), 2–3
  bone loss, upper extremity, 80–82

Platelet-rich plasma (PRP) *(Continued)*
  chronic lateral epicondylar tendinopathy, 3
  commercial PRP systems, 21
  Ehrenfest classification, 3t
  fracture healing, 2
  growth factors, 2–3
  hand surgery, 137
  for knee osteoarthritis, 3
  leukocyte-and platelet-rich fibrin (L-PRF), 22
  leukocyte-and platelet-rich plasma (L-PRP), 22
  muscle injuries, 23
  musculoskeletal conditions, 2
  osteoarthritis (OA), 23–24, 88–89
    cartilage regeneration, 101–102
    intraarticular injections, 102
    modulatory effect, 101
    procedure, 101
  partial anterior cruciate ligament (ACL) reconstruction, 114–115
  plantar fasciitis, 176
  platelet concentration, 20
  platelet count, 2
  preparation, 2–3, 20–21, 22t
  pure platelet-rich fibrin (P-PRF), 22
  pure platelet-rich plasma (P-PRP), 22
  randomized controlled trials (RCTs), 20
  rotator cuff, 23
  sports medicine
    preparation, 64
    processing method, 64–65
    in surgical procedures, 64
    white blood cells (WBC), 64
  sports medicine classification, 3t
  tendinopathy, 23
Poly D, L lactide-co-epsilon-caprolactone conduits (PCL), 149–150
Polyglycolic acid (PGA) conduits, 148–149
Poly-methylmethacrylate (PMMA) bone cement, 194
Postarthroscopic osteonecrosis, 131
Posterior cruciate ligament (PCL), 105–106
Public Health Service Act (PHSA), 12
Pulsed electromagnetic fields (PEMFs) therapy, 128, 207
"Pure Food and Drugs Act", 9–10
Pure platelet-rich plasma (P-PRP), 22

Q
Quadriceps autograft, 108

R
Reamer irrigator aspirator (RIA), 185–186
Recombinant bone morphogenetic proteins-2 (rhBMPs-2), 168–169, 179

Recombinant human PDGF, osseous healing, 178–179
Regenerative engineering
  bridge-enhanced ACL repair (BEAR), 204
  calcium carbonate, 205
  ceramics, 204–205
  collagen type I, 203–204
  delivery of care, 210
  external stimulation, 207–208
  fibers, 207
  innovations, 210
  IntegraTM, 202–203
  mesenchymal stem cell (MSC) applications, 208–210
  micro-CT analysis, 207–208
  nanofibers, 207
  polymer fibers, 203–204
  scaffolds, 203
  synthetic ACL grafts, 204
  three-dimensional printing (3DP) composite material, 206
  tissue regeneration
    biological and physical signals, 202
    tissue gaps/large scars, 201–202
    in vivo environment, 202
    wound healing, 201
  xenografts, 205–206
Regenerative Medicine Advanced Therapy (RMAT) Designation, 15
Reliable and Effective Growth for Regenerative Health Options that Improve Wellness" (REGROW) Act, 15
Remodeling phase, wound healing, 19–20
Replamiform ceramics, 168
Restorative cartilage procedures, 85
Reverse shoulder arthroplasty (RSA), 69
Rotator cuff augmentation
  large-to-massive rotator cuff tears, 69
  muscle transfer, 69
  patch interposition (PI)
    cellular augments, 71–72
    extracellular matrix patches, 71
    xenograft and synthetic augment, 71
  superior capsule reconstruction
    arthroscopic view, 70f
    MRI coronal view, 70f
    patient-reported outcomes, 69–70
    reverse shoulder arthroplasty (RSA), 69
Rotator cuff, platelet rich plasma (PRP), 23

S
Sarcoma, tyrosine kinase inhibitors, 193–194
Schwann cells (SCs), 141

Secondary osteonecrosis (SON)
  bone impaction grafting, 130
  bone marrow involvement, 129
  contralateral joint involvement, 129
  corticosteroid use and alcohol abuse, 129–130
  gradual onset of pain, 130
  joint-preserving techniques, 130
  MRI findings, 130
  risk factors, 129–130
  two staging classification systems, 130
Segmental nerve defects, 144–145
Single Assessment Numerical Evaluation (SANE) score, 77–78
Sintered ceramics, 168
Small molecules (SMs), 170
Spinal fusion
  augmentation, 165
  biology, 165
  bone grafting
    allograft bone, 167
    autograft bone, 166–167
    cancellous grafts, 167
    cellular allograft, 167–168
  growth factors, 168–169
  implant optimization, 169–170
  intervertebral disc regeneration, 171, 172f
  mesenchymal stem cells, 170
  osteogenic materials, 165
  osteoinductive agents, 165
  scaffolds, 170–171
  small molecules (SMs), 170
  small peptides, 171
  synthetic grafts, 168
Spontaneous osteonecrosis of the knee (SPONK)
  categories, 123
  classification and prognosis, 126, 127f
  clinical presentation and diagnosis, 126, 126f–127f
  etiology, 125
  incidence, 125
  medial meniscus tears, 125
  nonoperative management, 126–128
  surgical management, 128–129
Sports medicine
  autologous chondrocyte implantation (ACI), 65
  bone marrow aspirate concentration (BMAC), 65
  cell therapies, 65
  growth factors, 64
  platelet-rich plasma (PRP)
    preparation, 64
    processing method, 64–65
    in surgical procedures, 64
    white blood cells (WBC), 64
  tissue therapies, 65–66
Stem cell characteristics, 65

Stem cell therapy, 4–5
  osteoarthritis (OA)
    intraarticular injection, 102–103
    mesenchymal stems cells (MSCs), 102
  partial anterior cruciate ligament (ACL) reconstruction, 115–116
  peripheral nerve repair
    adipose-derived stem cells (ADSCs), 152
    amniotic fluid mesenchymal stem cells (AF-MSCs), 153
    bone marrow stem cells (BMSCs), 153
    embryonic stem cells, 151–152
    induced pluripotent stem cells (iPSCs), 152
    neural crest cells, 152–153
Sterility test guidelines, 51–52
Subchondral bone
  blood flow, 123
  dissected lateral femoral condyle, 124f
  mechanical and biological support, 123
  subchondral plate, 123
Subchondral bone lesions
  articular cartilage zones, 123
  cartilage lesions, 123
  osteonecrosis
    postarthroscopic osteonecrosis, 131
    secondary osteonecrosis (SON). See Secondary osteonecrosis (SON)
    spontaneous osteonecrosis of the knee (SPONK). See Spontaneous osteonecrosis of the knee (SPONK)
Subtalar bone block arthrodesis, 178
Superior capsule reconstruction
  arthroscopic view, 70f
  MRI coronal view, 70f
  patient-reported outcomes, 69–70
  reverse shoulder arthroplasty (RSA), 69
Synovial fluid, 86
Synovium-derived mesenchymal stem cells, 41
Synthetic bioactive growth factors, 4
Synthetic bone grafts, 4
Synthetic bone void fillers, 186
Synthetic conduits, peripheral nerve repair
  collagen conduits, 149
  fibrin matrix, 148
  poly D, L lactide-co-epsilon-caprolactone conduits (PCL), 149–150
  polyglycolic acid (PGA), 148–149
Synthetic grafts, 106–107, 109, 168
Synthetic patch augmentation, 71

T

Tendinopathy, platelet rich plasma (PRP), 23
Tendon allografts, 49–50
Terminal sterilization, 52
3D printing technology, 154–155
Tissue sterility, 51–52
Tissue therapies, sports medicine, 65–66
  acellular dermal matrix, 66
  American Association of Tissue Banks (AATB), 65–66
  amniotic membrane products, 66
  musculoskeletal human allograft tissue, 65–66
  particulated juvenile articular cartilage, 66
  sterilization methods, 66
Trabecular bone, 205
Transforming growth factor-beta (TGF-β), 21t
Transforming growth factor β1 (TGF-β1), 64
Transforming growth factor- β2 (TGF- β2), 27–29, 28t

U

Unicompartmental arthroplasty (UKA), 128–129
University of California at Los Angeles score (UCLA), 71

V

Vascular endothelial growth factor (VEGF), 20, 21t
  bone marrow aspirate concentrate (BMAC), 27–29, 28t
Viscosupplementation, 1

W

Western Ontario and McMaster Universities Osteoarthritis Index (WOMAC) scores, 88–89
Western Ontario Rotator Cuff score (WORC), 71

Tricalcium phosphate, hand surgery, 135
Trinity Evolution, 168
Two-phase preparation steps, platelet rich plasma, 22t

Western Ontario Shoulder Instability (WOSI) index, 77–78
Wound-healing process
  growth factors. *See* Growth factors
  healing process, 19–20
  inflammatory phase, 19–20
  maturation phase, 19–20
  platelet aggregation, 19–20
  proliferative phase, 19–20
  remodeling phase, 19–20

X

Xenografts, 49
  anterior cruciate ligament (ACL) reconstruction, 109–110
  patch augmentation, 71
  and synthetic augment, 71
Xiaflex, 137–138

Printed in the United States
By Bookmasters